OUTBREAK

Cases in Real-World Microbiology

OUTBREAK
Cases in Real-World Microbiology

Rodney P. Anderson

Department of Biological and Allied Health Sciences
Ohio Northern University
Ada, Ohio

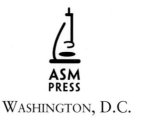

ASM
PRESS

WASHINGTON, D.C.

Address editorial correspondence to
ASM Press, 1752 N St. NW, Washington, DC 20036-2904, USA

Send orders to ASM Press, P.O. Box 605, Herndon, VA 20172, USA
Phone: (800) 546-2416 or (703) 661-1593
Fax: (703) 661-1501
E-mail: books@asmusa.org
Online: estore.asm.org

Library of Congress Cataloging-in-Publication Data

Anderson, Rodney P.
Outbreak : cases in real-world microbiology / Rodney P. Anderson.
p. ; cm.
Includes bibliographical references and index.
ISBN-13: 978-1-55581-366-6 (pbk.)
ISBN-10: 1-55581-366-6 (pbk.)
1. Epidemics—Case studies. 2. Communicable diseases—Case studies. 3. Medical
microbiology—Case studies.
[DNLM: 1. Disease Outbreaks—Case Reports. 2. Communicable Diseases—Case
Reports. 3. Disease Reservoirs—Case Reports. 4. Disease Transmission—Case
Reports. 5. Environmental Microbiology—methods—Case Reports. WA 105 A549o
2006] I. Title.

RA651.A68 2006
614.4—dc22
2005037791

10 9 8 7 6 5 4 3 2 1

Cover photo: Scanning electron micrograph of *Staphylococcus aureus*. Source: Beltsville
Electron Microscopy Unit, Beltsville Agricultural Research Center, U.S. Department of
Agriculture.

Cover and interior design: Susan Brown Schmidler

For Tami—always

Contents

Introduction

The science of microbiology is fascinating to those of us who have taken up the challenge of researching and teaching in this largely undiscovered and rapidly expanding field. One of the significant challenges faced by microbiology educators is to balance the need for providing a content foundation to students against the time required to demonstrate how microbiology affects their lives. The goal of *Outbreak: Cases in Real-World Microbiology* is to help students make the important connections between the content of the course, their everyday lives, and the ways in which microbiology impacts society as a whole. These real-world cases provide an opportunity for students to apply practical knowledge and to integrate their solutions to specific problems in cultures where customs, religion, public resources, and infrastructure impact the analysis.

Content

The outbreaks featured in each section are preceded by one or two tables listing the significant pathogens that can cause outbreaks. The cases presented in that section include only diseases caused by pathogens listed in the table(s). The diseases and pathogens chosen are those which are often covered in an introductory microbiology course. Limiting the pool of possibilities helps the students learn the basics thoroughly without having to consider the myriad of possible causes normally associated with a differential diagnosis. Each chapter ends with a set of descriptions of the diseases covered in the case studies. The descriptions are meant to be used by students for reference, if necessary, to gather the information needed to develop appropriate answers to the questions at the end of each outbreak. Each disease description presents information on (i) the causative agent of the disease, (ii) the pathogen's mode of transmission from its reservoir to a new host, (iii) pathogenesis, (iv) the clinical features of the disease, (v) clinical and laboratory diagnosis, (vi) treatment of the disease, and

(vii) general principles of prevention of the disease. Throughout each section, there is a balance between outbreaks that allow students to integrate and apply their knowledge and those that also require students to diagnose the pathogenic agent on the basis of lab test data and the clinical features of the disease.

Appendix A consists of several tables that outline the mechanisms of action and the use of some common antibacterial, antiviral, antifungal, and antiprotozoal agents. The material can be used for quick reference by students investigating how to treat a particular disease. The tables are an educational tool, not a medical guide. The drugs of choice for treating a particular microbe change as drug resistance spreads and as new agents are discovered and approved for use. This appendix presents the major classes of antimicrobial agents, some specific examples of common drugs that students may be familiar with, and a general outline of the diseases that the drugs have been useful to treat.

Appendix B directs students to specific reference material which provides information relevant to the study questions and encourages the students to apply the reference content to the cases they are studying.

Special features

The last two outbreaks in each section are designated "College Perspective" and "Global Perspective." The College Perspectives present outbreaks that directly impact the lives of students. The pathogens are typically spread easily in the college-age population, or the outbreaks focus on issues important to students. The Global Perspectives present outbreaks that occur in non-Western cultures. As a result, solutions developed by students for treatment and prevention require them to consider cultures in which differences in customs, religion, public resources, and infrastructure impact the analysis.

Case studies in the classroom

There are many ways in which case studies such as the outbreaks presented in this book can be integrated into a typical microbiology class. For example, they can be used as supplemental class readings and assignments to review application of content presented in class and to help students prepare for exams. They can be used to promote discussion to enhance lecture material. Students can become active participants in their learning by solving case studies that either review material already presented or introduce new material. Case studies can serve as the foundation for innovative approaches using cooperative learning groups. Cooperative learning groups can be used instead of lectures to allow students to investigate microbiological topics in depth.

Case studies help students develop application, integration, and analysis skills. They can also be used as assessment tools to evaluate a course's ability to develop integration and application skills. Therefore they can be helpful in preparing for professional admission exams such as the MCAT, NCLEX, and GRE.

As with much of life, the most challenging parts are also the most rewarding. With much of science, learning the content base, although often challenging, is just the beginning. The real objective is to integrate and apply scientific concepts and principles to make a difference in the real world. The best education provides students with such opportunities both in the classroom and through practical experiences.

Acknowledgments

I thank several individuals who took time out of their busy schedules to help with this project, especially Cara Calvo, who provided several needed cultures and images, and Graetel Anderson, who reviewed material for appropriate vocabulary level. I also thank the staff of and contributors to the Centers for Disease Control and Prevention's journals and image library. The journals and image library are a rich resource of information for educators and the public to use.

About the Author

Rodney P. Anderson received his Ph.D. in biological sciences from the University of Iowa in 1989. His doctoral work centered on protein synthesis mechanisms in *Escherichia coli*. After graduate school, he began his academic career at Ohio Northern University, where he continues to teach and conduct research with undergraduates in the Department of Biological and Allied Health Sciences. He teaches courses in microbiology for both majors and allied health students as well as courses in genetics. He has also introduced nonmajors to microbiology through interdisciplinary seminars in disease and society.

Dr. Anderson has been actively involved in microbiology education. He is a past chair of the American Society for Microbiology (ASM) Conference for Undergraduate Educators, which developed the core curriculum for undergraduate microbiology courses, and has organized and spoken at a number of education division symposia at the ASM General Meeting. Outreach activities have included Microbial Discovery Workshops for high school science instructors and science presentations at local elementary schools. His interest in microbiology education has resulted in a children's book, *The Invisible ABCs*, which will be published by ASM Press. *The Invisible ABCs* emphasizes the benefits of the microbial world to children, rather than the incomplete message that all microbes cause disease.

Dr. Anderson and his wife, Tami, are parents of two adult children, Isaac and Graetel, who are both pursuing careers in nursing. He loves classic cars, golfing, hunting, antiquing, and spending vacations parachuting and rock climbing with his children.

SECTION I

Outbreaks and Cases Emphasizing Concepts in Basic Microbiology

All interest in disease and death is only another expression of interest in life.

THOMAS MANN, Nobel laureate in literature (1929)

When one studies the fundamentals of microbial structures and their functions, it is often difficult to link this content to mechanisms of disease transmission and the pathogenesis of the microbe. The outbreaks and cases in this section have been chosen as examples of how basic microbial features enable pathogens to cause disease. For example, the structures of some cell walls influence a pathogen's ability to survive treatments that would kill other bacteria. *Mycobacterium tuberculosis*, the causative agent of tuberculosis (TB), has a waxy cell wall. As a result, it resists drying, so the cell is easier to transmit. The waxy wall is also an effective barrier to the diffusion of many antibiotics and disinfectants, making infection difficult to treat and control. In contrast, *Mycoplasma pneumoniae*, one causative agent of primary atypical pneumonia, lacks a cell wall. This reduces its ability to survive during transmission. As a result, long-term exposure is normally required to transmit the pathogen. The lack of a cell wall, however, makes *Mycoplasma* resistant to the antibiotics that target peptidoglycan synthesis. In general, gram-negative cells are more resistant to antiseptics and disinfectants than are gram-positive bacteria because the outer membrane provides an additional barrier to diffusion. In addition, *Pseudomonas aeruginosa*, a common hospital-acquired gram-negative pathogen, has very small porins, which further restrict diffusion, allowing it to survive some chemical treatments that effectively kill other pathogens.

Understanding microbial fundamentals is the basis for understanding the pathogenesis of disease. After entry, microbes must attach to host tissues, avoid or overcome host defenses, and cause damage, leading to disease. Adhesins are located on the exterior of the microbe and attach to specific host cell receptors. The site of attachment often determines where damage will occur. For example, *Neisseria gonorrhoeae* has adhesins at the ends of pili. These can attach to cells of the reproductive epithelium, leading to gonorrhea, a sexually transmitted disease (STD). However, the pathogen can also attach to tissues in the eye. This can occur during birth, leading to vertical transmission of the pathogen to cause ophthalmia neonatorum. The pathogen can also attach to host cells in the pharynx. Oral-genital contact results in *Neisseria gonorrhoeae*-caused pharyngitis.

Pathogens must also avoid or overcome host defenses to cause disease. Many structures enable some pathogens to survive defenses that typically destroy other microbes. Rotavirus has a relatively acid-stable capsid, allowing it to survive stomach acid effectively enough that ingestion of only a small number of viral particles will cause disease. *Staphylococcus aureus*, one of the most common pathogens that affect humans, is able to survive in high-osmotic environments, such as the nasal mucus, that kill most cells. *Bacillus anthracis* and *Streptococcus pneumoniae* produce antiphagocytic capsules that inhibit destruction by leukocytes. *Staphylococcus aureus* and *Streptococcus pyogenes* have cell wall proteins that also inhibit phagocytosis by leukocytes. As they are passed from host to host, influenza A and B viruses slowly accumulate mutations in the key antigens that our immune system recognizes. As a result of this antigenic drift, influenza viruses can reinfect a previous host and not elicit a host immune response. In addition, influenza A virus can undergo antigenic shifts when it recombines with an influenza virus from birds or swine. These genetically unique viruses are able to cause worldwide epidemics, since no one is immune. Other pathogens, such as human immunodeficiency virus (HIV), the causative agent of acquired immune deficiency syndrome (AIDS), and measles virus survive by overcoming host defenses. HIV leads to a collapse of all parts of the immune system. Measles virus destroys the T cells that destroy virus-infected cells.

More recently, the ability of bacteria to form biofilms has been recognized as leading to infection of indwelling catheters. The sticky coating surrounding cells contained in a biofilm allows the pathogen to attach to plastic and also restricts the diffusion of antibiotics, resulting in a drug-resistant persistent infection.

Many microbes destroy cells and tissues directly. Manifestations of disease are the result of functional loss of damaged cells and/or the resulting inflammatory response, causing fluid loss and edema. Some microbes cause indirect damage from the enzymes and toxins they release. For example, mutant *Escherichia coli* produces a cytotoxin that targets cells of the large intestine to cause bloody diarrhea, especially in young children. The toxin can also lead to a lethal complication, hemolytic-uremic syndrome (HUS). *Bordetella pertussis*, the causative agent of whooping cough, produces toxins that inhibit ciliary action and destroy cells of the respiratory tract. *Bacillus anthracis* produces a highly lethal toxin that causes tissue death at the site of infection. Various strains of *Staphylococcus aureus* and *Streptococcus pyogenes* produce a host of tissue-damaging enzymes: hemolysin, leukocidin, hyaluronidase, coagulase, streptokinase, and collagenase. The understanding of these general microbiology concepts has led to the development of new drugs and vaccines and changes in the way we treat and prevent the spread of certain microbes.

Table I.1 Microbial structures and their roles in pathogenesis

Structure or organelle	Function	Role in pathogenesis
Bacteria		
Biofilm	Attaches and connects an interdependent microbial community to a surface	Biofilms anchor a bacterial community to indwelling prosthetic medical devices and prevent diffusion of antibiotics and disinfectants into biofilm bacteria, which may result in resistance.
Capsule	Attaches bacteria to a surface or protects the bacteria from phagocytosis	Capsules can attach bacteria to host tissues or inhibit phagocytosis.
Cell wall	Prevents osmotic lysis, determines the shape of the bacteria, anchors flagella	Cell walls containing mycolic acid provide a waxy coating that inhibits the diffusion of most drugs. Cell wall proteins can attach to host cells or inhibit phagocytosis. Lipid A is a structural component of gram-negative bacteria and acts as an endotoxin. Other degradation components of the cell wall can induce an intense inflammatory response.
Pili	Attach bacteria to a surface or form a bridge for conjugation	Proteins on pili can attach to host cell tissues. Pili are used in conjugation and transfer antibiotic resistance genes to new bacterial pathogens
Flagella	Provide bacterial motility	Flagella are used by pathogens to swim to sites of infection, such as the bladder to cause a urinary tract infection.
Plasmids	Carry extrachromosomal information used for survival in different environments	Plasmids carry drug resistance genes that can be transferred to other cells through conjugation, transformation, or transduction.
Endospores	Found in *Clostridium* and *Bacillus*; dormant structures that can germinate in an appropriate environment	Endospores enable anaerobic bacteria to survive in aerobic environments until they have a suitable environment for growth. Endospores are resistant to antibiotics, disinfectants, heat, acidity, etc., which allows them to survive many bacterial-control actions. Endospores enable some bacteria to be dried and milled into weapons of mass destruction.
Viruses		
Envelope	Carries surface proteins that can be used to attach to the host cell	Envelope proteins may attach to host cell tissues. They can be key proteins for the immune system to target to destroy the virus and to develop immunity.
Capsid	Protects nucleic acid; also, external proteins can be used to attach to the host cell	External capsid proteins may attach to host tissues. They can be key proteins for the immune system to target to destroy the virus and to provoke a strong immune response.
Nucleic acid	Codes for the enzymatic and structural molecules of the virus	Accumulation of mutations in the genetic information can lead to genetic drift, which results in the virus being able to reinfect a previously infected host. Recombination between different related viruses can cause antigenic shifts. These lead to unique viruses that the human population has no immunity against.

Table I.2 Eukaryotic microbes and their roles in pathogenesis

Organisms	Characteristics	Role in pathogenesis
Fungi		
Molds and yeasts	Environmental decomposers	Some can degrade keratin-containing cells, which allows them to infect hair, skin, and nails. (Also, some produce antibiotics which can be used to treat bacterial infections.)
Protozoa		
Sporozoa	Unicellular, eukaryotic microbes with a complex life cycle involving spore formation	Complex life cycles enable pathogens to switch antigens to avoid host immune responses.
Flagellates, ciliates	Motile, eukaryotic microbes that absorb or ingest their food	Cyst formation provides resistance to stomach acids and bile. Motility enables them to move to suitable environments for infection.
Amoebae	Unicellular microbes that engulf their food using pseudopodia	Cyst formation provides resistance to stomach acids and bile. Defenses are impaired by amoeba-ingesting cells.

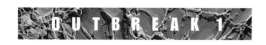

Multidrug-Resistant Tuberculosis Outbreaks

UNITED STATES

In 1930, Americans with TB numbered 3 million. There were over 600 sanatoriums with a capacity of 84,000 beds that dotted the American landscape. Even so, they could only treat less than 5% of those afflicted with "consumption," or active TB. John Bunyan's claim in 1680 that TB was "the Captain of all these men of death" still held true, with about 1 of every 10 deaths worldwide caused by TB. The treatment of fresh cold air and a rich diet did not affect the rate of death.

With the introduction of streptomycin by Selman Waksman in 1947 and the government's "war on tuberculosis," the number of cases of TB rapidly declined. Our triumph over TB once read like a paid advertisement for modern science; by the 1960s, powerful antibiotics and synthetic antitubercular agents had virtually eliminated TB in this country. In 1984, the Public Health Service reported that the number of TB cases reported annually had declined by 74% relative to 1953. It was widely believed that modern medicine had all but eradicated this potentially fatal disease. As a result, public health programs were terminated and significant biomedical research into drug development and vaccines was not funded as highly.

The wake-up call alerting the public to the resurgence of TB came between 1985 and 1993, when the number of cases reported in the United States began to increase steadily and dramatically, with 25,701 cases reported in 1990, 26,382 cases in 1991, and 26,673 cases in 1992. From 1985 through 1992, the rate of increase was 14%.

Worldwide, TB has made a comeback. In the United States, more than 10 million Americans carry the TB bacterium; worldwide, more than 3 million people die of TB every year. TB is the second most common cause of death by infectious disease each year. Most alarming of all, several new strains of *Mycobacterium tuberculosis* are proving resistant to treatment by the few drugs we know that can cure the disease. As a result of dangerous multidrug-resistant (MDR)

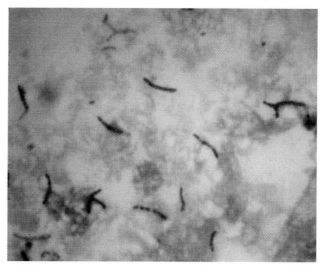

Figure 1.1 Acid-fast stain of *Mycobacterium tuberculosis* from a sputum sample.

5

TB, some individuals with TB are now treated in facilities that are locked and guarded. The patients are not free to leave. One mother who was suffering from an active case of MDR TB would not take her medications regularly. Fearing she would infect her children, her friends, and her community, the Public Health Department obtained a court order for her arrest. Seized and handcuffed at a laundromat, she was brought kicking and screaming to the TB ward for 12 months of intensive treatment.

The World Health Organization reports that the death rate of patients with MDR TB in the United States is approximately 70%. The typical interval from diagnosis to death in such cases is 4 to 16 weeks. Left untreated, 1 person with TB will infect 10 to 15 people per year. Drug-resistant TB has become a serious concern. In a recent survey in New York City, 33% of patients were infected with organisms resistant to at least one drug, and 19% were infected with organisms resistant to both isoniazid and rifampin, the two most effective drugs available for treating TB. When organisms are resistant to both isoniazid and rifampin, the course of treatment increases from 6 months to 18 to 24 months, and the cure rate decreases from nearly 100% to 60% or less.

The drug resistance problem appears to be worsening. For example, from 1982 to 1986, only 0.5% of new cases were resistant to both isoniazid and rifampin; by 1991, this proportion had increased to about 3.1%. Among recurrent cases, 3.0% were resistant to both drugs in 1982 to 1986, but in 1991, this proportion had more than doubled to 6.9%.

Of significant concern are recent outbreaks of MDR TB in institutional settings. Significant outbreaks of MDR TB have been reported in prisons from South Carolina to Azerbaijan. Virtually all these institutional epidemics involved organisms resistant to both isoniazid and rifampin, and some had organisms resistant to seven anti-TB drugs. Mortality among patients with MDR TB in these outbreaks was high, ranging from 72 to 89%, and the median interval between TB diagnosis and death was short, from 4 to 16 weeks.

QUESTIONS

1. What physical property of *Mycobacterium tuberculosis* makes it acid-fast?

2. Why does *Mycobacterium tuberculosis* require long-term drug therapy?

3. How does drug resistance develop in bacteria?

4. What types of laws are used to protect the public from individuals who could potentially spread a serious infectious disease?

5. Do you agree with locking up those who carry MDR TB and who are noncompliant with treatment? Explain your reasoning.

6. How would you stop the outbreak of MDR TB in institutional settings?

Outbreak of a Mycoplasmal Pneumonia

OHIO, 1993

From 15 June through 5 September 1993, an acute respiratory illness caused by *Mycoplasma pneumoniae* occurred among 47 (12%) of 403 staff members and clients of a sheltered workshop for developmentally disabled adults in Ohio. The disease was characterized by acute onset of cough and fever. The median age of the patients was 35 years (range, 20 to 60 years); 7 (15%) required hospitalization, and 31 (66%) had chest X rays showing fluid in the lungs—evidence of pneumonia. One workshop participant died on 30 June from complications of pneumonia. Specimens of blood, sputum, and nasopharyngeal secretions were analyzed in the clinical laboratory. The results of the Gram stain of a sputum sample were inconclusive; however, abundant cells that fight off infection (polymorphonuclear leukocytes) were observed. Serologic and microbiologic studies were negative for acute viral infections. No bacteria were present in the blood sample. An antigenic test was able to identify the pathogen as *Mycoplasma pneumoniae*.

QUESTIONS

1. List several viral and bacterial pathogens that can cause primary pneumonia. Describe several of their physical features.

2. Why is an institutional setting a common place for such an outbreak?

3. What physical property makes *Mycoplasma* different from all other pathogens that cause bacterial pneumonia? How does this contribute to its ability to cause disease (pathogenicity)?

4. To which group of antibiotics would *Mycoplasma pneumoniae* be resistant?

5. Explain how you would treat patients affected by the outbreak described.

6. How would you stop the outbreak described?

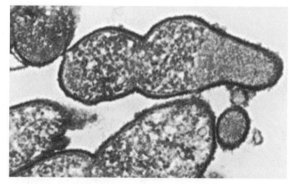

Figure 2.1 Transmission electron micrograph of *Mycoplasma*.

OUTBREAK 3

Hickman Catheter-Related Infections in a Hemato-Oncologic Department

THE NETHERLANDS,
1994 TO 1996

A study was done to evaluate the source of *Staphylococcus epidermidis*, the bacteria that predominantly causes Hickman catheter-related infections (CRIs). The analysis was done in several steps. First, samples of air from the patient's room were analyzed, along with skin cultures taken prior to insertion of the catheter. The bacteria from these samples were analyzed using molecular techniques (random amplification of polymorphic deoxyribonucleic acid [DNA]). The second step of the analysis was to analyze blood samples and catheters after the catheters had been inserted. Comparisons were made between the bacteria isolated before and after catheter insertion.

Cultures from different sites were taken regularly according to the following scheme. (i) Before skin disinfection with 0.5% chlorhexidine in 70% ethanol, cultures were taken from the skin at the insertion site and from air samples. (ii) After insertion, but prior to closure of the wound, two exit site cultures were taken. (iii) During hospitalization, serial cultures from the exit site and hub interiors and blood cultures drawn directly from both Hickman catheter channels were taken twice weekly. (iv) In the case of fever, extra cultures from the exit site and hub interiors plus at least two blood culture sets each via both Hickman catheter channels and a peripheral vein were taken. As long as fever persisted, these investigations were performed daily. (v) When indicated, the Hickman catheter was removed by a surgeon and the tip, tunnel, and hub segments were cultured separately.

The results of the analysis indicated that two genotypes of *Staphylococcus epidermidis* predominated in the isolates. These two closely related (clonal) types of *Staphylococcus epidermidis* were found in 13% (11 of 86) of air samples and 44% (33 of 75) of skin samples taken before the insertion of the catheter. After insertion of the catheter, the prevalence of these two clonal types increased: 53% (33 of 62) in catheters that did not show evidence of a clinical infection and 74% (139 of 188) in catheters associated with CRIs. Despite prompt treatment with vancomycin (a drug that typically is highly effective at killing a broad range of bacteria), 70% of the catheters infected with the two clonal types had to be removed to stop the infection. The *S. epidermidis* strains involved in CRI appeared to be from the skin flora in 75% of cases.

Coagulase is an enzyme produced by some bacteria that causes blood clots to form. A very common pathogen, *Staphylococcus aureus*, produces this enzyme (coagulase positive). However, the normally nonpathogenic relative *Staphylococcus epidermidis*, a coagulase-negative staphylococcus (CoNS), has become the most frequently isolated pathogen in intravascular CRIs. CoNS accounted for an estimated 28% of all nosocomial (hospital-acquired) bloodstream infections reported to the National Nosocomial Infections Surveillance System from 1986 through 1989. The emergence of CoNS as the primary pathogen causing CRI has been attributed to the increased use

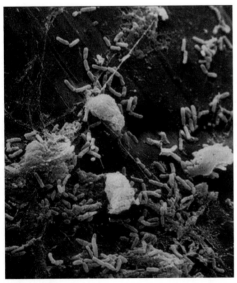

Figure 3.1 Scanning electron micrograph of a fouled catheter.

of prosthetic and indwelling devices, the increased use of parenteral nutrition (nutrients delivered intravenously), and the improved survival of people after their immune system fails (immunocompromised individuals). In addition, CoNS have been recognized as potentially true nosocomial pathogens rather than harmless culture contaminants not worthy of being reported by the laboratory to the attending physician.

Thirty-six different antibiotic susceptibility patterns were determined for CoNS: 71% of the strains isolated were resistant to methicillin, 89% were resistant to penicillin, 55% were resistant to gentamicin, 71% were resistant to ciprofloxacin, 87% were resistant to sulfamethoxazole-trimethoprim, 81% were resistant to erythromycin, 56% were resistant to clindamycin, 20% were resistant to rifampin, and 51% were resistant to tetracycline. All were susceptible to vancomycin. The majority of strains were resistant to five or more antibiotics.

Furthermore, most Hickman catheters were inserted at the end of the first week following a patient's admittance to the hematology department, according to the hemato-oncologic workup protocol. This probably explains why, at the time of Hickman catheter insertion, 44% of patients were already carrying these two clones on their skin.

QUESTIONS

1. Where is the probable source of the *Staphylococcus epidermidis* that causes the CRIs?

2. Outline the basic process of biofilm formation.

3. What physical properties make biofilm-forming bacteria difficult to treat in a clinical environment?

4. If *Staphylococcus epidermidis* is sensitive to vancomycin, why did 70% of the catheters have to be removed to stop the infection?

5. Describe several hypotheses formulated to account for the antimicrobial resistance of biofilm-related bacterial populations.

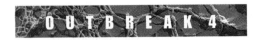

A Gang-Related Outbreak of Drug-Resistant Gonorrhea

COLORADO, 1991

In April 1990, the El Paso County (Colorado) Health Department recognized an outbreak of drug-resistant gonorrhea in Colorado Springs. A subsequent investigation by the El Paso County Health Department and the Colorado Department of Health eventually identified 56 cases of penicillinase-producing *Neisseria gonorrhoeae* that occurred from December 1989 through March 1991. Penicillinase is an enzyme produced by most penicillin-resistant bacteria. The enzyme degrades the penicillin to a form that is harmless to the organism.

To gather information about the outbreak, people were interviewed in STD clinics, in their homes, and at locations where they congregated (e.g., movie theaters, shopping malls, clubs, and bars). Network analysis was performed to characterize the sexual and social connections of those identified. The network analysis included 410 persons related through a densely connected set of social or sexual associations. This network included adolescents and young adults associated with street gangs. These gangs, which originated in Los Angeles and are associated with the crack cocaine trade in the United States, had not been observed in Colorado Springs before May 1988. The men in this subset were young (mean age, 21.5 years) and mostly black (87.2%), and the women were younger (mean age, 19.7 years) and more racially/ethnically diverse. During interviews, many women reported engaging in multiple risk behaviors associated with transmission of STDs (e.g., engaging in frequent sexual encounters with multiple sex partners, exchanging sex for crack cocaine, and heavily using crack cocaine). In comparison, fewer men reported heavy use of crack cocaine, but many reported having engaged in frequent sexual encounters and having had multiple sex partners. Two hundred persons with infections named 558 sex partners in the sociosexual network.

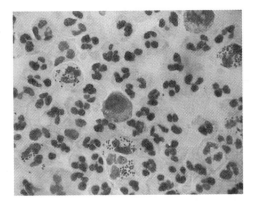

Figure 4.1 Gram stain of a pus sample.

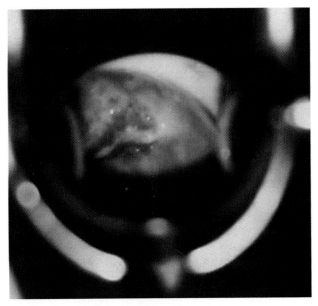

Figure 4.2 Pus discharge from the cervix.

Of the persons in the network, 83% were infected with one or more STDs. In addition, the bacterial pathogen (Fig. 4.1) was resistant to penicillins. This strain of drug-resistant *Neisseria gonorrhoeae* accounted for 70% of all the drug-resistant cases reported in Colorado Springs.

QUESTIONS

1. Besides *Neisseria gonorrhoeae*, list a bacterial, a viral, and a protozoal pathogen that the individuals who are part of the sociosexual network described are at high risk for acquiring.

2. What cell structure enables *Neisseria gonorrhoeae* to attach to the urethra and avoid being washed away?

3. How would you treat those affected by the drug-resistant gonorrhea?

4. How can this disease be prevented?

5. How would you propose to stop the outbreak described?

6. Why can't physicians simply increase the concentration of penicillins to overcome the infection?

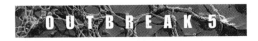

Skin Rash Caused by *Pseudomonas* and Associated with Pools and Hot Tubs

MAINE, 2000

Several cases of a skin rash (folliculitis) caused by *Pseudomonas aeruginosa* infection occurred among persons who had stayed at hotel A in Bangor, Maine, from 18 to 27 February 2000. The Maine Board of Health conducted a study comparing those who had the rash with those who did not have the rash (a case control study) among persons connected with a high school basketball tournament who stayed at hotels with swimming pools and/or hot tubs in Bangor during the outbreak. Those who were infected (case patients) had a rash for 7 days or less or a *Pseudomonas* infection of the outer ear (otitis externa) with onset between 18 February and 3 March. The nine case patients were matched by age and high school with healthy controls. The nine case patients had stayed at hotel A and spent time in either the hot tub or pool; seven spent time in both. The case patients were more likely than the controls to have spent time in the hot tub or to have used the pool.

The indoor pool and hot tub were located within 5 feet of each other and had separate filtration systems. Pool disinfectant and pH levels were monitored by an offsite contractor. The pool had an automated chlorination system that relied on an onsite probe to measure chlorine and pH levels. Chlorine and pH levels were maintained manually in the hot tub. During the outbreak, free-chlorine levels were tested daily and repeatedly registered <1.0 milligram (mg)/liter, less than the state-required level of 1 to 3 mg/liter, in the pool and hot tub. The pool and hot tub were crowded during the outbreak, and free-chlorine levels were very low to zero after the 25 and 26 February weekend; no measurements were recorded over the weekend.

The facilities had been cleaned thoroughly before the environmental investigation in March. *Pseudomonas aeruginosa* was isolated from the top of the pool filter and from the draining ear of a child aged 6 years who used the pool.

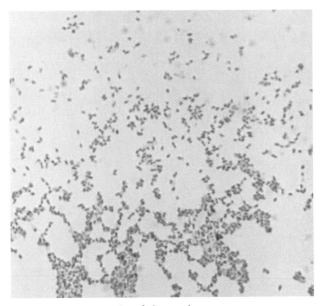

Figure 5.1 Gram stain of the pathogen.

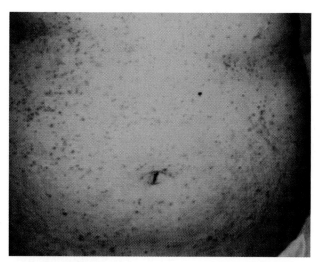

Figure 5.2 Folliculitis.

QUESTIONS

1. What other diseases can be caused by *Pseudomonas aeruginosa*?

2. What physical characteristics of *Pseudomonas aeruginosa* make it resistant to disinfection and antibiotics?

3. How would you treat those infected with *Pseudomonas*?

4. How would you prevent future outbreaks in hotel A?

5. Do you think the investigators should have controlled for cuts and abrasions in this athletic population?

6. Do you consider this a biofilm-related outbreak?

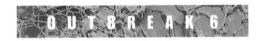

Human Anthrax Linked to an Outbreak in Livestock

NORTH DAKOTA, 2000

In May 2000, four cattle were found dead on a North Dakota farm. From 6 July through 24 September 2000, 157 animals died on 31 farms on which 62 persons were involved with animal care, vaccination, specimen processing, or carcass disposal.

On 19 August 2000, a 67-year-old resident of eastern North Dakota participated in the disposal of five cows that had died. On the day of disposal, he placed chains around the heads and hooves of the animals and moved them to a burial site. He reported having worn leather gloves throughout transportation and disposal.

On 23 August, he noticed a small bump on his left cheek at the angle of his jaw. On 25 August, the lesion had enlarged, and he sought medical attention. He denied fever, malaise, headache, itching, or difficulty swallowing. On examination, the lesion was approximately the size of a quarter and was surrounded by a purple ring. The patient did not have a fever or appear ill. The physician reported a firm, nontender, superficial nodule with an overlying 0.5-cm black eschar (scab). No drainage was noted, and neither wound nor blood cultures were obtained. The patient was placed on antibiotics.

On follow-up examination on 28 August, the eschar had enlarged to 1 cm. As a result, laboratory tests (Fig. 6.1 and 6.2) were completed on a sample of the infected area.

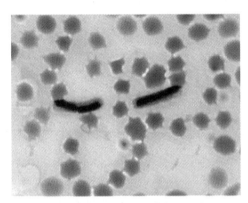

Figure 6.1 Capsule stain of the pathogen.

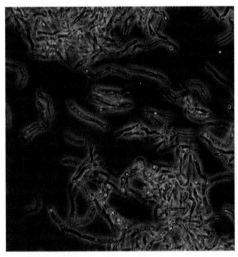

Figure 6.2 Phase-contrast micrograph of endospores.

QUESTIONS

1. What pathogen causes anthrax?

2. Describe the expected progress of the disease if it remains untreated.

3. What structural features of the pathogen enable it to avoid phagocytosis?

4. What effect do the toxins the pathogen produces have on the tissues they affect?

5. What feature of the pathogen enables it to resist drying and temperature changes and to survive for long periods in the environment?

6. How would you treat this man's disease?

7. How would you manage the animal outbreak?

8. How did this infection probably originate?

9. How would you alter the process of transport and burial of diseased animal carcasses?

10. Considering the nature of this pathogen, is burial of the dead animals an adequate public health measure?

11. What is the longevity of the spores of this pathogen in soil?

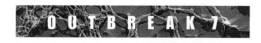

A Multidrug-Resistant *Salmonella* Outbreak in Veterinary Clinics

IDAHO, 1999

The Centers for Disease Control and Prevention (CDC) received reports in 1999 from the Idaho Department of Health and Welfare about an outbreak of diarrhea among employees and clients of a small-animal veterinary clinic. Ten of the 20 persons at the clinic had abdominal cramps. The median age of the ill persons was 31 years, the median duration of illness was 7 days, and four persons sought medical care. The index patient (the first patient to become ill) reported caring for several kittens with diarrhea 1 or 2 days before the onset of illness. Stool specimens were not cultured from the ill kittens, and they all died.

All 10 ill employees ate meals in the clinic yet had no common exposures outside the clinic. Fecal samples taken from those infected were cultured. Further tests identified the pathogen as *Salmonella*, a facultatively anaerobic (i.e., able to live with or without oxygen), gram-negative, motile, rod-shaped bacterium.

Drug resistance testing indicated the pathogen was resistant to multiple antibacterial agents. Of five isolates tested at a clinical laboratory, all were resistant to ampicillin, ceftriaxone, cephalothin, chloramphenicol, clavulanic acid-amoxicillin, gentamicin, kanamycin, streptomycin, sulfamethoxazole, and tetracycline.

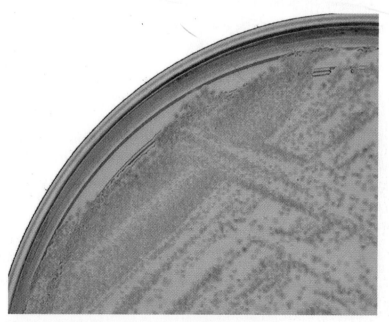

Figure 7.1 Pathogen growth on MacConkey agar.

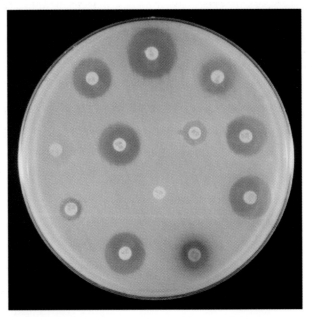

Figure 7.2 Kirby-Bauer assay for drug resistance.

QUESTIONS

1. Besides *Salmonella*, list several viral, bacterial, and protozoal causes of diarrhea.

2. Describe three ways that bacteria can acquire resistance to antibiotics. Given the number of drugs this strain of *Salmonella* was resistant to, what was the most probable mechanism for its acquisition of the antibiotic-resistant genes?

3. Describe the reservoir(s) for this pathogen and its typical mode of transmission.

4. What recommendations would you make to prevent outbreaks such as this from occurring at other veterinary clinics?

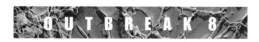

A Pertussis Outbreak

COLORADO, 2000

On 6 January 2000, a full-term, white, non-Hispanic female infant aged 3 months was evaluated by her pediatrician for a runny nose and cough of 7 days duration. A test for respiratory syncytial virus (a common cause of bronchitis in infants) was negative. On 17 January, the infant returned with persistent symptoms that had progressed during the preceding 2 or 3 days to include paroxysmal cough (near-continuous coughing), breathing difficulty, fever, and vomiting after a spasm of coughing. Cyanosis (lack of oxygen resulting in a blue color to the skin) and intercostal retractions (indicating the infant was struggling to inhale enough air) were noted. The infant became increasingly irritable and had a temperature of 104°F (40°C). A chest radiograph revealed marked pneumonia. Blood samples and specimens of nasopharyngeal secretions were collected and analyzed by the laboratory.

The infant's mother reported a cough illness with onset 3 to 4 weeks before the infant's cough onset; the infant's sibling, aged 3 years (who had received four DTP vaccinations to protect against diphtheria, tetanus, and pertussis), also had a mild cough illness.

Laboratory analysis indicated the infant's leukocyte count was 129,000 (normal, 5,000 to 20,000). *Bordetella pertussis*, a slow-growing, gram-negative, fastidious bacillus (a rod-shaped bacterium that grows only on specially supplemented growth media) was isolated from nasopharyngeal secretions.

On 22 January, the infant was placed on mechanical ventilation. After the infant suffered multisystem organ failure and severe hemorrhage of the frontal lobe of the brain, support was withdrawn, and the infant died on 25 January.

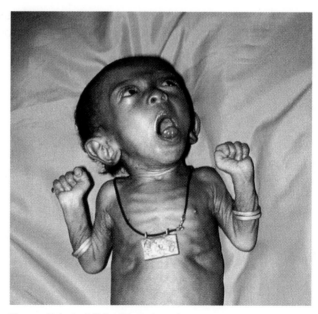

Figure 8.1 A child with pertussis.

QUESTIONS

1. What were the key risk factor(s) for the infant to become severely affected while the mother and sibling experienced only milder versions of the disease?

2. How does a vaccine prevent disease?

3. What part of a bacterial pathogen is typically used as an antigen in this vaccine?

4. Describe what antibiotic would have been appropriate to treat the ill infant. What antibiotic (if any) would be used to treat close contacts?

5. How would you stop this disease from spreading?

6. What are several reasons some parents do not have their children vaccinated?

Vancomycin-Resistant *Staphylococcus aureus*

DETROIT, 2002

Vancomycin-resistant *Staphylococcus aureus* (VRSA) was isolated from a swab obtained from a catheter exit site of a Michigan resident aged 40 years with diabetes, peripheral vascular disease, and chronic renal failure. The patient received dialysis at an outpatient facility (dialysis center A). Since April 2001, the patient had been treated for chronic foot ulcerations with multiple courses of antimicrobial therapy, some of which included vancomycin. In April 2002, the patient underwent amputation of a gangrenous toe and subsequently developed methicillin-resistant *Staphylococcus* bacteremia (bacteria circulating in the bloodstream) caused by an infected dialysis catheter. The infection was treated with vancomycin, rifampin, and removal of the infected graft. In June, the patient developed a suspected catheter exit site infection, and the temporary dialysis catheter was removed; cultures of the exit site and catheter tip subsequently grew *Staphylococcus* bacteria that were resistant to oxacillin and very high concentrations of vancomycin. Laboratory tests to identify the pathogen were completed.

Initially, the Wayne State University professor who directed the microbiology laboratory at the Detroit Medical Center hoped the laboratory report was in error. When he retested the bacteria for vancomycin resistance and again got an off-the-chart reading, he immediately notified the CDC in Atlanta, Georgia, which sent a team to investigate the VRSA.

A week after catheter removal, the exit site appeared to have healed; however, the patient's chronic foot ulcer appeared to be infected. This time, vancomycin-resistant *Enterococcus faecalis* was recovered from a culture of the ulcer. The infection responded to outpatient treatment consisting of aggressive wound care and systemic antimicrobial therapy.

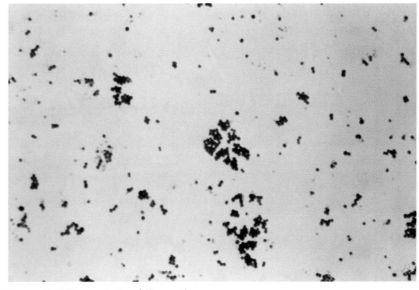

Figure 9.1 Gram stain of the pathogen.

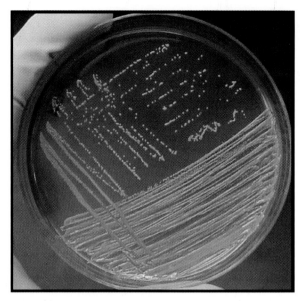

Figure 9.2 Growth on mannitol salt agar.

The infection was the first of its kind in the world and a defeat in the fight against growing antibiotic resistance. The discovery also provided more evidence that the Detroit area has become an incubator for resistant strains. In the 1970s, many area intravenous drug users mixed antibiotics, including methicillin, with heroin. It was a misguided attempt to avoid infection from dirty needles that caused rapidly increasing methicillin resistance. Subsequently, the resistant bacteria infected hospital patients and others in the community, requiring vancomycin (as a last resort) to be widely used in comparison to its use in other areas of the country.

Staphylococcus aureus is a common pathogen that infects about 400,000 U.S. hospital patients a year. *Staphylococcus aureus* can live innocuously in the nose of a healthy person. About 5 to 10% of healthy people carry it asymptomatically. About 400 people were identified in the Detroit area who had regular contact with the patient infected with VRSA: hospital workers and patients, members of the women's choir, and women who had gone to the same nail salon as the patient.

QUESTIONS

1. Explain a possible mechanism for *Staphylococcus aureus* to acquire vancomycin resistance from *Enterococcus*.

2. Besides the conditions mentioned, what other diseases can *Staphylococcus aureus* cause?

3. What physical properties make *Staphylococcus aureus* a common hospital-acquired pathogen?

4. Explain why VRSA is a serious heath risk to the population of Detroit.

5. How would you prevent further spread of VRSA in the Detroit area?

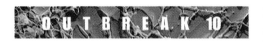

An Influenza Outbreak on a Cruise Ship

NORTHERN EUROPE, 2000

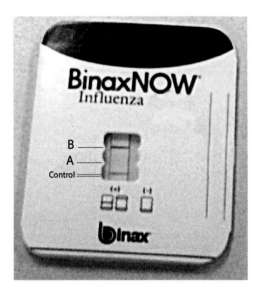

Figure 10.1 Enzyme-linked immunosorbent assay (ELISA) for influenza B.

Between 23 June and 5 July 2000, an outbreak of respiratory illnesses occurred on the *MS Rotterdam* (Holland America Line and Windstar Cruises) during a 12-day Baltic cruise from the United Kingdom to Germany via Russia. The ship carried 1,311 passengers, primarily from the United States, and 506 crew members from many countries.

On 26 June, nine crew members presented to the ship's infirmary with acute respiratory infection (ARI), including a cough, sore throat, and fever of 100.0°F (37.8°C) or more. All had developed symptoms during the preceding 24 hours. Three crew members with high fevers were started on rimantadine therapy (an anti-influenza virus drug) for clinically suspected influenza A virus infection.

To characterize and control the suspected outbreak among crew members, the ship's medical staff implemented a respiratory illness protocol that included surveillance for cases of respiratory illness. Medical and demographic information, including country of residence, cabin number, and crew duties (if applicable), was collected from ill patients. By 29 June, 38 crew members and 26 passengers had been seen in the infirmary for ARI.

The most likely index patient was a 78-year-old U.S. passenger who boarded the ship ill with ARI after visiting London, England. She remained in her cabin except for occasional meals and did not seek medical attention until the fifth day of the cruise (28 June). Two crew members with ARI, who were seen in the infirmary on 25 and 26 June, were her cabin and dining room stewards. Both had worked, socialized, or shared cabins with other crew members who became ill. A total of 64 (13%) crew members and 54 (4%) passengers were identified with ARI during the cruise.

Direct fluorescent antibody tests were positive for influenza B virus but negative for influenza A virus and bacterial pathogens.

QUESTIONS

1. Besides influenza viruses, list three different pathogens that could have caused the outbreak and several of their important physical characteristics.

2. Explain several reasons why having influenza does not make you immune to the disease in the future.

3. How can the risk of outbreaks like this be reduced on cruise ships?

4. Describe an appropriate way to treat the disease to give individuals the best chance of recovering from the illness.

5. From the case study, estimate the incubation period for influenza B.

6. What is the difference between the common usage of the term "flu" and an infection by an influenza virus?

OUTBREAK 11

An AIDS Outbreak Traced to a Single Infected Male

NEW YORK, 1997

As of July 1997, six sexually transmitted infections in young women who reported sexual contact with the same man (the index patient) were detected at health service clinics in a rural county in upstate New York. During the next several months, other sexual contacts of the man were discovered by public health officials. For this investigation, female sex partners of the index case individual were considered primary contacts, and male sex partners of infected primary contacts were considered secondary contacts. Blood specimens from consenting persons were forwarded to the CDC for identification and DNA sequence analysis.

Forty-seven primary contacts were identified, and they reportedly had had vaginal sex with the index case individual: 13 (31%) of 42 tested HIV positive. From these 13 primary contacts, 84 secondary contacts were identified; 1 of 50 tested had acquired HIV infection. One of three infants born to infected women was also infected. There was no evidence that the index case individual or the infected primary contacts had had same-sex or needle-sharing contacts.

The DNA analyses of the pathogens by the CDC indicated a high degree of relatedness among the pathogens infecting the primary contacts, suggesting they were all infected by the index case individual. The single infected secondary contact was probably infected by a source not related to this cluster.

Median ages at first exposure through sexual intercourse with the index case individual were similar for the infected women (17.8 years; range, 13 to 22 years) and uninfected women (17.7 years; range, 14 to 24 years). The infected women had significantly more exposures to the index case individual (median, three exposures; range, two to six exposures) than the uninfected women (median, one exposure; range, one to two exposures.

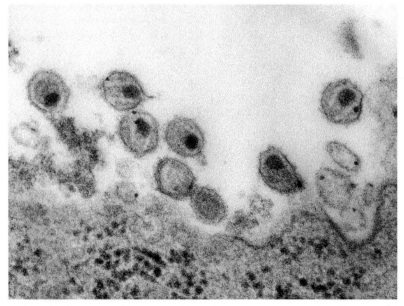

Figure 11.1 Virus budding from a host cell.

Clinical symptoms of the infection were not observed in all individuals. Those who were ill had weight loss, fever, persistent lymphoadenopathy (swollen lymph nodes), diarrhea, and night sweats. The pathogen was identified as an enveloped virus with a spherical capsid and ribonucleic acid (RNA) as the genetic information (Fig. 11.1).

QUESTIONS

1. What potential complications are the infected individuals at risk for if they are not treated?

2. What characteristics of HIV enable it to avoid immune system defenses?

3. What characteristics of HIV require treatment with multiple antiviral agents?

4. Describe how you would prevent this epidemic from spreading.

5. Should the index case individual be located and informed of his status?

6. Should the index case individual be threatened with legal prosecution if he persists in having unprotected sex with partners (particularly minors)?

7. Are the primary contacts who tested HIV negative safe from infection?

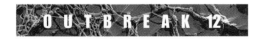

A Rubella Outbreak

ARKANSAS, 1999

Between 7 September and 26 October 1999, a total of 12 cases of a fever and rash outbreak were identified in three Arkansas counties. On 7 September, a pregnant woman aged 23 years presented to a public health clinic in Fort Smith, Sebastian County, Arkansas, with a rash of small flat red spots and fever. The woman was from Mexico and had lived in Arkansas for 1 year before the onset of illness. She later delivered a stillborn infant with pathologic findings compatible with intrauterine viral infection. Her exposure to the virus was from a household contact with a Mexican male aged 20 years. Both patients worked in a poultry-processing plant in Fort Smith.

The rubella virus was identified through laboratory testing for a rising titer of antibodies to the virus using a latex bead agglutination test. The virus is a positive-sense RNA virus with an enveloped polyhedral capsid.

Outbreak investigators interviewed household and workplace contacts of the woman. An additional 10 cases were confirmed by laboratory testing. Among the 12 confirmed case patients, the median age was 23 years; 10 (83%) were Hispanic, 9 (75%) were born outside the United States (in Mexico or El Salvador), and 6 (50%) were women.

All six female patients were pregnant, and one became infected during the first trimester of pregnancy. The pregnant patients exposed 155 women in the clinic waiting room as they were obtaining prenatal care. Of the 155 women, only 46 (32%) reported a complete history of childhood vaccination.

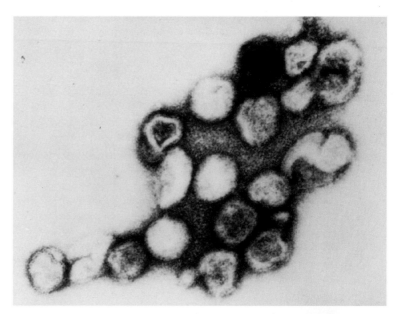

Figure 12.1 Transmission electron micrograph of the pathogen.

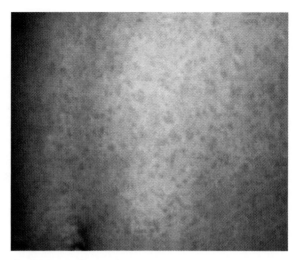

Figure 12.2 Skin rash.

QUESTIONS

1. Describe the clinical features of rubella. How does it differ from measles (rubeola)?

2. Describe the pathogenesis of this disease in adults.

3. What property of the virus makes it particularly dangerous to pregnant women?

4. In order to minimize the number of cases of the disease, how would you manage the outbreak?

5. How does a rubella infection in a pregnant female affect the fetus?

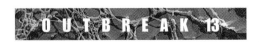

An Outbreak of Rotaviral Gastroenteritis among Children

JAMAICA, 2003

In late May 2003, the Jamaican Ministry of Health (MoH) identified a sharp increase in the number of acute gastroenteritis (AGE) cases reported throughout the country, accompanied by increases in AGE-associated hospital admissions and deaths among children. The greatest increase in AGE cases was observed among children aged <5 years in parts of Kingston and St. Andrew. During June and July, 12 AGE-associated deaths were reported among children aged <8 years. The MoH began an investigation to determine the etiology of the outbreak, ascertain risk factors for illness and death, and identify appropriate control measures.

Interviews with primary caregivers suggested that 8 of the 12 deaths were attributable to diarrhea. These eight deaths occurred among children aged 4 months to 3 years. All eight children had watery diarrhea and vomiting that began 1 to 5 days before death. All had visited a public or private health care provider at least once for treatment. Five children had received oral rehydration therapy for their diarrheal illness; three received no oral rehydration therapy during their clinic visits. Three children were treated with antibiotics, two with antidiarrheals, and three with antiemetic injections to prevent vomiting.

Tests of 43 stool specimens collected during June and July for *Salmonella*, *Shigella*, *Vibrio cholerae*, and *Escherichia coli* O157:H7 were negative. However, the pathogen responsible for the outbreak and the deaths observed was identified by latex agglutination and ELISAs as rotavirus. Rota-virus is a nonenveloped virus with a polyhedral capsid and double-stranded RNA. It was found in 54 (50%) of the 109 stool specimens collected from children aged <5 years as part of the MoH investigation.

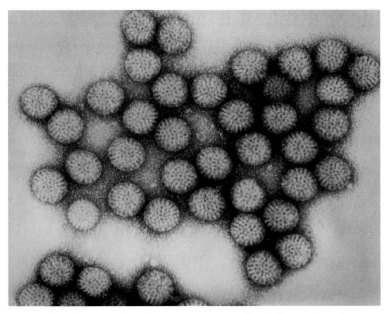

Figure 13.1 Transmission electron micrograph of the viral pathogen.

QUESTIONS

1. What physical property enables rotavirus to survive until it reaches the small intestine, where infection occurs?

2. How does rotavirus cause diarrhea?

3. Why did this pathogen not primarily affect the adult population?

4. How would you treat those who were ill from the pathogen?

5. How would you contain this outbreak and prevent future similar outbreaks?

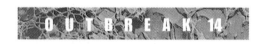

A *Cryptosporidium* Outbreak in a Day Camp

FLORIDA, 1995

In July 1995, the Alachua County Public Health Unit in central Florida was notified of an outbreak of gastroenteritis among children and counselors at a day camp on the grounds of a public elementary school. The camp operated from 12 June through 4 August and enrolled 98 children (age range, 4 to 12 years) and 6 counselors.

Of the 104 people attending the camp, 77 had symptoms (abdominal pain [74%], nausea [73%], diarrhea [71%], vomiting [57%], and fever [43%]), with onset between 20 July and 15 August, including 72 of the children and 5 of the counselors. Follow-up phone calls to 67 of 79 households of those who attended the camp indicated that 24 household members had onset of gastrointestinal (GI) symptoms between 20 July and 23 August.

Water sources for the camp included an outdoor drinking fountain, a sink inside the trailer that served as camp headquarters, and portable coolers. The coolers were filled at either a kitchen sink inside the school or an outdoor faucet with an attached hose and spray nozzle used for washing garbage cans.

Virtually all people at the camp reported drinking water from one of the camp sources during the 3 weeks before the outbreak. Water treatment plant samples were repeatedly negative. Outdoor-faucet samples were positive for fecal coliforms, gram-negative bacteria that are normally found in feces; other school sites were negative or below detectable limits for fecal coliforms. The area around the outdoor faucet was not fenced, and feces of unknown origin were observed on several occasions near the faucet and attached hose.

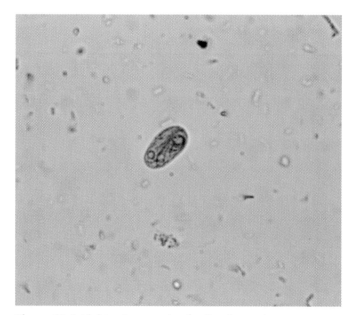

Figure 14.1 Light micrograph of a fecal sample.

Stool samples from those affected were tested. Microscopic examination indicated the presence of acid-fast cysts, indicating *Cryptosporidium parvum* as the pathogen responsible for the outbreak.

QUESTIONS

1. Besides *Cryptosporidium*, list several viral, eukaryotic, and bacterial pathogens that could account for the outbreak of diarrhea.

2. What physical feature of *Cryptosporidium* makes it resistant to chlorination and other types of disinfection processes?

3. How can future outbreaks be prevented?

4. Describe how you would treat those who were most severely affected by the pathogen.

5. How would you account for the 24 reported cases among family members between 20 June and 23 August?

An *Escherichia coli* O111:H8 Outbreak among Teenage Campers

TEXAS, 1999

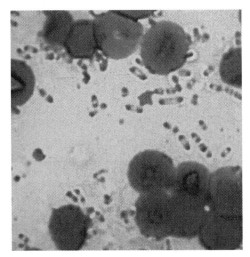

Figure 15.1 Gram stain of the pathogen.

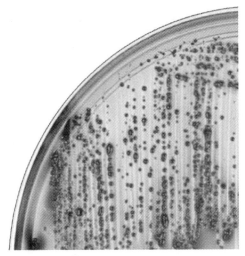

Figure 15.2 Growth on MacConkey agar.

In June 1999, the Tarrant County Health Department reported to the Texas Department of Health that a group of teenagers attending a cheerleading camp from 9 to 11 June became ill with nausea, vomiting, severe abdominal cramps, and diarrhea, some of which was bloody. Two teenagers were hospitalized with hemolytic-uremic syndrome (HUS) (a syndrome where the blood cells are being broken down), and two others underwent appendectomies.

The campers were interviewed for medical histories and symptoms and about their food and beverage consumption at the camp. No campers reported having a diarrheal illness or contact with a person with diarrhea during the 2 weeks before the start of camp. Sanitarians inspected the cafeteria and the plumbing system in the dormitory where the campers resided. Food handlers and other kitchen staff were interviewed about food preparation practices, menus, and the delivery schedules and suppliers for food items served to campers. The food handlers submitted stool specimens and rectal swabs for testing. Several food items from the cafeteria were cultured. In all instances, no pathogens or procedural errors were identified. Also, inspection of the camp's water systems showed no evidence of plumbing cross-connections or failures that might have led to exposures to contaminated water or waste.

Investigation of the outbreak revealed that the diarrhea was correlated with consuming ice from large trash-can-style lined barrels that the camp provided in the dormitory lobby for filling water bottles. Campers reported dipping their drink containers and arms, hands, and heads into the ice. They also reported observing floating debris in the ice barrels. Testing of ice from the ice machines used to fill the barrels for fecal contamination was negative. Culture analysis of feces samples from the patients grew pathogenic *E. coli*. Identification was completed by testing antigens on the cell wall (O111) and flagella (H8). ELISA tests for Shiga toxin were positive.

QUESTIONS

1. Describe the rationale for the different aspects of the initial investigation to identify the pathogen.

2. Describe the benefits of nonpathogenic *E. coli* in the GI tract.

3. How do Shiga toxin-producing strains of *E. coli* cause bloody diarrhea and HUS complications?

4. Describe the probable route(s) of transmission of the pathogen during the outbreak.

5. Describe how you would manage the care of the ill individuals.

6. What recommendations would you make to camp authorities to prevent future outbreaks?

An Outbreak of Lethal Viral Pneumonia

THAILAND, 2004

From mid-December 2003 to mid-February 2004, a total of 23 laboratory-confirmed human cases of a highly pathogenic strain of avian influenza were identified. The cases were reported in eight different Asian countries, including China, Japan, Thailand, and Vietnam. The outbreak caused worldwide concern for several reasons. Although the number of cases was small, the mortality of the resulting pneumonia was extremely high: 78% of all those infected died. The pathogen was identified as a genetically unique virus that had not previously been found to infect humans. As a result, no one was immune. Therefore, if the disease was highly contagious, it could result in a deadly pandemic. Finally, the pathogen was found to infect previously healthy children and adults rather than those who were already in poor health.

Details of the transmission from poultry to humans were investigated in Thailand. Of the five case patients, four reported deaths of poultry owned by their family, and two of those four reported touching an infected chicken. The fifth patient reported having played near a cage containing infected chickens.

Patient symptoms included fever, cough, sore throat, runny nose, and muscle aches. All of the patients experienced shortness of breath and reported to the hospital 2 to 6 days after the onset of fever and cough. After admission, the patients were appropriately treated with broad-spectrum antibiotics for community-acquired pneumonia. Laboratory tests indicated there was no evidence of secondary bacterial infection. All of the patients had respiratory failure and died 1 to 4 weeks after the onset of symptoms.

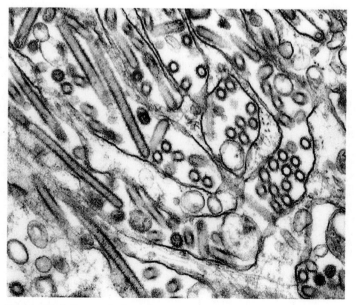

Figure 16.1 Transmission electron micrograph of the viral pathogen.

Laboratory tests identified the pathogen as influenza A virus, an enveloped virus with a polyhedral capsid and eight different segments of single-stranded RNA as genetic information. Antigen testing indicated that the hemagglutinin (H) and neuraminidase (N) proteins embedded in the envelope were H5 and N1, respectively.

QUESTIONS

1. How does influenza A virus occasionally produce unique antigenic combinations that can lead to pandemics?

2. How would you treat those infected with the virus?

3. Is this particular variant of the virus transmitted person to person?

4. How would you have contained this outbreak?

5. Suggest an explanation for why bird flu outbreaks have been reported mostly in Asian countries.

Acquired Immune Deficiency Syndrome (AIDS)

AIDS is now the number one killer disease in sub-Saharan Africa, surpassing malaria. It is estimated that 29.4 million people are currently living with HIV/AIDS in sub-Saharan Africa. That is two-thirds of the HIV/AIDS cases reported globally. According to the Joint United Nations Program on HIV/AIDS, an estimated 3.5 million adults and children in sub-Saharan Africa became infected with HIV in 2002. In that year, 2.4 million people died of AIDS-related illness in Africa. What sets AIDS apart, however, is that it kills so many adults in the prime of their working and parenting lives, which decimates the work force, impoverishes families, orphans millions, and shreds the fabric of communities. Of the 13 million children orphaned by AIDS worldwide, 10 million live in sub-Saharan Africa.

In at least 10 African countries, prevalence rates among adults exceed 10%. In several of the countries with the highest adult infection rates, life expectancy has now dropped to less than 40 years, with a child being born today having over a 50% chance of dying of AIDS.

Cause of the disease

The cause of AIDS is HIV, an enveloped virus with a polyhedral capsid and single-stranded RNA as its genetic information. HIV is called a retrovirus because it has an enzyme, reverse transcriptase, that catalyzes the copying of single-stranded RNA to double-stranded DNA.

Transmission

Reservoir

Humans are the only reservoir of HIV.

Mode of transmission

Horizontal: The virus is spread by direct intimate contact as an STD or as a blood-borne pathogen via the parenteral route.

Vertical: The virus can be spread to newborn children during birth, when there is a potential for maternal and placental blood exchange to occur.

Pathogenesis

Entry

Entry requires blood-to-blood or semen-to-blood exchange.

Attachment

The protein on the outside of the HIV envelope (gp160) binds to T4 lymphocytes, neurons, and macrophages, which carry the CD4 receptor protein.

Avoiding host defenses

The virus is an intracellular pathogen, so it can avoid circulating antibodies. In addition, HIV can form a provirus, in which the viral DNA has been incorporated into the host cell chromosome. In a proviral state, the viral genome as DNA can be dormant for extended periods until it is stimulated to complete its normal replication cycle.

Overcoming defenses

The pathogen destroys CD4$^+$ lymphocytes, which activate both the antibody-mediated immune system (B cells and antibodies) and the cell-mediated immune system (T cells and cytotoxic T cells). Also, the viral reverse transcriptase is very error prone as it synthesizes its genetic information, resulting in a heterogeneous mix of mutant viruses and allowing it to quickly adapt to changing defenses and antiviral agents.

Damage

Damage is direct, as infected cells lose their functions and die. Indirect damage results from loss of immune functions, resulting in a person with AIDS acquiring a number of opportunistic infections (infections that are easily defeated by a person with a healthy immune system).

Exit

HIV exits through the blood, semen, or breast milk of infected individuals.

Clinical features

After the primary infection by HIV, a person will experience a mononucleosis-like illness. After recovery, there is a long period (about 10 years on average) during which the virus continues to replicate and damage the tissues and cells of the immune system but there is little clinical expression of the disease. Following the asymptomatic period, those with HIV infection begin to experience chronic systemic problems, including weight loss, persistent fever, persistent lymphadenopathy (swollen lymph nodes), persistent diarrhea, and night sweats. AIDS is characterized by an HIV infection causing a T4 lymphocyte count of less than 200 cells/ml, resulting in chronic systemic signs and symptoms plus an opportunistic infection. *Pneumocystis jaroveci* is the most common cause of death among people with AIDS. It is a fungal pathogen that causes pneumonia in people who are severely immunocompromised.

Diagnosis

Specimen
A blood sample is used as a specimen.

Test
Initially, an ELISA is used to screen for serum antibodies to HIV. If the first test is positive, HIV infection is confirmed through a second sample using Western blotting to identify HIV-specific proteins or polymerase chain reaction (PCR) analysis to identify HIV-specific DNA sequences.

Treatment
AIDS usually is treated with a "triple cocktail" composed of two inhibitors of the reverse transcriptase enzyme and one inhibitor of the HIV protease. Both enzymes are unique to HIV-infected cells. The reverse transcriptase inhibitors are nucleoside analogs that have a high affinity for reverse transcriptase. They are missing the –OH group that normally links nucleotides during DNA synthesis. The protease inhibitor has a unique structure that allows it to bind specifically to HIV protease and prevents it from cleaving a large virus polypeptide precursor, thus preventing viral maturation.

Prevention

Sexual transmission
- Abstinence and monogamy (one partner for life) prevent the transmission of all STDs.
- Consistent and correct latex condom use is an effective way to prevent the spread of AIDS.
- General risk can be decreased by limiting the number of different sexual partners and not having intercourse with individuals who are at high risk for acquiring STDs, e.g., commercial sex workers.
- Public education may also work to induce changes in high-risk sexual behavior.
- The spread of HIV can be reduced in a community by screening high-risk groups and providing easy and free treatment programs.

Blood-to-blood transmission
- Pregnant women who are infected should take anti-HIV medications to prevent spread to the newborn infant.
- Intravenous-drug users should not share needles.
- The blood supply must be screened to eliminate HIV-contaminated blood.
- Contacts of HIV⁺ blood donors must be traced.
- Hemophiliacs should be supplied with recombinant blood-clotting factors.
- Health care workers should wear gloves and masks and use needle disposal devices.

Breast milk-to-infant transmission
- Prohibit breast feeding of infants by HIV-positive mothers.

Anthrax
Anthrax is found in three potentially fatal forms: cutaneous anthrax results from an infection of the skin of humans and animals that have come in contact with anthrax endospores, GI anthrax results in serious damage to the GI tract when animals eat infected food, and inhalation anthrax results in life-threatening pneumonia. In today's world, inhalation anthrax is most likely an indication of the use of biological weapons.

Cause of the disease
Bacillus anthracis, a bacterial pathogen, is a large, aerobic, nonmotile, gram-positive rod that forms an antiphagocytic capsule. Members of the genus *Bacillus* are capable of forming spores that can survive long periods of harsh conditions.

Transmission
Humans can become infected by coming into contact with spores from animals infected with *Bacillus anthracis* that enter through the skin, mucous membranes, or respiratory tract. The most common means of infection for humans is via contact with spores found on animal products, such as hides, bristles, or wool.

Reservoir
Bacillus anthracis is found in soil where animals that have died of anthrax have decomposed.

Mode of transmission
Cutaneous anthrax is transmitted by direct contact with endospore-contaminated material—infected tissue, the carcass of a dead animal, or contaminated soil. GI anthrax is transmitted by ingestion of contaminated food. Inhalation anthrax is transmitted by airborne particles less than 5 μm in diameter. This normally requires the technologically demanding process of preparing the endospores for use as a biological weapon.

Pathogenesis

Entry
The endospores enter the body by way of the skin, mucous membranes, or respiratory tract.

Attachment
The spores germinate and attach to the tissues that they have entered.

Avoiding host defenses
The pathogen produces an antiphagocytic capsule that enables it to avoid phagocytosis.

Damage
The pathogen produces two toxins: the edema factor causes large amounts of fluid to be lost from the capillaries, while the lethal factor causes cell death, leading to necrosis (dead tissues) and hemorrhaging.

Exit
The pathogen is not typically spread person to person, since infection is normally from the soil reservoir.

Clinical features
Symptoms vary depending on how the disease was contracted, but in all cases, symptoms usually arise within 7 days of infection.

Cutaneous
Skin infection begins as a raised, itchy bump that looks similar to an insect bite. Within 1 to 2 days, the bump develops into a painless black ulcer (an eschar), usually 1 to 3 cm in diameter. Also, lymph nodes in the area begin to swell. In about 20% of untreated cases, the pathogen enters the bloodstream and causes a fatal infection.

Inhalation
Symptoms initially resemble those of a common cold. After several days, the symptoms progress to severe breathing problems and shock. Pulmonary anthrax usually results in death in 1 to 2 days after the onset of symptoms.

GI
The major symptom is inflammation of the intestinal tract. Initial signs of nausea, loss of appetite, vomiting, and fever are followed by abdominal pain and severe diarrhea. Intestinal anthrax is lethal in about 40% of cases.

Diagnosis
Clinical features aid in the diagnosis. The spreading, necrotic eschar indicates cutaneous anthrax. Inhalation anthrax is characterized by overwhelming pneumonia.

A chest X ray shows not only fluid in the lungs, but also a widening of the mediastinal cavity (the space between the lungs, where the heart and major blood vessels are located) caused by large amounts of fluid lost from the infected mediastinal lymph nodes.

Bacillus anthracis can be identified by a rapid hemagglutination test. However, diagnosis must be confirmed by a positive blood culture showing gram-positive, endospore-forming rods.

Treatment
A number of antibiotics given in large doses are effective. Ciprofloxacin is approved by the Food and Drug Administration (FDA) to treat anthrax. It is a fluoroquinolone and kills *Bacillus anthracis* by inhibiting DNA gyrase activity, thus preventing DNA replication of the pathogen.

Prevention
- People in high-risk occupations are given a series of anthrax immunizations that lead to immunity. Animals can also be vaccinated.
- Infected animals should be isolated.
- Carcasses of dead animals should be incinerated.

Biofilm Formation and Control
The Centers for Disease Control and Prevention and the National Institutes of Health estimate that 65 to 80% of all chronic infections can be attributed to microbial biofilms. Many of these chronic infections are caused by organisms such as *Candida albicans*, *Pseudomonas aeruginosa*, *E. coli*, *Staphylococcus epidermidis*, and *Staphylococcus aureus*.

Structure
Bacterial biofilms consist of microorganisms attached to a surface and embedded in a slimy layer of extracellular polysaccharides. Mature biofilms have a complex organization. The extracellular polysaccharide matrix forms columns and knob-shaped pillars with an interdependent community of bacteria embedded. These structures contain channels and large spaces that allow the flow of liquid through the film to efficiently carry nutrients and oxygen to the cells and remove waste products.

Although a mature biofilm is a complex microbial ecosystem of interdependent bacteria, its formation requires only two essential steps: reversible attachment and irreversible attachment. Reversible attachment occurs when planktonic (free-swimming) bacteria adhere to dissolved organic material that has adhered to a surface. External portions of the bacteria (such as pili or flagella) temporarily adhere to organic material left behind by the decomposition or excretion of organisms. Attachment may stimulate the bacterial cells to secrete a sticky polysaccharide that forms a matrix around the cells and glues them to the surface irreversibly.

Function

The bacterial cells secrete a polysaccharide matrix that aids the cells in surviving hostile environments. Environmentally stressful conditions, such as desiccation or changes in pH and temperature, are modified by the biofilm matrix.

The biofilm can provide protection from some predatory protozoa. The matrix of the biofilm also acts to collect and concentrate essential nutrients found in the environment surrounding the biofilm. Besides the normal mechanisms for drug resistance, bacteria in biofilms can be protected by the extracellular matrix, which can restrict the diffusion of antibiotics and disinfectants, enabling the biofilm bacteria to survive conditions that effectively kill planktonic bacteria.

Benefits of biofilms

Biofilms have been used for decades in trickle tanks to treat sewage wastewater. Sewage is trickled through a large tank containing tons of rocks coated with biofilms. As the water trickles between the rocks, the aerobic bacteria within the biofilm digest the organic material in feces and other wastes to purify the water before it is released.

Problems caused by biofilms

Many industries continually fight the growth of biofilms to attempt to minimize damage to surfaces in contact with water. Metal water pipelines in cooling towers and heat exchangers are continuously corroded by biofilms. Thick biofilms also reduce water flow. Since biofilms adhere to plastic, they often form on inserted prosthetic medical devices and catheters, causing chronic infections. Often, removal of the medical device is the only solution to get rid of the infecting microbes. Biofilms also initiate the colonization of marine invertebrates on ships and submerged structures, leading to continuous damage in the marine industry. Biofilms can also ferment nutrients to acid end products. These acids cause cavities in teeth (plaque is a biofilm on your teeth) and quickly corrode cement pipes used as storm drains and sewer pipes.

Treatment and control

Biofilms can be more resistant to antibiotics and disinfectants if the matrix restricts diffusion of the chemicals. Medical devices are sometimes constructed with a coating of chemicals that inhibit biofilm formation.

High concentrations of chlorine or cationic surfactants are used to control biofilm growth in pipelines. Regular treatment is needed because of constant regrowth of the biofilms.

Cryptosporidiosis

Cryptosporidiosis is a self-limited diarrheal illness in healthy individuals, mostly children. Only recently, cryptosporidiosis has been recognized as a cause of self-limited diarrhea in persons with a normal immune system and severe prolonged diarrhea in patients with AIDS.

Cause of the disease

Cryptosporidiosis is caused by *Cryptosporidium parvum*, a eukaryotic protozoal pathogen that has a complex life cycle, including the formation of sporozoa and thick-walled oocysts that are acid-fast during staining, indicating that the cysts have a waxy coating.

Transmission

Reservoir

C. parvum can be carried by humans and a wide range of animals, including cattle, cats, deer, and horses.

Mode of transmission

C. parvum is spread by the oral-fecal route through contaminated drinking water, recreational water, and foods that have been contaminated.

Pathogenesis

Entry

Ingestion of approximately 100 oocysts in fecally contaminated material.

Attachment

The epithelial cells of intestinal villi.

Avoiding host defenses

Oocysts have an acid resistance capsule that allows them to pass through the low pH of the stomach without damage and proceed into the intestines, where they attach.

Damage

After ingestion of oocysts, asexual release of sporozoites is initiated. Sporozoites attach to and penetrate the intestinal mucosa, where they mature into other forms of the parasite and rupture the infected cells. Damaged tissue and inflammation prevent water absorption, causing diarrhea.

Exit
Infective thick-walled oocysts are excreted through feces.

Clinical features
Symptoms may last about 1 to 3 weeks and appear 2 to 10 days after infection; they include loose, watery diarrhea; stomach cramps; and a slight fever. In immunocompromised patients (those whose immune systems function poorly), *Cryptosporidium* infection leads to chronic watery diarrhea with severe cramps, weight loss, a low-grade fever, and severe dehydration.

Diagnosis
Sample
A feces sample is obtained.

Tests
Acid-fast staining and detection of acid-fast oocysts by microscopy.

Treatment
Those with a healthy immune system will recover in 1 to 3 weeks without treatment. Oral fluids and electrolytes help to prevent dehydration from diarrhea.

In immunocompromised patients, such as AIDS patients, paromomycin is often used to inhibit growth of the pathogen. Although paromomycin inhibits eukaryotic protein synthesis, it is not absorbed by the GI tract, so oral administration preferentially inhibits *Cryptosporidium* in the GI tract.

Prevention
- Practice good hygiene.
- Wash hands thoroughly with soap and water (after using the toilet, changing diapers, handling animals, or cleaning up feces; before eating or preparing food; and after handling anything contaminated with fecal matter).
- Avoid drinking untreated water from lakes, streams, pools, hot tubs, or other water sources. Thick-walled oocysts can survive extreme environments, including high levels of chlorination.
- Peel or rinse fruits or vegetables that are to be eaten raw to prevent ingestion of food that may be contaminated with feces.
- Drink bottled water without ice when traveling to places with poor sanitation.
- Boil contaminated water for at least 10 minutes or filter the water to remove any bacterial, protozoal, or viral pathogens.

Enterohemorrhagic *E. coli*
Even though *E. coli* is a normal resident of the large intestine, where the bacterium does not cause disease, some strains are among the most frequent causes of many common bacterial infections, including urinary tract infections, diarrhea, and other clinical infections, such as neonatal meningitis and pneumonia. The urinary tract is the most common site of infection by *E. coli*, which accounts for more than 90% of all uncomplicated urinary tract infections. The O157:H7 and O111 variants of *E. coli* are enterohemorrhagic and cause bloody diarrhea that can be complicated by HUS.

Cause of the disease
E. coli, a gram-negative bacterial pathogen, is part of the normal flora of all healthy individuals. However, mutant strains, like *E. coli* O157:H7, which carries the H7 antigen on its flagella and the O157 antigen on the O oligosaccharide of the lipopolysaccharide of the outer membrane, and O111 cause hemorrhagic diarrhea.

Like nonpathogenic *E. coli*, the pathogen is a facultative anaerobe with peritrichous flagella, and it ferments lactose. However, the O157:H7 variant does not ferment sorbitol, as does the usual nonpathogenic strain.

Transmission
Reservoir
Cattle can carry *E. coli* O157:H7 in their intestines and appear healthy.

Mode of transmission
Transmission is by the oral-fecal route through ingestion of contaminated meat and through anything contaminated with cow feces, including unpasteurized cider, and petting zoos in fairs.

Pathogenesis
Entry
During the slaughter of cattle, the bacteria can be mixed into the meat. Eating inadequately cooked beef can transmit *E. coli* O157:H7. It can also be found on cow's udders and can be transmitted by drinking unpasteurized milk.

Attachment
The pathogen adheres to mucous surfaces in the gut via fimbriae.

Avoiding host defenses

Initial infection is restricted to the epithelium of the intestine, so the pathogen is not initially exposed to circulating antibodies and cells of the immune system.

Damage

The pathogen produces Shiga-like toxins, which cause cell death along the intestinal mucosa, and the endotoxin, leading directly to capillary damage. Vascular damage in the colon by the Shiga-like toxins allows inflammatory mediators into the circulation. Mediators then initiate HUS.

Exit

The pathogen exits in the feces.

Clinical features

Clinical features include severe bloody diarrhea, abdominal cramps, and potentially HUS, a serious complication in which red blood cells are destroyed and the kidneys fail. HUS has 50% mortality in children under 5 years of age.

Diagnosis

Specimen

A fecal swab or stool sample is used as a specimen.

Test

Tests are isolation of *E. coli* that does not ferment sorbitol on sorbitol MacConkey agar and detection of O157 and H7 antigens by ELISA.

Treatment

Most people recover in 5 to 10 days without any antibiotic or other treatment. For serious infections, antibiotics are given after testing for antibiotic-resistant properties of the pathogen. HUS is treated with blood transfusions and kidney dialysis.

Antidiarrheal agents may make the symptoms worse, because preventing bowel movements allows the pathogen to grow to high concentrations within the GI tract, potentially causing more damage and increasing the risk of serious complications.

Prevention

- Cook all meat thoroughly.
- Do not drink unpasteurized milk or juices.
- Wash hands carefully and frequently to reduce risk.

Gonorrhea

Worldwide, approximately 200 million new cases of gonorrhea occur each year. In developed countries, the incidence of gonorrhea is declining, due to public health initiatives. In the United States, there are about 600,000 new infections per year with many more suspected to occur but not be reported. The incidence of penicillinase-producing *N. gonorrhoeae* is rising and is expected to make the treatment of gonorrhea in the future more difficult.

Cause of the disease

Neisseria gonorrhoeae, a bacterial pathogen, is a gram-negative diplococcus that uses fimbriae to adhere to host cell surfaces.

Transmission

Reservoir

Symptomatic men and women and asymptomatic women are the reservoirs.

Mode of transmission

Horizontal: Direct contact as an STD. The pathogen is sensitive to drying and temperature changes and requires direct intimate contact.

Vertical: Newborn infants can develop conjunctivitis that may lead to blindness after being exposed to *N. gonorrhoeae* during birth.

Pathogenesis

Entry

Sexual contact is the means of entry.

Attachment

Adhesins on bacterial fimbriae attach to tissues of the reproductive tract, the oral cavity, the conjunctiva of the eye, and the rectum. Although in women the cervix is usually the initial site of infection, the pathogen can be carried on sperm cells and spread to and infect the uterus and fallopian tubes.

Avoiding host defenses

Attachment prevents the bacteria from being washed away by urine or vaginal discharges. In addition, the pathogen produces immunoglobulin A protease, which degrades the antibodies associated with mucosal immunity.

Damage

Replication of the pathogen causes direct tissue damage, which induces a large inflammatory response.

Exit

The pathogen exits through pus discharge.

Clinical features

Incubation

The incubation period is 2 to 10 days after sexual contact with an infected partner.

Females

Infection is asymptomatic in 50% of females. Symptomatic infections cause a painful or burning sensation when urinating and vaginal discharge that is yellow or bloody. Advanced symptoms can cause abdominal pain, bleeding between menstrual periods, vomiting, fever, and pelvic inflammatory disease, a mixed infection of the upper reproductive tract that can lead to abscesses, chronic pain, ectopic pregnancy (when an embryo begins development outside of the uterus, such as in the fallopian tube), or infertility.

Males

Symptoms are pus discharge from the penis and a burning sensation during urination that may be severe.

Gonorrhea also increases the risk of HIV infection because it causes tissue damage that allows semen-to-blood exchange. Prevention and early treatment of gonorrhea are critically important.

Diagnosis
Specimen

A swab or pus sample is taken from the cervix, penis, throat, or rectum.

Tests

Cultural: Growth on modified Thayer-Martin medium.

Noncultural: PCR using *N. gonorrhoeae*-specific primers or Gram stain of pus to detect gram-negative diplococci in leukocytes.

Treatment

Some strains of *N. gonorrhoeae* produce β-lactamase, so penicillin-resistant cases of gonorrhea are common. A typical treatment is a single intramuscular dose of ceftriaxone, a β-lactamase-resistant β-lactam antibiotic.

It is not unusual for gonorrhea to be complicated by a chlamydial infection; therefore, doctors usually prescribe a combination of antibiotics.

Prevention

- Abstinence and monogamy prevent the transmission of all STDs.
- Consistent and correct latex condom use is an effective way to prevent the spread of *N. gonorrhoeae*.
- General risk can be decreased by limiting the number of different sexual partners and not having intercourse with individuals who are at high risk for acquiring STDs, e.g., commercial sex workers.
- Physicians are required to notify their state department of public health when gonorrhea is identified in one of their patients. The public health department does contact tracing, in which they follow up with infected individuals to identify and recommend treatment for previous sexual partners. In this way, asymptomatic carriers can be identified and treated before they experience complications or spread the pathogen to other sexual partners.
- Antimicrobial agents are routinely added to the eyes of newborns to prevent conjunctivitis and blindness from *N. gonorrhoeae*.
- The spread of gonorrhea can also be reduced in a community by screening high-risk groups and providing easy and free treatment programs. Public education may also work to induce changes in high-risk sexual behavior.

Influenza

Worldwide, pneumonia is the number one cause of death from infectious disease, causing about 3 million deaths per year. Influenza virus is the most common cause of viral pneumonia.

Millions of people are typically infected by an influenza virus each year in the United States. Influenza is the leading reason for a physician's visit among all infectious diseases. Depending on the strain of influenza circulating and the effectiveness of the vaccine, there are about 20,000 to 40,000 deaths from influenza each year. During the winter months, when the annual influenza epidemic peaks, pneumonia caused by influenza viruses causes 10% of all deaths.

Cause of the disease

Influenza is caused by the influenza A, B, and C viruses. Influenza A and B viruses cause the most serious illnesses.

Influenza A and B viruses are enveloped viruses belonging to the family *Orthomyxoviridae* ("myxo" is Greek for mucus). The viruses have a polyhedral capsid and multiple segments of single-stranded, negative-sense RNA for genetic information. The virus is classified based on two different proteins embedded in the envelope: hemagglutinin (H protein) and neuraminidase (N protein).

Transmission
Reservoir

The reservoirs for influenza A virus are birds and a variety of mammals, including humans and swine. The reservoir for influenza B virus is primarily humans.

Mode of transmission

The influenza viruses are spread by respiratory droplets produced during coughing and sneezing. It can also be spread via fomites, i.e., touching contaminated objects and then touching your nose or eyes.

Pathogenesis

Entry

The virus enters by fomites or inhaling mucus droplets carrying the pathogen.

Attachment

The virus uses the H protein to attach to the ciliated respiratory epithelium.

Avoiding host defenses

The pathogen is intracellular, and infection is restricted to the surface of the respiratory tract, resulting in the pathogen initially avoiding circulating antibodies and cells of the immune system.

Both influenza A and B viruses can undergo antigenic drift, in which they accumulate point mutations in the H and N proteins. With time, these key antigens change their structures sufficiently that the immune response from previous infections of a host will not provide immunity. Influenza A virus undergoes antigenic drift more rapidly than influenza B virus.

Influenza A virus can also undergo antigenic shifts. These occur when a human and an animal virus recombine in a single host. The resulting recombinant virus is unique and can cause worldwide pandemics.

Damage

Influenza viruses destroy the tissue lining the respiratory epithelium. The tissue damage induces an inflammatory response that accounts for the clinical features of the disease. Tissue damage also makes an infected host more susceptible to secondary bacterial pneumonia.

Exit

The virus exits through respiratory droplets.

Clinical features

The average incubation period for influenza is 2 days. The disease usually starts suddenly and may include the following symptoms: fever (usually high), headache, fatigue (which can be extreme), cough, runny or stuffy nose, body aches, and sore throat. Diarrhea and vomiting can also occur but are more common in children. Influenza results in pneumonia and death primarily as a result of the infection compromising the normal defenses of the respiratory tract, increasing the risk for secondary bacterial infections. Approximately 36,000 deaths resulting from influenza occurred per year in the United States from 1990 to 1999. Older adults (>65 years old) account for ≥90% of deaths attributed to influenza.

Diagnosis

Specimen

A throat swab, nasal wash, or nasal swab is used as a specimen, depending on the type of test used.

Test

Rapid diagnostic tests detect influenza viruses within 30 minutes.

Treatment

There are three approved antivirals for treating influenza A virus infections (amantadine, rimantadine, and oseltamivir). Amantadine prevents entry of the virus into the host cell. The others prevent release of the virus from the host cell. All are effective at reducing the severity and duration of influenza if given within the first 48 hours after the appearance of clinical signs and symptoms. Symptomatic therapy includes bed rest, drinking plenty of fluids to prevent dehydration, and using analgesics to reduce pain and fever. (Aspirin is not used as a pain reliever because of an increased risk of Reye's syndrome in children and adolescents.)

Prevention

- The influenza vaccine consists of inactivated and attenuated live viruses that are prepared from the two dominant variants of influenza A virus and the one dominant version of influenza B virus from the previous year. As a result, the vaccine is effective if the virus does not undergo significant genetic drift or an antigenic shift.

- Other prevention strategies include covering the mouth when coughing or sneezing, avoiding others with the flu, frequent and thorough washing of hands, and avoiding touching the eyes and nose.

Mycoplasmal Pneumonia

Mycoplasmal pneumonia, also referred to as primary atypical pneumonia or "walking pneumonia," is common in all age groups over 4 years of age. Only about 3% of infections with *Mycoplasma pneumoniae* result in pneumonia, with most of the rest causing upper respiratory tract infections. The incubation period averages 3 weeks, in contrast to those of other bacterial pneumonias and influenza, which generally develop in a few days. Transmission of *Mycoplasma* requires prolonged exposure to an infected individual; consequently, epidemics of mycoplasmal pneumonia tend to occur more frequently within closed populations, such as military and institutionalized populations, including those in prisons and colleges.

Cause of the disease

Mycoplasma pneumoniae, a bacterial pathogen, is a very small, wall-less organism that is pleomorphic (able to assume many different forms).

Transmission

Reservoir

Mycoplasma pneumoniae has worldwide distribution. Its reservoir is infected humans.

Mode of transmission

Direct contact and prolonged exposure are typically required to spread *Mycoplasma pneumoniae*. The droplet mode of transmission is a minor mechanism.

Pathogenesis

Entry

The pathogen enters the respiratory system after prolonged, close exposure to an infected host.

Attachment

The pathogen adheres to the tissues of the respiratory tract epithelium.

Avoiding host defenses

Gliding motility facilitates penetration of the pathogen through the mucus of the respiratory tract. The pathogen lodges between microvilli and cilia, preventing phagocytosis.

Damage

Tissue damage is caused by mycoplasmal metabolites, such as hydrogen peroxide and superoxide radicals and ammonia, causing death of cells lining the respiratory tract.

Exit

The pathogen exits the respiratory tract in mucus droplets.

Clinical features

About two-thirds of the respiratory infections by *Mycoplasma pneumoniae* result in bronchitis. Onset of pneumonia occurs slowly about 2 to 3 weeks after infection. There is a gradual onset of fever, headache, and a constant, nonproductive cough. As the disease progresses, rales (cracking sounds in the lungs indicating fluid) are detected, and chest X rays reveal fluid accumulation in one or more lobes of the lungs.

Diagnosis

Although *Mycoplasma pneumoniae* can be grown and identified in the laboratory using special growth media and special stains, extremely slow growth can delay diagnosis up to 4 weeks. Consequently, specific diagnosis of the pathogen may not be completed before treatment is required. Pneumonias that respond to antibiotics and are not caused by *Streptococcus pneumoniae* are classified as primary atypical pneumonias. They can be caused by pathogens such as *Mycoplasma pneumoniae* or *Chlamydia pneumoniae*.

Treatment

The tetracyclines and erythromycin are effective at treating the disease but do not inhibit shedding of the organism. Both tetracyclines and erythromycin inhibit protein synthesis on 70S ribosomes.

Prevention

- Avoid close contact with acutely ill individuals.
- Wash hands frequently and thoroughly.

Pertussis

Pertussis is an endemic disease worldwide. It is the eighth leading cause of death from infectious disease, accounting for about 400,000 deaths annually. Although there is a vaccine that effectively prevents pertussis in children, neither acquisition of the disease nor vaccination provides complete or lifelong immunity. In parts of Europe, the frequency of pertussis increased when the percentage of those vaccinated dropped to as low as 30%.

The CDC estimates that only 5 to 10% of pertussis cases are recognized and reported. In reported studies, 12 to 32% of adults with prolonged cough (1 to 4 weeks) have been found to have pertussis.

Cause of the disease

Pertussis is caused by *Bordetella pertussis*, a bacterial pathogen. *B. pertussis* is a gram-negative coccobacillus. It is fastidious, requiring special media to grow in the laboratory.

Transmission

Reservoir

B. pertussis is found only in humans. In the vaccine era, asymptomatic carriers transmit the pathogen.

Mode of transmission

Pertussis is highly communicable. It is transmitted by airborne particles and mucus droplets.

Pathogenesis

Entry

The pathogen enters the respiratory tract by inhalation of infective droplets.

Attachment

The pathogen attaches to the ciliated respiratory epithelium.

Avoiding host defenses

The pathogen produces a toxin that inhibits ciliary action, so the pathogen is not swept out of the respiratory tract. Since the infection is limited to the epithelial surface, the pathogen initially avoids circulating antibodies and cells of the immune system.

Damage

Pertussis toxin causes tissue death of the respiratory epithelium. The damage allows the pertussis toxin to enter the bloodstream, where it induces the systemic effects of the disease.

Exit

The pathogen exits by coughing and sneezing of the host.

Clinical features

After infection, there is a 5- to 10-day incubation period.

There are three stages of the disease in children. Adolescents and adults have milder disease.

The prodromal stage (the initial symptomatic period) lasts from 1 to 2 weeks and includes only mild cold-like symptoms.

The second stage lasts from 1 to 6 weeks and is characterized by a progressively worsening cough. The cough progresses to paroxysm, in which 5 to 20 forcible hacking coughs are produced in 15 to 20 seconds, terminating with production of mucus or vomiting. The sudden inspiration of air produces a characteristic whooping. Death can result from lack of oxygen caused by the paroxysmal coughing.

The third stage is convalescence, but the cough persists for several months.

Diagnosis

Clinical

Paroxysmal coughing is observed.

Laboratory

Specimen: Cough plate.

Test: Growth on a selective medium containing charcoal. A slide agglutination test is used to identify the pathogen.

Treatment

Erythromycin is used. It kills the pathogen and eliminates carriage in the nasopharynx. Erythromycin is a macrolide that prevents completion of protein synthesis on 70S ribosomes by stimulating the dissociation of peptidyl-transfer RNA (tRNA).

Supportive measures in the hospital are important to prevent death.

Prevention

- The DTaP vaccine is safe and effective at preventing pertussis.
- Infants under 2 years old who have not been immunized can be given immune serum globulin.
- Close contacts of individuals who have pertussis should be given prophylactic erythromycin and a booster immunization.

Pseudomonas aeruginosa Skin Infections

Pseudomonas aeruginosa is a common opportunistic pathogen (a disease-causing microbe that infects those with a compromised immune system) and nosocomial pathogen. It is very common in patients with diabetes and burns. It is also the second most common cause of nosocomial pneumonia. Relatively recently, *Pseudomonas* folliculitis has emerged as a community-acquired skin infection. The infection is caused by bacterial colonization of hair follicles after exposure to contaminated water from whirlpools, hot tubs, swimming pools, water slides, bathtubs, etc.

Cause of the disease

P. aeruginosa, a bacterial pathogen, is gram negative and rod shaped and has a monopolar flagellum. It produces a blue-green pigment, pyocyanin. The outer membrane of the cell has small porins, which can restrict the diffusion of many disinfectants and antibiotics into the cell. The pathogen also acquires plasmids that carry antibiotic resistance genes.

Transmission

Reservoir

P. aeruginosa is normally a common inhabitant of soil and water and is sometimes present on humans but typically does not cause disease in those with healthy immune systems.

Mode of transmission

The pathogen can be spread in the droplet mode by the respiratory route or by direct contact with an infected individual. It is also a common contaminant of hospitals due to its resistance to disinfection. It is spread by fomites, such as respiratory equipment, food, sinks, taps, and mops.

Pathogenesis

Entry

The pathogen enters by several different routes and from a variety of environmental sites.

Attachment

The fimbriae of *Pseudomonas* adhere to the epithelial cells of the respiratory tract, burn wounds, or postoperative wounds and spread to other epithelial cells.

Avoiding host defenses

The pathogen has an antiphagocytic capsule and can form biofilms.

Damage

Pseudomonas produces two extracellular proteases (elastase and alkaline protease), which together cause the inactivation of some components of the immune response; two hemolysins, which destroy erythrocytes, and a cytotoxin, which kills a variety of cells; and two extracellular toxins, one that impairs phagocyte function and one that mimics the cytotoxic effects of the diphtheria toxin.

Exit

The pathogen exits via respiratory secretions, fomites, or direct contact.

Clinical features

P. aeruginosa can cause folliculitis and often affects those with an immunosuppressed system (burn victims, postoperative patients, hospital residents, AIDS patients, and those with cystic fibrosis). Folliculitis is characterized by a red, itchy, pustular rash. The pus can be a blue-green fluid and can have a fruity smell.

Diagnosis

Specimen

A sample of pus is obtained.

Tests

P. aeruginosa is commonly isolated on blood agar plates and further characterized by Gram staining, an inability to ferment lactose, fruity odor, and the ability to grow at 42°C. It also forms green colonies on tryptic soy agar plates.

Treatment

P. aeruginosa is resistant to many antibiotics because its small porins restrict diffusion, and it often carries plasmids with antibiotic resistance genes. Infections are often treated with a combination of antibiotics selected from a group of antipseudomonal penicillins and cephalosporins: imipenem, meropenem, and ciprofloxacin.

Prevention

- Nosocomial infections can be prevented by proper hospital isolation procedures, aseptic techniques, and careful cleaning and monitoring of respirators, catheters, and other instruments.

- Topical therapy of burn wounds and postoperative patients with antibacterial agents can dramatically reduce incidence.

- Health care workers should follow strict infection control procedures.

- Waterborne outbreaks can be prevented with adequate chlorination of pools and hot tubs.

Rubella

Although there is a highly effective childhood vaccine to prevent rubella, studies have shown that 10 to 20% of the U.S. population is susceptible to the disease. As a result, outbreaks still occur among susceptible adults. From 1996 to 1999, 15 outbreaks were reported. Most of these outbreaks were reported on college campuses, at military installations, in prisons, and in workplaces, including health care environments. Pregnant women who are infected by the rubella virus are at risk for giving birth to children with serious birth defects. Although the burden of congenital rubella syndrome is not well characterized in all countries, more than 100,000 cases are estimated to occur each year in developing countries alone.

Cause of the disease

The disease is caused by rubella virus, an enveloped virus with single-stranded, positive-sense RNA and a polyhedral capsid.

Transmission

Reservoir

Humans serve as the reservoir. Nearly one-half of individuals infected with the virus are asymptomatic.

Mode of transmission

Horizontal: Droplet mode through coughing and sneezing.

Vertical: Transplacental infections occur in 90% of women infected by the virus during the first trimester. Transmission also occurs during the second trimester, but there is less damage to the fetus.

Pathogenesis

Entry

Inhalation of infected droplets via the respiratory route is the means of entry.

Attachment

The pathogen attaches to the epithelial cells of the respiratory tract.

Avoiding host defenses

The virus replicates intracellularly and therefore initially avoids circulating antibodies and cytotoxic T cells.

Damage

The virus replicates locally (in the epithelium and lymph nodes), leading to viremia and spread to other tissues. As a result, disease symptoms develop. In congenital rubella, the virus infects the placenta and then spreads to the fetus. The risk to a fetus is highest in the first few weeks of pregnancy and then declines in terms of both frequency and severity, although there is still some risk in the second trimester.

Exit

The virus is shed from the respiratory tract for 1 week preceding the rash and 2 weeks after the rash appears. Therefore, many are infected before it is recognized that the person has rubella.

Clinical features

A 2-week incubation period is followed by a mild fever, mild respiratory symptoms, and a pink rash of macules and papules that appear first on the face and then the neck, trunk, and extremities. The rash disappears after 3 days. In adults, acute short-lived arthritis is associated with the disease.

Congenital infections during the first trimester, when organogenesis occurs, result in serious abnormalities, such as deafness, congenital heart disease, growth retardation, encephalitis, and mental retardation.

Diagnosis

The clinical presentation can be used to diagnose rubella. An indirect ELISA measuring a rise in anti-rubella virus antibody concentrations can be used to confirm the illness.

Treatment

There is no specific therapy for rubella or congenital rubella.

Prevention

In 1969, a highly effective attenuated live rubella virus vaccine was developed. It provides lasting immunity and is given as part of the normal measles-mumps-rubella vaccination series.

Salmonellosis

Salmonellosis is one of the most common bacterial infections in the United States. It is estimated that more than 2 million cases occur each year. The incidence of *Salmonella* infection is greatest among children, with outbreaks also common among individuals who are institutionalized and residents of nursing homes. Nations with an adequate public health infrastructure report frequencies of gastroenteritis similar to those in the United States. Gastroenteritis is far more common in areas where sanitation is inadequate than in areas with adequate sanitation.

Cause of the disease

The disease is caused by *Salmonella*, a bacterial pathogen. The genus *Salmonella* is divided into more than 2,000 serotypes (different strains within a serovar grouping) on the basis of differences in cell wall and flagellar antigens. These serotypes are divided into several different serovars, including *Salmonella enterica* serovar Typhi (which causes typhoid fever) and *Salmonella enterica* serovar Enteritidis (a diverse group of bacteria with over 2,000 serotypes that cause diarrhea). They are gram-negative rod-shaped bacteria that are facultatively anaerobic. They are motile by peritrichous flagella (surrounding the cell), and they produce H_2S from the metabolism of proteins.

Transmission

Reservoir

The pathogen is found in the GI tracts of humans and other animals.

Mode of transmission

The pathogen is spread by the oral-fecal route, e.g., ingesting contaminated food or water.

Pathogenesis

Entry

The pathogen enters via the ingestion of fecally contaminated food, often undercooked beef, poultry, eggs, or dairy products.

Attachment

The pathogen attaches to the mucosal epithelium of the small intestine.

Avoiding host defenses

Initially, the infection is restricted to the epithelial tissue, where the pathogen is not exposed to circulating antibodies or cells of the immune system.

Damage

Salmonella disrupts the epithelial tissue and invades the lamina propria of the small intestine, where it causes an inflammatory response, resulting in fluid loss that causes diarrhea.

Exit

The pathogen exits through feces.

Clinical features

The incubation period is 18 to 24 hours and is followed by diarrhea, abdominal cramps, and fever.

Diagnosis

Specimen

A feces sample from an infected person serves as a specimen.

Test

Cultural: Growth on selective agar, such as *Salmonella*/*Shigella* agar. Since *Salmonella* does not ferment lactose, colonies are colorless, except for a black center resulting from H_2S production.

Noncultural: Widal agglutination testing identifies O and H antigens.

Treatment

Many cases are self-resolving and last only 5 to 7 days, so that no extensive treatment is needed. In cases of severe dehydration (especially in infants and the elderly), fluid and electrolyte replacement may be necessary. Antibiotics are given if the disease spreads from the intestinal tract, resulting in a systemic infection. Typical antibiotics include amoxicillin and trimethoprim-sulfamethoxazole.

Prevention

- Public water and sewage treatments are effective.
- Thoroughly wash produce, meat, and poultry. Completely cook beef, poultry, and eggs before eating them.
- Wash hands before and after handling food and after using the restroom.
- Avoid cross-contamination of clean food and utensils with raw meat.
- Do not drink unpasteurized milk.

Staphylococcus aureus Skin Infections

Staphylococcus aureus is a very common pathogen. About 10% of individuals are colonized persistently with *S. aureus*. Health care workers, persons with diabetes, and patients on dialysis all have higher rates of colonization. The nose is the predominant site of colonization. *Staphylococcus aureus* is a very versatile pathogen and can cause skin infections, such as folliculitis, furuncles, impetigo, wound infections, and scalded-skin syndrome. In addition, it can cause septic bursitis, septic arthritis, toxic shock syndrome, endocarditis (infection of the inner wall of the heart tissue), osteomyelitis (infection of the bone), pneumonia, food poisoning, infections related to prosthetic devices, and urinary tract infections, and it is the leading cause of nosocomial infections.

Besides being a versatile pathogen, *S. aureus* has shown an extraordinary ability to acquire resistance to antibiotics. Currently, less than 5% of clinical isolates remain sensitive to penicillin, and over half of methicillin-resistant isolates are sensitive only to vancomycin.

Etiology

S. aureus, a bacterial pathogen, is a gram-positive coccus in clusters that is coagulase positive (causes blood plasma to clot) and catalase positive (breaks down H_2O_2 using the enzyme catalase). It is nonfastidious (able to grow on simple laboratory media) and is a facultative anaerobe (capable of both anaerobic and aerobic growth) and can tolerate high-salt environments.

Transmission

Reservoir

S. aureus is found in humans and other animals and can contaminate food. It is typically found as part of the perineum and skin, under fingernails, and within the nose.

Mode of transmission

The pathogen can be passed from person to person via respiratory droplets or direct contact or by fomites, contaminated environmental surfaces and patient care equipment in hospitals. The pathogen survives drying and temperature changes, so it is common in hospital settings (a nosocomial pathogen).

Pathogenesis

Entry

S. aureus can cause boils by infecting hair follicles or enter the body through breaks in the skin. It also complicates infections by other pathogens, such as by causing secondary pneumonia in someone with a primary influenza virus infection.

Attachment

S. aureus can attach to a variety of mammalian tissues by attaching to plasma proteins and components of the extracellular matrices of a variety of cells (fibronectin and collagen).

Avoiding host defenses

S. aureus produces a protein (protein A) that binds antibodies in such a way that the pathogen is not targeted for destruction by cells of the immune system. Some strains also have antiphagocytic capsules.

Damage

S. aureus contains more mechanisms for causing tissue damage than any other pathogen. The damaging enzymes are coagulase, which causes blood clotting; lipases, which hydrolyze cellular lipids; hyaluronidase, which breaks down the extracellular matrices of bone and cartilage; staphylokinase, which dissolves blood clots; and a nuclease that can break down DNA and RNA. The toxins produced include hemolysins, which cause erythrocyte lysis; leukocidins, which destroy leukocytes; delta toxin, which acts like a detergent to solubilize cell membranes; six types of enterotoxins that cause food poisoning; epidermolytic toxin, which causes scalded-skin syndrome; and toxic shock syndrome toxin, which causes a life-threatening drop in blood pressure. The damage produced by enzymes and toxins is complicated by inflammation, causing edema (swelling) and a local fever.

Clinical features

S. aureus is a very common and versatile pathogen. Some common diseases it causes are boils, impetigo, folliculitis, cellulitis, pneumonia, endocarditis, osteomyelitis, toxic shock syndrome, and food poisoning.

Diagnosis

A specimen from the infected site is obtained and grown on blood agar (it forms golden colonies and destroys surrounding erythrocytes) or mannitol salt agar (*S. aureus* survives the high concentration of salt and ferments mannitol to an acid product, causing the medium to turn yellow).

Treatment

If possible, treatment is determined after the clinical laboratory has characterized the pathogen's antibiotic-sensitivity profile. *S. aureus* is very adaptable and has developed resistance to nearly every antibacterial medicine used to treat infections. Once useful medicines no longer can be used against most strains of *S. aureus*. Ninety per cent of hospital isolates of *S. aureus* are resistant to most of the β-lactams. In some cities, over 50% of isolates are resistant to the β-lactams that are resistant to degradation by β-lactamase, the enzyme that is produced by most β-lactam-resistant cells. These variants are termed methicillin-resistant *Staphylococcus aureus* because a mutation alters the enzyme that is normally inhibited by the β-lactams. Therefore, methicillin-resistant *S. aureus* strains are resistant to all but a few of the β-lactams.

In addition, *S. aureus* has developed resistance to vancomycin, a medicine often viewed as the drug to use when most other drugs fail. Both vancomycin-intermediate and vancomycin-resistant strains of *S. aureus* have been identified and are spreading.

Prevention

- Proper hygiene is most important in preventing the spread of *S. aureus*.

- Frequent and thorough hand washing prevents the pathogen from being carried or spread on the hands.

- In a hospital setting, health care workers should change gloves prior to contact with a new patient. Contaminated surfaces in the hospital (stethoscopes, blood glucose monitors, weighing scales, and electronic thermometers) should be disinfected with 70% isopropyl alcohol and chlorine compounds.

Tuberculosis

Worldwide, about 2 billion persons are infected with the TB bacillus. New cases number about 8 million yearly, and annual mortality worldwide is estimated at 3 million. This accounts for 7% of total worldwide mortality and places TB as the number two cause of death by infectious disease (behind pneumonia). Approximately 1 in 10 new cases of TB involves a resistant strain, and 1 in 100 involves a strain that is MDR. TB is fatal for up to 50% of untreated patients, and MDR-TB cases have a reported fatality rate of more than 70%

Cause of the disease

TB is caused by a bacterial pathogen, *Mycobacterium tuberculosis*, an acid-fast, rod-shaped streptobacillus. It is aerobic and grows very slowly. The waxy cell wall restricts the diffusion of many chemicals, making the pathogen resistant to disinfectants and many antibiotics.

Transmission

Reservoir

Infected humans are the reservoir for *M. tuberculosis*.

Mode of transmission

The pathogen is transmitted by the airborne and droplet modes. The bacteria are resistant to temperature change and drying and survive as suspended particles in the air for several hours.

Pathogenesis

Entry

Airborne particles or respiratory droplets containing *M. tuberculosis* are inhaled.

Attachment

The organism attaches to alveolar macrophages after entering the lungs.

Avoiding host defenses

The organism is engulfed by alveolar macrophages but avoids fusion with lysosomes, resulting in the pathogen being protected within the host cell.

Damage

Replication within the macrophage results in cell lysis. Other macrophages are drawn to the site of infection and layer around the infected cells, forming tubercles or small granulomas. The tubercles can block alveoli and bronchioles. If the immune system cannot contain the mycobacteria in the tubercles, the pathogen spreads to other organs. Many of the clinical manifestations are caused by chemicals released as the immune system responds to the infection.

Clinical features

Approximately 10% of infected people go on to develop TB disease. The lungs are the most commonly affected organ.

Clinical signs and symptoms of pulmonary TB include a bad cough that produces bloody sputum, chest pain, chronic fever, weakness or fatigue, chills, night sweats, weight loss, and loss of appetite.

Diagnosis

Clinical

Diagnosis of a person with suspected TB is made by using a Mantoux tuberculin skin test. A Mantoux skin test is performed by injecting a small amount of purified protein derivative or tuberculin under the skin of the inside forearm. The test is read 48 to 72 hours later; if the site of injection shows an area of swelling and redness larger than 15 millimeters in a healthy person, the test is considered positive. A positive skin test is followed up with a chest radiograph. TB is indicated by small granulomas in the lungs. A negative result on the chest X ray indicates the person is free of disease but at sometime in the past has been exposed to *Mycobacterium tuberculosis* and developed an immune response.

Laboratory

Specimen: A sputum sample is obtained.

Test: The test is acid-fast staining to detect acid-fast bacilli or polymerase chain reaction to detect *M. tuberculosis*-specific DNA.

A positive culture for *M. tuberculosis* confirms the diagnosis, although diagnosis may also be made based simply on the clinical presentation of the patient.

Treatment

Because the pathogen grows so slowly and has a waxy cell wall, long-term therapy is required with antibiotics that can penetrate the pathogen.

Treatment with isoniazid for 6 to 12 months is commonly used for people diagnosed with *M. tuberculosis* infection to prevent development of TB.

Active TB is typically treated with a combination of four drugs—isoniazid, rifampin, pyrazinamide, and either ethambutol or streptomycin—for anywhere from 6 to 24 months. The combination of drugs is used to prevent *Mycobacterium* from becoming resistant to any single drug.

Prevention

- *Mycobacterium bovis* bacillus Calmette-Guérin (BCG) vaccine is used for prevention in countries with a high rate of TB.

- Health care workers and others who work where TB is common must be skin tested regularly to ensure that they are not infected.

- Isolation of those with active TB prevents the spread of the disease to others.

- For those exposed to someone with active TB, drug prophylaxis with isoniazid can be used to prevent development of active TB.

Viral Gastroenteritis

Rotavirus is the most common cause of severe diarrhea among children, resulting in the hospitalization of approximately 55,000 children each year in the United States and the death of over 600,000 children annually worldwide. The CDC estimates that 23 million cases of acute gastroenteritis in the United States are due to norovirus (Norwalk-like virus) infection, and it is now thought that at least 50% of all foodborne outbreaks of gastroenteritis can be attributed to noroviruses. Among the 232 outbreaks of norovirus illness reported to the CDC from July 1997 to June 2000, 57% were food borne, 16% were due to person-to-person spread, and 3% were waterborne. In 23% of the outbreaks, the cause of transmission was not determined. In the study, common settings for outbreaks included restaurants and catered meals (36%), nursing homes (23%), schools (13%), and vacation settings or cruise ships (10%).

Cause of the disease

Several viral pathogens cause acute gastroenteritis in humans. Common pathogens include rotavirus and noroviruses.

Rotavirus has a unique wheel-like appearance (hence its name). It is a nonenveloped virus with an icosohedral capsid (20-sided polyhedral shape) and has 11 segments of double-stranded RNA.

Noroviruses are a group of small, polyhedral, nonenveloped viruses using single-stranded RNA as genetic information.

Transmission

Reservoir
Infected humans are the reservoir for the pathogen.

Mode of transmission
The pathogen is spread via the fecal-oral route or through contaminated fomites.

Pathogenesis

Entry
The viral pathogen enters via the consumption of contaminated food or water or through contact with contaminated surfaces.

Attachment
One of the outer capsid proteins binds to receptors on the surface of the epithelium of the small intestine.

Avoiding host defenses
The viruses are acid resistant, allowing them to survive the acidity of the stomach. They are also intracellular pathogens that infect epithelial cells lining the intestines. This allows the initial infecting viruses to be hidden from circulating antibodies or cells of the immune system.

Damage
Damage is direct as a result of the lytic cycle of the virus destroying infected cells. The tissue damage also induces an inflammatory response. Diarrhea is caused by the tissue damage inhibiting the ability of the villi to absorb fluids and the fluid lost during the inflammatory response.

Exit
The viral pathogen exits in the feces.

Clinical features

The disease is often called the "stomach flu," although it is not caused by any of the influenza viruses. The main symptoms of viral gastroenteritis are watery diarrhea and vomiting. Infants infected with rotavirus often experience projectile vomiting. The affected person may also have headache, fever, and abdominal cramps (stomach ache). In general, the symptoms begin 1 or 2 days following infection with a virus that causes gastroenteritis and may last for 1 to 10 days, depending on which virus causes the illness.

Diagnosis

Specimen
A stool sample is taken.

Test
Viral gastroenteritis caused by rotavirus can be diagnosed by rapid antigen detection. Noroviruses are diagnosed by reverse transcriptase PCR.

Treatment

Normally, the disease is self-limiting, requiring only oral rehydration therapy to prevent dehydration. However, about 1 in 40 children with rotavirus gastroenteritis requires hospitalization for intravenous fluids. The CDC recommends that families with infants and young children keep a supply of oral rehydration solution (ORS) at home at all times and use the solution when diarrhea first occurs in the child. ORS is available at pharmacies without a prescription. Follow the written directions on the ORS package, and use clean or boiled water.

Prevention
- An effective vaccine was approved in 1998; however, it is now no longer recommended for infants in the United States because of data that indicated a strong association between the vaccine and intussusceptions (bowel obstructions) among some infants during the first 1 to 2 weeks following vaccination.
- Wash hands with soap and water after using the toilet or changing diapers and before eating or preparing food.

Outbreaks of Diseases of the Respiratory Tract

The biggest disease today is not leprosy or tuberculosis, but rather the feeling of being unwanted.

MOTHER TERESA, Albanian-born Roman Catholic missionary in India

Infections of the respiratory system are the most common reason for requiring a visit to a physician, accounting for an average of 79 physician visits per 100 persons each year. Infections of the respiratory tract are also the leading cause of death by infectious disease worldwide. Pneumonia and tuberculosis (TB) are the number one and two causes of death, respectively, resulting in about 6 million to 7 million deaths per year.

The containment of a respiratory outbreak can be complicated by a pathogen's ability to survive outside the body. For example, some cold-causing viruses can remain infective on an environmental surface for several hours. This makes classroom desks and doorknobs potential fomites, nonliving intermediates that can be contaminated with the pathogen, for the spread of disease. Consequently, two important ways to decrease the spread of respiratory pathogens are to wash the hands frequently and to avoid touching the eyes. Pathogens on the hands can be inoculated into the eyes and drain into the nose. There, they can attack the respiratory tract and initiate an infection.

The primary method of spread for respiratory tract pathogens is via airborne particles and mucus droplets. As a result, respiratory pathogens are highly contagious and spread rapidly through a community. Outbreaks of respiratory pathogens are common in colleges. Students who occupy college residence halls are sharing rooms with one or more other students and are in contact with hundreds of people at sporting events and recreational facilities and in classrooms. As a result, the number of opportunities for transmission of respiratory pathogens is greatly increased, especially during cold-weather periods, when students are more restricted to indoor activities. Annual outbreaks of colds, influenza, strep throat, and bronchitis are common.

Although several thousand microbes are inhaled each day, the defenses of the respiratory system are very efficient and regularly prevent infection and disease. Mucus is secreted by goblet cells within the respiratory epithelium. This mucus traps most microbes before they travel deep into the respiratory tract and helps to inhibit attachment of microbes to host cell receptors. Microbes that are trapped in the mucus are swept out of the respiratory system by cilia on the surface of the pseudostratified epithelium. The mucus is swallowed, and the microbes are destroyed in the digestive system. In addition, the mucus has a high concentration of dissolved solutes. The hypertonic environment created inhibits the growth of most cellular microbes—bacteria, fungi, and protozoa. In the alveoli of the lungs, macrophages are present to phagocytize microbes that escape the defenses of the upper respiratory system.

Microbial pathogens have evolved strategies to bypass these defenses. Adhesins on the surfaces of microbes allow pathogens to attach to receptors on epithelial cells so that the microbes are not swept out of the respiratory tract. These adhesins are highly specific and at times limit infections to only parts of the respiratory tract. For example, rhinoviruses attach to receptors located in the upper respiratory tract and are thus limited to causing the common cold. Influenza A virus, however, attaches all along the respiratory mucosa and can cause a wide range of respiratory diseases from a common cold to life-threatening pneumonia. *Bordetella pertussis,* the causative agent of whooping cough, produces a toxin that inhibits ciliary action, thus preventing it from being swept out by the cilia.

Microbes that can survive in the alveoli of the lungs are the most dangerous, causing a life-threatening infection that blocks gas exchange. *Streptococcus pneumoniae* has an antiphagocytic capsule that inhibits phagocytosis by alveolar macrophages. Strains with a capsule cause pneumonia, while those without a capsule are nonpathogenic. *Mycobacterium tuberculosis,* the causative agent of tuberculosis, a chronic infection of the lungs, and *Legionella pneumophila,* the causative agent of Legionnaires' disease, avoid being digested after being phagocytized by alveolar macrophages.

The outbreaks presented in this section emphasize the serious nature of respiratory tract infections, the difficulty of consistently and effectively implementing basic disease control measures, and the rapid spread of microbes that travel through the air.

Table II.1 Selected outbreak-causing respiratory pathogens

Organism	Key physical properties	Disease characteristics
Bacteria		
Bordetella pertussis	Fastidious, gram-negative coccobacillus	Whooping cough in unvaccinated individuals
Chlamydia pneumoniae	Obligate intracellular bacterium; very small size; gram negative	Pneumonia, bronchitis
Corynebacterium diphtheriae	Gram-positive, club-shaped bacillus	Diphtheria in unvaccinated individuals
Streptococcus pyogenes	Gram-positive streptococcus; beta-hemolytic on blood agar; group A surface antigen	Strep throat, scarlet fever, rheumatic fever
Legionella pneumophila	Fastidious, gram-negative bacillus	Pneumonia (Legionnaires' disease)
Mycobacterium tuberculosis	Acid-fast bacillus found in chains or cords; waxy cell wall important in survival and resistance to drugs and disinfectants	Tuberculosis
Mycoplasma pneumoniae	Wall-less bacterium; variable shape	Walking or "atypical" pneumonia
Streptococcus pneumoniae	Gram-positive diplo- or streptococcus; alpha-hemolytic on blood agar; catalase-negative	Otitis media, sinusitis, conjunctivitis, lobar pneumonia
Viruses		
Adenovirus	Nonenveloped polyhedral capsid with double-stranded DNA	Pharyngitis, bronchiolitis, pneumonia, conjunctivitis
Epstein-Barr virus	Enveloped polyhedral capsid with double-stranded DNA	Mononucleosis
Hantavirus	Enveloped helical capsid with single-stranded RNA	Hantavirus pulmonary syndrome, zoonotic disease carried by rodents
Influenza viruses (A, B, and C)	Enveloped helical capsid with multiple pieces of single-stranded RNA	Influenza, pneumonia, predisposes to secondary bacterial pneumonia
Mumps virus	Enveloped helical capsid with single-stranded RNA	Mumps in unvaccinated individuals
Parainfluenza virus	Enveloped helical capsid with single-stranded RNA	Croup, bronchiolitis, pneumonia, laryngitis
Respiratory syncytial virus	Enveloped helical capsid with single-stranded RNA	Cough, wheezing bronchiolitis, and pneumonia primarily in infants
Rhinoviruses	Noneveloped polyhedral capsid with single-stranded RNA	Common cold
Rubella virus	Enveloped polyhedral capsid with single-stranded RNA	German measles; can cause significant birth defects when pregnant women are infected
Rubeola virus	Enveloped helical capsid with single-stranded RNA	Measles in unvaccinated individuals; pneumonia and encephalitis complications; sixth-leading cause of death from infectious disease worldwide
Varicella-zoster virus	Enveloped polyhedral capsid with double-stranded DNA	Chicken pox in unvaccinated individuals; shingles as a latent manifestation

A Legionellosis Outbreak

BARCELONETA, SPAIN, 2000

In a fishing neighborhood in Barceloneta, Spain, on the Mediterranean waterfront, 33 people were hospitalized in respiratory distress. Four of the victims were in serious condition. The area was predominantly inhabited by elderly people. The youngest victim was 49, while the oldest was 92. The common signs and symptoms were fatigue, malaise, high fever, shortness of breath, and coughing. Examination revealed rales (crackling sounds heard when breathing, indicating fluid in the lungs) and bilateral shadowing in the lungs on X ray (indicating fluid accumulation in both lungs).

City health officials carried out bacterial analyses of a ventilation system in the neighborhood located in a seaside building that used a water tower as part of the cooling system for air conditioning. They isolated *Legionella pneumophila,* a gram-negative, rod-shaped bacterium.

QUESTIONS

1. Besides *Legionella*, list four possible microbial causes of pneumonia.
2. How is *Legionella pneumophila* transmitted?
3. Describe an appropriate way to manage the disease.
4. How would you prevent future outbreaks of the disease?
5. How is legionellosis diagnosed?

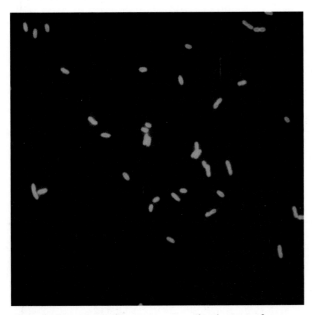

Figure 17.1 Direct fluorescent antibody assay for *Legionella.*

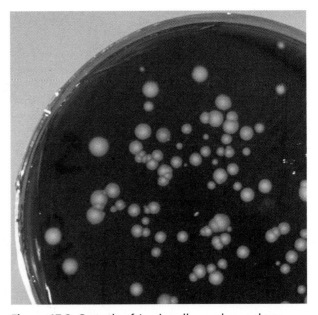

Figure 17.2 Growth of *Legionella* on charcoal agar.

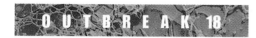

An Outbreak of Respiratory Syncytial Virus Infection

ARVIAT, CANADA, 1998

The hamlet of Arviat, formerly known as Eskimo Point, is a primarily Inuit community of 1,700 people located on the southwestern shore of Hudson Bay. In 1998, an outbreak of respiratory syncytial virus (RSV) sent 50 sick babies from Arviat to hospitals in the south. For 2 weeks, the waiting room at the small clinic staffed by Arviat's nurses had up to 70 sick people looking for treatment, half of them with coughing, crying infants. Nurses worked around the clock with no backup to care for the ill and to decide which children to send out, in medevac batches of three, to Churchill or Winnipeg, Manitoba. The disease was characterized initially as a cold or influenza, but the children then developed coughing, fast breathing, wheezing, and difficulty breathing.

Laboratory tests of respiratory fluids were positive for RSV, an enveloped virus with a helical capsid and single-stranded ribonucleic acid (RNA).

Arviat's nursing station was built in 1938 and was no longer adequate for the town's population. There was no resident physician in the community or hospital facilities to treat seriously ill patients. Community leaders had called for better medical services for Arviat, including a full-time doctor, a suggestion that the hard-pressed Keewatin Regional Health Board had not yet acted on. In 1998, Arviat saw its population of 1,700 grow by 75 new babies. With a growth rate of more than 4% a year, Arviat was one of the fastest-growing communities in the region.

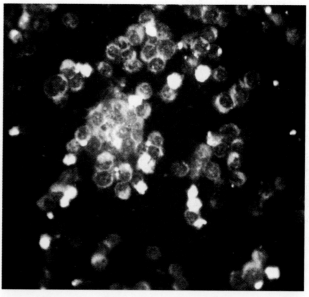

Figure 18.1 Direct fluorescent antibody assay for respiratory syncytial virus.

Even though the population was small, overcrowding was common. It was not unusual for many individuals to live in very small homes. In addition, the public schools and community center were considered too small. With 82 new Nunavut government jobs slated for Arviat, the community's population was expected to jump to more than 2,000 residents, which would only worsen the problems with overcrowding.

City officials worried that the outbreak would be compounded in the following week by hundreds of Christians from around Nunavut and Nunavik who traveled to the area to attend the "Holy Spirit Crusade." Arviat's mayor was concerned that sitting elbow to elbow in the heat would make a great incubator for disease.

QUESTIONS

1. How is RSV transmitted?

2. Why are children most seriously affected by RSV?

3. How would you treat individuals affected by this disease?

4. What public health actions should have been taken to stop the outbreak and prevent future occurrences?

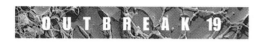

A Tuberculosis Outbreak in a Prison Housing Inmates Infected with HIV

SOUTH CAROLINA, 1999 AND 2000

An outbreak of drug-susceptible TB occurred in a state correctional facility housing human immunodeficiency virus (HIV)-infected inmates in 1999 and 2000. Before entry, inmates were tested for HIV status. They were then segregated in three dormitories of one prison, with each dormitory partitioned into right and left sides. On admission to the facility, all inmates were also screened for TB infection and disease with a tuberculin skin test and chest radiography.

In early July 1999, a 34-year-old HIV-infected man housed in a dormitory (dormitory A) was taken to the prison hospital with a 2-week history of fever, abdominal pain, and cough. His chest radiograph was normal; however, sputum specimens were not obtained for culture, and no acid-fast staining was done to detect acid-fast bacilli (AFB). As a result, he was not placed in respiratory isolation. The inmate was returned to the prison in mid-July without a definitive diagnosis. In mid-August 1999, the man was evaluated at a community hospital. A laboratory test result was positive for AFB in his sputum (Fig. 19.1), and he was diagnosed with active pulmonary TB (Fig. 19.2). Later that year, the medical student who examined the inmate during the initial hospitalization developed active TB with cavities within the lungs.

A contact investigation of dormitory A inmates identified 31 current or former inmates who had signs and symptoms of active TB. They were transferred from dormitory A to the hospital for respiratory isolation and medical evaluation. The exposed group comprised 323 men who had spent from 1 to 152 days (median, 135 days) in dormitory A during the period. Of the 31 case patients, 27 (87%) resided on the right side of dormitory A during the exposure period; 4 (13%) resided on the left.

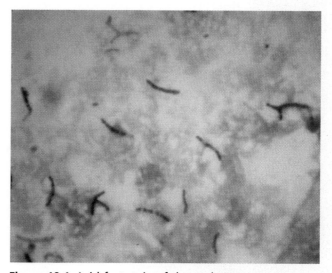

Figure 19.1 Acid-fast stain of the pathogen.

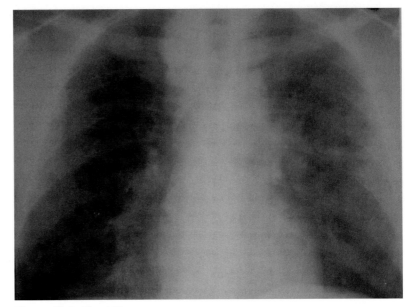

Figure 19.2 Chest X ray.

All case patients were non-Hispanic black men born in the United States and were infected with HIV. The median age was 36 years (range, 23 to 56 years). All of the isolates of the pathogen tested were identical based on deoxyribonucleic acid (DNA) fingerprinting analysis. Five case patients had TB diagnosed after being released from prison; all five were released before the source case patient had TB diagnosed in August.

QUESTIONS

1. What is a tuberculin skin test?

2. What does a positive test indicate?

3. What characteristic of AFB makes them difficult to treat?

4. What characteristics of *Mycobacterium tuberculosis* result in the requirement for long-term multidrug therapy?

5. What type of results would be expected in a chest X ray of a person who had active TB?

6. How did the inmates living on the opposite side of dormitory A contract TB?

7. How does a person's HIV status influence the risk of acquiring TB?

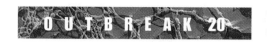

An Otitis Media Outbreak in a Child Care Center

GEORGIA, 2000

On 18 December 2000, public health officials in southwestern Georgia contacted the Georgia Division of Public Health about a child aged 11 months hospitalized for otitis media. Eight days before hospitalization, a culture of drainage obtained from the child's middle ear revealed a gram-positive coccus arranged in chains. The bacteria were resistant to penicillin, clindamycin, erythromycin, trimethoprim-sulfamethoxazole, and tetracycline. The child attended a local child care center.

The child care center was located in a rural county (1999 population, 6,318) in southwestern Georgia and served approximately 54 children (age range, 9 months to 10 years). The children were divided into two groups on the basis of age (<18 months and >18 months), and the two groups had separate rooms. Nasopharyngeal (NP) swabs were collected and sent to the Centers for Disease Control and Prevention for identification and antimicrobial susceptibility testing.

NP swabs were obtained from 5 of the 12 children who had shared a room at the child care center with the child who was hospitalized; NP swabs were also obtained from 17 of the 42 children from the other room. The pathogen was grown on blood agar under anaerobic conditions. Alpha-hemolytic colonies (Fig. 20.1) were Gram stained (Fig. 20.2). The bacterium was isolated from 90% of the NP cultures; of these, 79% were nonsusceptible (having intermediate or high-level resistance to more than one antibiotic or class of antibiotics) to penicillin.

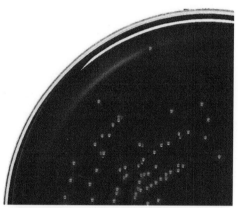

Figure 20.1 Growth of the pathogen on blood agar.

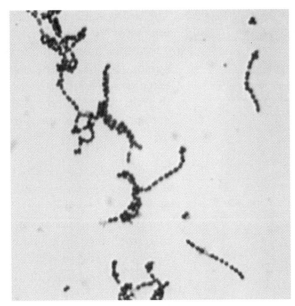

Figure 20.2 Gram stain of the pathogen.

Eighty-two percent of the children in the child care center had had an illness for which they received antibiotic treatment during the 2 months preceding administration of the questionnaire.

QUESTIONS

1. What pathogen was most likely affecting the children at the child care center? What other disease(s) can this pathogen cause?

2. How would you treat those infected with the multidrug-resistant pathogen?

3. Why are children in day care and their mothers particularly susceptible to infections by drug-resistant pathogens?

4. How would you have stopped this outbreak and reduced the risk of similar outbreaks in the future?

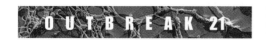

An Outbreak of a Rash

VENEZUELA AND COLOMBIA, 2001 AND 2002

In January 2002, a girl aged 7 months received medical care at a local hospital. Her illness started with a fever and the appearance of a macular rash (a rash of flat red spots) (Fig. 21.1). She infected a nurse, who then transmitted the disease to several other contacts, some of whom visited a popular tourist site in Falcón, Venezuela. Of the 165 persons who were infected during this outbreak, 52% had visited the same tourist site.

The first rash case in Zulia, Colombia, occurred in a woman aged 27 years who was an auxiliary nurse in a physician's office that provided care to residents of Falcón. The nurse had onset of the rash on 25 October 2001 and subsequently infected four other persons. During the next 3 months, the outbreak spread to all municipalities in Zulia; 2,074 cases had been confirmed as of 24 July 2002. For several chains of transmission, the index case (the first case which initiates an outbreak) individual was a health care worker. Beginning in February 2002, the outbreak spread to 14 additional states in Venezuela, including 4 states bordering Colombia. By July 2002, Venezuela had reported 6,380 cases.

In 2000, routine measles, mumps, and rubella vaccination coverage in Venezuela was 84%. By September 2001, estimated coverage had decreased to 58% and was lower in Venezuelan states near the border with northern Colombia (e.g., 44% in Falcón and 34% in Zulia).

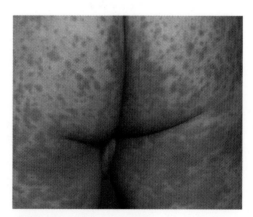

Figure 21.1 Macular rash.

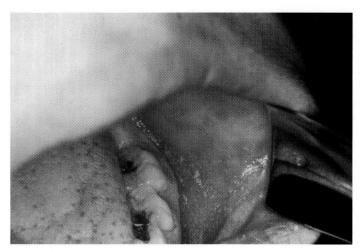

Figure 21.2 Koplik's spots on the buccal mucosa.

Affected persons first experienced a fever lasting about 2 to 4 days that peaked at about 104°F (40°C). This was followed by a cough, runny nose, and the outbreak of a macular rash that began at the hairline and then proceeded down throughout the body. In addition, tiny white dots surrounded by a red halo appeared on the inflamed mucosa inside the cheeks (Koplik's spots) (Fig. 21.2). The rash lasted about 5 days.

QUESTIONS

1. What was the disease?

2. Name the pathogen and describe several of its physical characteristics.

3. Describe how you would treat a patient who contracted this disease.

4. In order to minimize the number of cases of the disease, how would you have managed the outbreak?

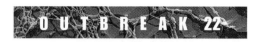

An Outbreak of a Rash at a Camp for HIV-Infected Children

CONNECTICUT, 1997

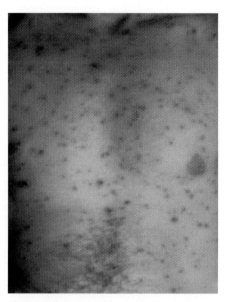

Figure 22.1 Vesicular rash.

In the summer of 1997, the Centers for Disease Control and Prevention were notified of an outbreak of an infectious rash among attendees at a summer camp for HIV-infected children. The camp was composed of 110 campers and 96 staff. Of the 96 staff, 92 were resistant to the infection as a result of immunity from previous exposure. Of the 110 campers, 79 were resistant to the infection. The most likely index case individual was a child who came to camp with an active infection that was not detected by the staff. The pathogen infected 11 of the 31 susceptible children (36%) and two of the four susceptible adults. Cases occurred among children in 5 of 15 cabins.

The disease initially caused a vesicular rash on the scalp, head, and trunk, which progressed to the extremities. Other signs and symptoms included fever, headache, fatigue, sore throat, anorexia (loss of appetite), irritability, and the rash causing intense itching. Two children were hospitalized with high fever and encephalitis. One other child developed cellulitis (an infection of the tissue under the skin). Diagnosis of the rash was made from clinical signs and symptoms—no laboratory tests were completed.

QUESTIONS

1. Identify the disease, name the pathogen, and describe several of its physical characteristics.

2. Describe how you would have treated the most seriously ill individuals.

3. Explain how secondary bacterial cellulitis can be a complication of the initial disease.

4. How could an outbreak like this be contained and prevented in the future?

5. How did HIV status complicate the presentation or diagnosis of this disease?

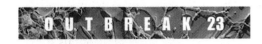

A Diphtheria Outbreak

NEWLY INDEPENDENT STATES OF
THE FORMER SOVIET UNION, 1998

In 1990, a diphtheria epidemic began in Russia. It spread to all of the remaining newly independent states (NIS) of the former Soviet Union by the end of 1994. More than 150,000 cases and 5,000 deaths were reported in the NIS from 1990 to 1998. The risk of diphtheria infection is still present in all countries of the former Soviet Union. Diphtheria is caused by the bacterial pathogen *Corynebacterium diphtheriae*.

The dire state of Russia's public health system created what President Vladimir Putin called a national emergency: between 1990 and 1994, life expectancy at birth had fallen by over 5 years to 58.5 years, the lowest level in the developed world. Only one child in five was born healthy, according to official statistics, which many experts said understated the problem. The death rate rose by 20%, an increase with no modern precedent.

After the collapse of the former Soviet Union, doctors no longer had the medicine, equipment, or money to deal with standard health care. Many physicians at the time were pessimistic about any improvements in the near future. Almost half of the 1990 medical school graduating class (doctors who are practicing throughout Russia today) could not even read an electrocardiogram on the day they got their diplomas, according to the Russian Academy of Sciences. On average, doctors earn less money than drivers or babysitters—about $145 each month.

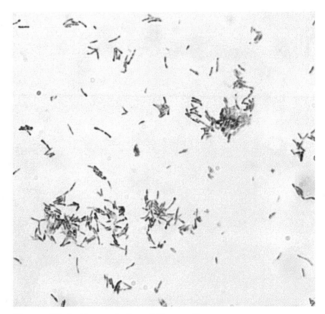

Figure 23.1 Gram stain of the pathogen.

Russia budgets slightly less than 1% of its resources to health care, about the same as the poorest African nations. Recently, the Russian Health Ministry said that half of the country's 21,000 hospitals did not have hot water, a quarter had no sewage systems, and several thousand had no water at all.

The collapse of the previous economic system and civil wars in parts of the former Soviet Union have seriously impaired the social and health situation. In some of the newly independent states, over 65% of the population has been estimated to be below the poverty level. Health services are free of charge only for emergency situations; otherwise, drug treatment and hospital care must be paid for by the patient.

QUESTIONS

1. What are the clinical features of diphtheria?

2. How can the disease be fatal?

3. How would you prevent the disease from spreading to tourists and travelers to the NIS?

4. How is diphtheria usually prevented?

5. Why are infants particularly at risk for acquiring diphtheria?

6. How would you have arrested this outbreak?

An Outbreak of Mononucleosis

PUERTO RICO, 1990

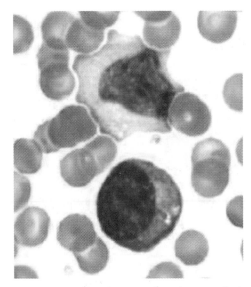

Figure 24.1 Blood smear showing atypical lymphocytes.

From 11 September through 7 October 1990, an outbreak of disease occurred at a community hospital in Puerto Rico. The disease was characterized by pharyngitis (inflammation of the pharynx and tonsils), fever, headache, fatigue, and lymphadenopathy (swollen lymph nodes).

Fifty-seven persons (including outpatients, inpatients, and staff) tested positive. Among persons for whom the duration of illness was known, 24 were ill for 1 to 15 days (mean, 9 days); 1 person was ill for 27 days. Two local newspapers and a television station reported that the hospital had detected an epidemic of mononucleosis in the surrounding community. Subsequently, outpatients treated in the emergency room requested tests, and persons from other towns came to the hospital for testing.

QUESTIONS

1. Identify and describe the pathogen that caused the disease.
2. What are the normal incubation period and mode of transmission for the disease and the typical age of those affected by the disease?
3. What white blood cells are infected by the pathogen?
4. How would you have stopped the outbreak?
5. What treatment is normally provided for those affected by the disease?

Note: A complete investigation of the outbreak revealed errors in interpretation of the laboratory results. Consequently, this case represents only a pseudo-outbreak of mononucleosis.

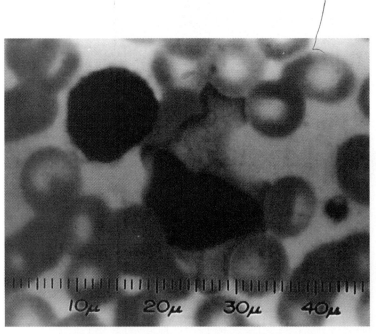

Figure 24.2 Blood smear showing atypical lymphocytes. μ, micrometers.

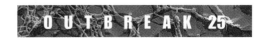

OUTBREAK 25

A Pneumonia Outbreak in a Nursing Home

NEW JERSEY, 2001

On 24 April 2001, nine cases of pneumonia among residents of a nursing home were investigated by the Department of Health of Hamilton Township, New Jersey. Illness onset among the residents occurred from 3 to 24 April. Four residents died. Pneumonia was characterized by one or more lobes filled with fluid and pleural effusions (pus in the pleural space) (Fig. 25.1).

The nursing home was a 114-bed facility that employed approximately 200 staff, including nurses, restorative aides, and other administrative and support personnel. None of the employees was known to have pneumonia during this period.

Seven of the residents lived in the same wing of the nursing home. All nine patients had blood cultures that grew alpha-hemolytic colonies on blood agar (Fig. 25.2). Sputum samples were Gram stained to identify the pathogen, a gram-positive streptococcus. All isolates were penicillin sensitive and resistant to erythromycin.

QUESTIONS

1. Name the pathogen causing the outbreak, and describe several of its physical characteristics.

2. Describe how you would treat a patient who contracted this disease.

3. What physical property does this pathogen have that enables it to avoid phagocytosis by the macrophages in the lungs?

4. In order to minimize the number of cases of the disease, how would you have managed the outbreak?

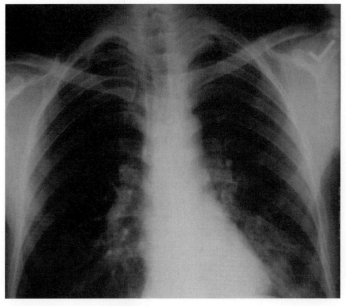

Figure 25.1 Chest X ray.

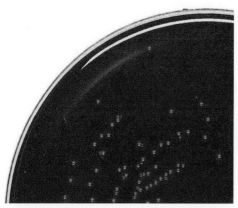

Figure 25.2 Growth of the pathogen on blood agar.

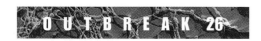

Past and Future Pandemics of Influenza A

WORLDWIDE, 1918 TO PRESENT

The "golden age of microbiology" began with Louis Pasteur and his development of the anthrax and rabies vaccines and saving of the French wine industry. It continued with Robert Koch, who established the germ theory of disease and discovered the causative agents of anthrax, cholera, and tuberculosis. The first time the new field of microbiology collided with a major epidemic was the influenza pandemic of 1918, probably the world's worst epidemic of all time.

Some modern epidemiologists estimate that the influenza pandemic caused 50 to 100 million deaths, with about one-half occurring among men and women in their 20s and 30s. "The flu" killed 8% of all young adults then living. The 2-year epidemic spread rapidly, with two-thirds of deaths occurring in 24 weeks and over half occurring from mid-September to early December 1918.

Past and present plagues fall far short of the influenza pandemic of 1918. The flu killed more people in 24 weeks than acquired immune deficiency syndrome (AIDS) has killed in 24 years. It killed more people in a year than the black death of the Middle Ages killed in a century.

In 1997, the partial sequences of five influenza virus genes were recovered from the preserved lung tissue of a U.S. soldier who died from influenza in 1918. The sequence data now suggest that the hemagglutinin gene (which codes for the H antigen) of the 1918 virus was a composite of a stretch of nucleotides from a pig virus flanked by nucleotides from a human virus.

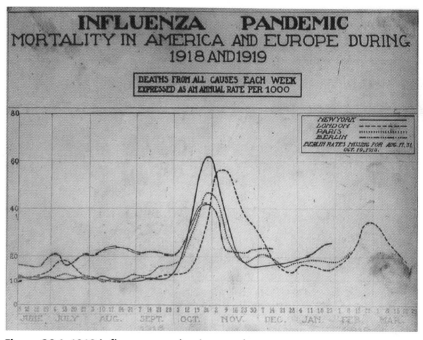

Figure 26.1 1918 influenza pandemic record.

The current version of the bird flu virus also has a unique combination of H and N antigens (H5N1) found in no other version of the virus. Fortunately for the world, this version of the influenza A virus has not been effectively spread via respiratory droplets. For most cases, it has been spread by direct contact with infected birds. Like the 1918 version, this new strain appears to result in extremely high mortality. Over 50% of those who are infected die.

In an interview with author Michael Spector (in the 28 February 2005 issue of *The New Yorker*), Scott Dowell, the director of the Centers for Disease Control and Prevention's Thailand office, stated, "the world just has no idea what it's going to see if this thing comes. When, really. It's when. I don't think we can afford the luxury of the word 'if' anymore. . . . The clock is ticking. We just don't know what time it is."

John S. Marr, the former director of the Bureau of Preventable Diseases and a principal epidemiologist in the New York City Department of Public Health, is also concerned about a future influenza pandemic. He stated, "the spread of the 'Spanish Flu' in 1918–19 took four months to circle the world. A new strain of influenza could cause a pandemic in four days. . . . Sadly, many people believe that 'flu,' a household word, is nothing much to be concerned about, but a new strain could kill tens of millions of people quite easily, within weeks. That is the one I worry about."

When Tommy Thompson, the Secretary of Health and Human Services, announced his resignation in December 2004, he cited a bird flu epidemic as one of the greatest dangers the United States faces. Governmental estimates of the cost of an influenza epidemic have been made. Without large-scale immunization, the estimates of the total economic impact in the United States of an influenza pandemic ranged from $71.3 billion to $166.5 billion.

QUESTIONS

1. How can a virus that primarily attacks birds be changed into a pathogen that effectively infects humans?

2. Given the increase in worldwide travel and population relative to the 1918 influenza pandemic, could a human version of this influenza virus that was spread by respiratory droplets be contained? Explain your reasoning.

3. Given the advances in vaccine production and medicine (relative to the 1918 influenza pandemic), could modern health care prevent tens of millions of deaths if the current bird flu was effectively spread by respiratory droplets? Explain your reasoning.

A Pharyngitis Outbreak in the Marine Corps

SAN DIEGO, CALIFORNIA, 2002

An outbreak of an infectious disease sent more than 100 recruits to the hospital at San Diego's Marine Corps Recruit Depot in 1 week. Fifty Marines were hospitalized with an upper respiratory tract infection. One was in critical condition, and one died. The outbreak was confined to four of the base's seven companies. All of the ill recruits arrived for training before the outbreak.

Sore throat was the most common symptom, but more serious complications developed. Major General Jan Huly, commander of the Marine Corps Recruit Depot, stated that no one expects casualties in recruit training. Huly said, "We take every one of those deaths personally, as if there were some way we could have prevented it, and we're going to find a way we can prevent it."

The initial onset of the clinical signs and symptoms of the disease included fever, pharyngitis, and headache. Later signs included exudative tonsillitis (creamy yellow pus produced on the tonsils). Some suffered from complications, such as peritonsilar abscesses, in which the infection invaded deeper tissue, or a high fever and bright-red rash.

Gram stains revealed gram-positive cocci (Fig. 27.1). Other laboratory tests of sputum samples and throat swabs showed beta-hemolytic colony growth on blood agar (Fig. 27.2). Antigen tests indicated that the pathogen carried group A antigens on its surface.

QUESTIONS

1. Given the laboratory test results, identify the pathogenic agent and the disease it causes.

2. How would you have treated those affected by the disease?

3. If the disease is not treated, what potential serious complications can result?

4. How could this outbreak have been quickly arrested?

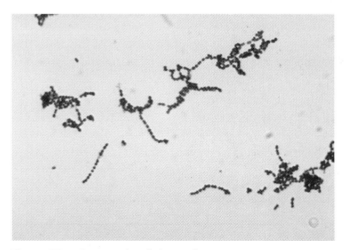

Figure 27.1 Gram stain of the pathogen.

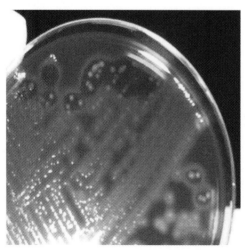

Figure 27.2 Growth of the pathogen on blood agar.

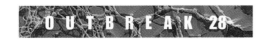

A Measles Outbreak among Kosovar Refugee Children

ALBANIA, 1999

Extensive ethnic conflict in the Kosovo region of the Federal Republic of Yugoslavia and an organized bombing campaign by the North Atlantic Treaty Organization led to mass population displacement in 1998 and early 1999. In April 1999, approximately 500,000 Kosovar Albanians fled into the Yugoslavian Republic of Montenegro and the neighboring countries of Albania, Bosnia-Herzegovina, and the former Yugoslav Republic of Macedonia (FYROM).

Of the estimated 130,000 refugees who fled to the FYROM, approximately 65,000 were housed in seven refugee camps. A major public health concern in the camps was the prevention of vaccine-preventable diseases. Vaccination against preventable microbial diseases is a major public health priority in the acute phase of any emergency involving large-scale displacement of a population. In past emergencies, up to 50% of deaths were attributed to vaccine-preventable disease.

In response, the FYROM Ministry of Health, in collaboration with the United Nations International Children's Emergency Fund and the International Medical Corps, planned a mass vaccination campaign. The campaign needed to overcome several significant obstacles. First, there were substantial fluctuations in the population. On a weekly basis, thousands of refugees were both leaving and entering the camps as they fled additional fighting, looked for relatives, tried to return to their homes, or sought better living conditions. For example, in the Macedonian camps, 44,417 refugees left and 46,492 refugees arrived in 1 week. Secondly, vaccination at the time of entry was not feasible. There was a lack of access to refugees at the camp borders, and the timing of their arrival and movement in the camps was unpredictable. Finally, there was concern that vaccination immediately upon entering the camps would be psychologically traumatic to children.

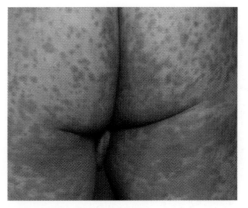

Figure 28.1 Macular rash.

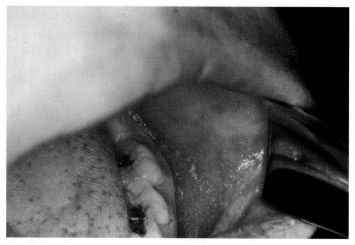

Figure 28.2 Koplik's spots on the buccal mucosa.

An outbreak of measles occurred in one of the camps that had a large population of undernourished children. Examination of those affected showed a high fever, a macular rash, and Koplik's spots on the inside of the cheeks (the buccal mucosa).

QUESTIONS

1. To what complications were the undernourished children especially susceptible?

2. How is the pathogen transmitted?

3. Why is this pathogen of significant concern?

4. How would you have prioritized the expenditure of funds and resources in order to minimize the number of deaths caused by measles and other vaccine-preventable diseases?

5. List five vaccine-preventable diseases that could have been a threat to the health of the refugee population.

Chicken Pox

Chicken pox affects 3 million children annually in the United States and is responsible for about 500,000 physician visits a year. About 12,000 people are hospitalized for chicken pox each year in the United States, and approximately 100 people die each year as a result of rare but serious complications of the disease. Chicken pox is primarily a pediatric disease, with 90% of the population infected as children.

Cause of the disease

Varicella-zoster virus (VZV), a member of the herpesvirus family, is the causative agent of chicken pox. It is an enveloped virus with a polyhedral capsid that contains double-stranded DNA as genetic information.

Transmission

Reservoir

Infected humans are the reservoir for the pathogen.

Mode of transmission

The virus is spread via the droplet mode during coughing and sneezing or by direct contact with infected lesions.

Pathogenesis

Entry

The virus enters by the respiratory route via mucus droplets.

Attachment

Protein in the envelope of the virus attaches to the epithelium of the respiratory tract.

Spread

Infected leukocytes carry the virus to lymphoid tissues. Virus released from lymphoid tissue is disseminated throughout the blood and lymph. The virus is carried through the blood to sites outside of capillaries under the skin.

Avoiding host defenses

VZV is an intracellular pathogen which initially avoids destruction by circulating antibodies and cells of the immune system. After a primary infection, a provirus is formed in the dorsal root ganglia of sensory neurons (the cell bodies of nerve cells near the spinal cord). A provirus forms when a virus incorporates its DNA into the chromosome of the host cell. In this state, the provirus can remain dormant. If it becomes active, secondary outbreak of shingles can occur.

Damage

The virus induces the formation of syncytia (large multinucleated fused cells) under the skin, induces programmed cell death, and causes a local inflammatory response.

Clinical features

Incubation

The incubation period is 10 to 23 days.

The distinguishing feature of chicken pox is a vesicular rash on the scalp, head, and trunk that progresses to the extremities. Other signs and symptoms include fever, headache, fatigue, sore throat, anorexia, irritability, and pruritus (itching). The vesicles turn pustular (filled with pus), form a crust and a scab, and then heal.

A secondary outbreak of VZV infection called shingles can also occur and typically affects the elderly. Shingles results when the dormant provirus becomes active, causing a vesicular or pustular rash to break out along the ends of the nerve that the virus infected. Shingles causes intense pain.

Treatment

The primary treatment for chicken pox is supportive care. Over-the-counter medications are often used: antihistamines to reduce itching, calomine lotion to help dry up vesicles, and ibuprofen or acetaminophen to reduce fever. Fluids and electrolytes are given to prevent dehydration from the fever. It is also important to monitor and treat secondary bacterial infections.

Rare complications, such as herpes encephalitis, are treated with acyclovir, a herpesvirus-specific antiviral agent. Acyclovir is a nucleoside analog of guanosine that blocks DNA synthesis in herpesvirus-infected cells.

Prevention

- An effective vaccine is available.
- Unvaccinated individuals should wash their hands regularly, avoid touching their eyes and nose where possible, and avoid contact with infected individuals. Infected individuals can help prevent spread by covering their mouths when coughing and sneezing.

- For shingles, early injection of local anesthetic following breakout results in pain relief and accelerated healing.

Diphtheria

Although diphtheria was under control in much of Asia through widespread use of an effective childhood toxoid immunization, political turmoil from the fall of the former Soviet Union has had dramatic effects on public health. As a result of the collapse of the health care structure, vaccination programs were interrupted. Consequently, in the early 1990s, a dramatic increase occurred in the number of cases reported in the newly independent states of the former Soviet Union. From 1990 to 1996, more than 110,000 cases of diphtheria with 2,900 fatalities were reported by the Russian Federation.

Cause of the disease

The pathogen, *Corynebacterium diphtheriae*, is a gram-positive, club-shaped bacillus that can produce a potent cytotoxin when carrying a prophage with the *tox* gene.

Transmission

Reservoir

Symptomatic and asymptomatic carriers serve as reservoirs of the pathogen.

Mode of transmission

The pathogen is spread in the droplet mode via inhalation of mucus droplets.

Pathogenesis

Entry

The pathogen is principally spread from person to person via the respiratory tract.

Attachment

C. diphtheriae attaches to the epithelial tissue of the tonsils and the pharynx.

Avoiding host defenses

C. diphtheriae infects the epithelial layer and initially avoids circulating antibodies and cells of the immune system.

Damage

The toxin that is produced by bacteriophage-infected organisms inhibits cellular protein synthesis. It also causes programmed cell death of surrounding cells, leading to damage in the pharynx. This allows entry into the bloodstream, causing damage to internal organs.

Clinical features

The disease begins with pharyngitis. The cytotoxin causes tissue death, leading to a bluish-gray and then black membrane of necrotic (dead) tissue on the soft palate (diphtheric membrane). The intense inflammatory response results in extensive swelling of the cervical lymph nodes, giving a bull neck appearance. The toxin enters the blood and lymph vessels, causing the systemic effects of the disease, including low-grade fever, exhaustion, electrocardiographic changes, and possibly cardiac failure. The toxin can also damage motor neurons, causing paralysis of the soft palate, resulting in the regurgitation of fluids, and paralysis of muscles and the diaphragm.

Diagnosis

Clinical

Physical features include a bull neck appearance from enlarged cervical lymph nodes and the presence of the diphtheric membrane, a bluish-gray membrane on the pharynx that becomes black and necrotic.

Laboratory

Specimen: Pharyngeal swab of any discolored areas or ulcerations.

Cultural tests: Growth on serum tellurite agar is selective for *Corynebacterium*, giving characteristic gray to black colonies. Gram stain of isolated colonies shows multiple club-shaped forms that look like Chinese characters. The production of toxin, detected by using immunoelectrophoresis, is required to demonstrate that *Corynebacterium* is pathogenic.

Treatment

Due to the serious nature of the illness and the rapid progression of the disease, an antitoxin, produced in horses, is administered as soon as diphtheria is suspected, without waiting for laboratory confirmation. The antitoxin inactivates the toxin in the bloodstream.

The antibiotic typically chosen to eliminate the pathogen is penicillin or erythromycin.

Prevention

- To prevent diphtheria, a highly effective vaccine is administered to children—the DTaP (diphtheria, tetanus, and pertussis) vaccine. The vaccine contains a denatured toxin that stimulates a protective immune response but is not pathogenic.
- Diphtheria is a highly contagious disease that requires urgent isolation to reduce the risk of spreading the infected bacillus.

Legionnaires' Disease

A serious pulmonary infection attacked 235 people who were attending a convention of the American Legion in Philadelphia, Pennsylvania, during the U.S. bicentennial celebration in July 1976—hence the name Legionnaires' disease and that of its causative organism, *Legionella pneumophila*. Since then, Legionnaires' disease has become recognized as the most common cause of atypical pneumonia in hospitalized patients. It is the second most common cause of community-acquired bacterial pneumonia.

Cause of the disease

The pathogen that causes Legionnaires' disease is *Legionella pneumophila*, a bacterial pathogen. It is a gram-negative aerobic bacillus that contains a capsule and has fastidious growth requirements.

Transmission

Reservoir

L. pneumophila is free-living in soil and stagnant water (25 to 42°C). *Legionella* can contaminate large air conditioning systems that use water in cooling towers.

Mode of transmission

Transmission is by inhalation of aerosolized droplets containing *Legionella*. The pathogen is not spread person to person. Most infections occur in patients who have compromised immunity and pulmonary function.

Pathogenesis

Entry

Inhalation of aerosols containing *Legionella* is the means of entry.

Attachment

Legionella attaches to the alveolar sacs.

Avoiding host defenses

Legionella is phagocytized by alveolar macrophages but avoids destruction by preventing fusion with lysosomes. *Legionella* replicates inside the macrophage and causes cell lysis.

Damage

Legionella causes direct damage through cell lysis and indirect damage by inducing an inflammatory response and producing damaging enzymes and toxins. After lysing macrophages, the bacteria spread and continue to cause damage and inflammation, resulting in bronchial hemorrhaging and abscesses.

Clinical features

Most infections are asymptomatic or produce only mild symptoms. The incubation period is between 2 and 10 days, normally 5 or 6 days. Symptoms include fever and chills, a nonproductive cough, difficulty breathing, confusion, headache, and muscle pain.

Diagnosis
Clinical

The clinical finding is evidence of pneumonia, including rales and a chest X ray showing fluid in the lungs.

Laboratory testing

Sample: A sputum or urine sample is obtained.
Cultural testing: The bacterium grows slowly on a buffered cysteine-containing charcoal yeast extract (BCYE) agar.
Noncultural testing: Indirect immunofluorescence microscopy and commercial rapid microagglutination tests are used.

Treatment
Antibiotics

Macrolides, such as erythromycin, have been commonly used to treat *Legionella* infection.

Clinical

Respiratory therapy is often required for seriously ill patients.

Prevention

- Regular maintenance and adequate chlorination of ventilation systems and other potential reservoirs
- Maintaining water reservoir temperature at >60°C or <20°C
- Avoiding water stagnation
- Avoiding smoking and excessive alcohol consumption, which can lower resistance to the pathogen

Measles

Measles is probably the greatest killer of children in history. Despite the availability of an effective vaccine that was developed more than 30 years ago, the measles virus still affects 50 million people annually and causes more than 1 million deaths. Worldwide, measles is the sixth leading cause of death by infectious disease. The highest incidence of measles is observed in developing countries. However, it still occurs infrequently in the United States and other industrialized nations.

Cause of the disease

Measles virus is a member of the paramyxovirus family. It is an enveloped virus with a helical capsid which contains single-stranded RNA with a negative-sense polarity as genetic information.

Transmission

Reservoir

The reservoir of the virus is symptomatic humans.

Mode of transmission

The virus is transmitted via the airborne and droplet modes. Airborne virus particles are stable for 2 hours when suspended in air but are quickly inactivated after landing on surfaces.

Pathogenesis

Entry

The virus enters through inhalation of airborne particles or mucus droplets.

Attachment

Envelope proteins attach to the CD46 receptor on host cells in the respiratory epithelium.

Spread

The virus is carried by leukocytes to subepithelial and local tissues, multiplies in lymphoid tissues, and disseminates via the bloodstream throughout the body.

Damage

The measles virus directly damages the host cells it infects. Most of the damage is done to the mucosal surface of the respiratory tract. Besides the direct damage, infection by the virus causes cells to fuse together into giant cells (syncytia). These cells can further restrict gas exchange and complicate measles pneumonia. As a result of damage to the defenses of the lungs, secondary bacterial infections are common. After initial infection, the virus travels to lymphoid tissue, causing a secondary viremia, which spreads the pathogen to tissues under the skin. The resulting inflammatory response initiates the rash formation.

Exit

The pathogen exits via the respiratory route. The virus continues to be shed for 3 or 4 days once the rash is gone.

Clinical features

The incubation period is typically 10 to 14 days, followed by an acute respiratory illness, including runny nose, fever, conjunctivitis, and cough. The fever rises steadily until the appearance of the rash 2 to 4 days later. A maculopapular rash (red, slightly raised spots) begins on the face and spreads down to the trunk and outward toward the extremities. Koplik's spots (pinpoint blue-white spots on a red background) appear on the inside of the cheeks (the buccal mucosa) of the mouth 1 or 2 days before the rash appears.

Serious complications, such as pneumonia and encephalitis, occur in about 4% of cases.

Diagnosis

Clinical features are used to diagnose the disease. Koplik's spots (a maculopapular rash spreading from the head down), fever, and conjunctivitis indicate measles.

Treatment

There are no antiviral medications to inhibit the measles virus.

Treatment is symptomatic and commonly includes bed rest, intake of fluids and electrolytes to replace those lost from the fever, and over-the-counter medications for fever and headache, such as acetaminophen or ibuprofen. Aspirin is not used as a pain reliever because of an increased risk of Reye's syndrome in children and adolescents.

Prevention

- There is a highly effective live attenuated (immunogenic but not pathogenic) measles vaccine, given most commonly to children as part of the MMR vaccine, which protects against measles, mumps, and rubella.

- People who are infected should be isolated due to the highly contagious nature of the disease.

Mononucleosis

Development of mononucleosis is associated with socioeconomic status. The poor are typically infected when young and develop only a mild disease. However, higher socioeconomic groups are more likely to become infected as adults or adolescents. In colleges in the United States, 35 to 85% of students are seropositive as entering first-year students, with a 10% rate of acquiring an Epstein-Barr virus (EBV) infection each subsequent year.

Cause of the disease

EBV is a herpesvirus. It has an envelope with a polyhedral capsid and double-stranded DNA as genetic information.

Transmission

Reservoir

Infected humans are the reservoir of the virus; symptomatic and asymptomatic individuals can shed virus for months after the disease.

Mode of transmission

The virus is transmitted by direct contact with infected saliva or contaminated fomites.

Pathogenesis

Entry

The route of entry is oral, via direct contact with infected saliva.

Attachment

Proteins in the envelope of EBV attach to receptors on the epithelium of the oropharynx and to B lymphocytes.

Avoiding host defenses

EBV is an intracellular pathogen that is not initially exposed to circulating antibodies and other cells of the immune system.

Damage

Immunological "civil war," in which activated T lymphocytes attack infected B lymphocytes, results in the production of cytokines, which produce the systemic symptoms.

Exit

Virus is shed in saliva from infected epithelial cells and lymphocytes in salivary glands and the pharynx.

Clinical features

Children

Infections are most often asymptomatic.

Adolescents and adults

Mononucleosis: A 4- to 7-week incubation period is followed by a fever for 1 to 3 weeks, tonsillitis, swollen lymph nodes (lymphadenopathy), enlarged liver and spleen (hepatosplenomegaly), and extreme fatigue.

Diagnosis

The presence of atypical lymphocytes in the blood indicates mononucleosis.

Treatment

Antibiotics are not effective against a viral disease and can cause complications, such as a rash caused by penicillin. Therefore, mononucleosis is treated with support-ive care, including bed rest, ibuprofen or acetaminophen to reduce fever, throat lozenges for sore throat, and fluids and electrolytes to prevent dehydration.

Prevention

- Prevention is very difficult, because EBV is such a ubiquitous pathogen, which is shed for long periods by asymptomatic carriers.
- Risk can be decreased by frequent hand washing.

Otitis Media (Middle Ear Infection)

Otitis media is common, with 50% of children having an episode before their first birthday and 80% of children having one by their third birthday. An estimated $3 billion to $4 billion is spent each year on care of patients with acute otitis media and related complications.

Cause of the disease

Acute otitis media frequently occurs with respiratory infections, as the nasal membrane and the Eustachian tube become swollen and congested.

Bacteria are responsible for most (~85%) cases of acute otitis media. *Streptococcus pneumoniae, Haemophilus influenzae, Moraxella catarrhalis, Streptococcus pyogenes,* and *Staphylococcus aureus* are common bacterial causes.

Transmission

Reservoir

Pathogens that cause upper respiratory tract infections that lead to middle ear infections are found in many environments. Those at highest risk are young children in day care.

Mode of transmission

The pathogens are transmitted through respiratory droplets and fomites, such as tissues and children's toys.

Pathogenesis

Entry

Acute otitis media is caused by bacteria (or viruses) that enter the nose or throat and ascend the Eustachian tube to reach the middle ear. Since the Eustachian tube in young children is short, pathogens are more likely to be able to spread to the middle ear than in older children and adults.

Attachment

The pathogens can attach to the tissues of the pharynx or nasal cavity.

Avoiding host defenses

Infection is restricted to the epithelium, an environment that is initially protected from circulating antibodies and cells of the immune system.

Damage

Children's Eustachian tubes are easily blocked by swelling caused by the infection, leading to a buildup of fluid, pus, and mucus, which causes pressure and pain in the middle ear.

Clinical features

Older children often complain about ear pain, ear fullness, or hearing loss. Younger children may demonstrate irritability, fussiness, or difficulty in sleeping, eating, or hearing. They may pull at their ears. Fever may be present in a child of any age. These symptoms are frequently associated with signs of upper respiratory infection, such as a runny or stuffy nose or a cough. Severe ear infections may cause the eardrum to rupture.

Diagnosis

Most children have at least one episode of otitis media before entering school.

Clinical

A physician examines the ears with an otoscope. This allows the doctor to check for redness and fluid behind the ear drum.

Treatment

For viral pathogens, antibiotics are not effective. Symptomatic therapy using over-the-counter medications can help reduce the pain and congestion. If the infection is caused by bacteria, antibiotics may be prescribed. Common antibiotics used to treat otitis media include the following.

Amoxicillin

Amoxicillin is a semisynthetic penicillin that blocks cell wall formation and is highly effective in treating susceptible gram-positive cocci (e.g., *Streptococcus pneumoniae*).

Amoxicillin and potassium clavulanate

The addition of potassium clavulanate inhibits the activity of a pencillinase produced by many penicillin-resistant bacteria (e.g., *Staphylococcus aureus*).

Azithromycin

Since allergic reactions to β-lactams are common, the macrolide azithromycin serves as an alternative. Macrolides block protein synthesis and are effective against both gram-positive cocci and many gram-negative bacterial pathogens.

Prevention

- Breast feeding helps to pass immunoglobulin A, an antibody class that prevents otitis media, from mother to child.
- If bottle feeding is necessary, the child should be held in an upright position. This prevents pooling of milk in the child's throat, which leads to a buildup of bacteria that can travel into the baby's ear.
- Children who spend time in large groups, such as day care centers, develop more frequent colds and therefore more earaches. Frequent hand washing and disinfection of toys can help reduce the spread of the pathogens.
- Secondhand tobacco smoke is also associated with otitis media and should be avoided.

Respiratory Syncytial Virus Bronchiolitis and Pneumonia

Respiratory syncytial virus is the most common cause of lower respiratory tract infections in children and the leading cause of hospitalization for infants younger than 1 year. Each year, RSV disease results in more than 125,000 hospitalizations, and about 2% of these infants die.

Cause of the disease

Respiratory syncytial virus is an enveloped virus with a helical capsid and single-stranded RNA with negative-sense polarity.

Transmission

Reservoir

The reservoir for RSV is infected humans.

Mode of transmission

Transmission occurs via the droplet mode and fomites. The pathogen is commonly spread through respiratory secretions or through close contact with infected persons or contaminated objects.

Pathogenesis

Entry

Infection occurs through contact of infectious material with the mucous membranes of the eyes, mouth, or nose or inhalation of droplets from an infected person's cough or sneeze.

Attachment

The envelope contains surface proteins (G proteins) which attach to tissues in the nasopharynx, bronchioles, and alveoli.

Avoiding host defenses

RSV initially avoids host defenses as an intracellular pathogen. Although the immune system defenses are able to destroy the pathogen, reinfection by RSV is common.

Damage

RSV infection causes fusion of infected cells. These large, multinucleate cells (syncytia), along with cellular debris, can cause direct damage by blocking gas exchange in the bronchioles.

Clinical features

Symptoms begin most frequently with a runny nose, sneezing, coughing, and fever, much like the common cold. The infection can spread to the lower respiratory tract, causing difficulty breathing and cyanosis (a blue color due to lack of O_2). In premature infants, RSV has a high mortality.

Laboratory diagnosis

Sample

A sample is obtained by nasal washings.

Test

Tests include direct detection with monoclonal antibodies targeted to unique RSV antigens using immunofluorescence (direct fluorescent antibody assay) or enzyme-linked immunosorbent assay and detection of RSV RNA using polymerase chain reaction.

Treatment

Most cases of RSV infection are mild, and no treatment is necessary other than the treatment of symptoms using over-the-counter medications. Common treatments include ibuprofen or acetaminophen to reduce fever and cough syrups to suppress coughing and relieve sore throat symptoms.

Most children recover naturally from RSV infection in 8 to 15 days, although a small proportion of children, usually under 6 months of age, require hospitalization for respiratory support due to reduced gas exchange from the RSV infection. For premature infants, a monoclonal antibody is used to provide passive immunity.

Treatment of severe pediatric cases can include the antiviral medication ribavirin. Ribavirin is a nucleoside analog of guanosine that inhibits RSV replication by preventing capping of messenger RNA (mRNA) in virus-infected cells. Uncapped mRNA is not translated.

Prevention

- RSV is unstable in the environment (it survives only 2 to 3 hours) and is readily inactivated with soap or disinfectants. The best prevention is careful and frequent hand washing and good hygiene practices, such as disposal of tissues used to clean nasal secretions, frequent disinfection of toys, and not sharing cups, glasses, eating utensils, etc.

- Isolating children with RSV will not significantly reduce transmission of the disease, because viral shedding occurs 3 or 4 days before symptoms are visible, allowing spread during the early stages of illness.

Strep Throat

The pathogen of strep throat causes 15% of all adult pharyngitis and about 30% of pediatric cases. One in 400 cases of untreated strep throat can be expected to result in acute rheumatic fever, a serious complication of infection with the pathogen. Approximately 20% of asymptomatic children are long-term carriers of the strep throat pathogen.

Cause of the disease

Streptococcus pyogenes, a bacterial pathogen, is a gram-positive coccus arranged in chains and pairs. It has a fermentative metabolism and an antiphagocytic capsule made of hyaluronic acid. It produces a toxin, hemolysin, that lyses erythrocytes. The pathogen contains the group A antigen on its surface and produces beta-hemolysis on blood agar.

Transmission

Reservoir

Infected humans and asymptomatic carriers are reservoirs of the virus.

Mode of transmission

Transmission is by the droplet mode via secretions sprayed from the air passages by sneezing or coughing, usually spreading the infection via the respiratory route. The organism may also be transmitted by fomites.

Pathogenesis

Entry

The pathogen enters via respiratory droplets or by contaminated fomites.

Attachment

The pathogen attaches to the mucosal cells of the upper respiratory tract. The bacterial F protein attaches to fibronectin receptors found on the pharyngeal cells.

Avoiding or overcoming host defenses

The capsule of *S. pyogenes* inhibits phagocytosis; streptolysins are cytotoxic to white blood cells.

Damage

Enzymes (protease, DNase, hemolysins, and streptokinase) secreted by *S. pyogenes* contribute to tissue damage. The tissue damage causes an intense inflammatory response. In addition, peptidoglycan fragments and teichoic acids induce a cytokine response. Cytokines are signaling proteins that also stimulate an inflammatory response.

Clinical features

Strep throat is characterized by fever, sore throat (pharyngitis), swollen lymph nodes, and pus discharge from the tonsils (exudative tonsillitis). Headache is usually associated with older adolescents and adults.

While these symptoms may be common for strep throat, many other bacterial and viral infections demonstrate similar signs. For this reason, it is very important to contact a physician to determine the definite cause of illness. Proper treatment is effective at preventing several serious complications that can result from strep throat.

Complications

Complications include peritonsilar abscesses resulting from invasion of the pathogen into deeper tissue; scarlet fever from the release of a toxin that indirectly causes a blanching bright red rash, followed by the surface of the skin peeling (desquamatization); rheumatic fever; rheumatic heart disease; and kidney failure (acute glomerulonephritis).

Diagnosis

Because it is not possible to tell if pharyngitis is viral or bacterial by clinical means, a throat swab and culture or antigenic test is the best way of confirming the presence of group A streptococci. Since it is not cost-effective to take a throat culture from every patient, it is usually done only if a child has all of the classical clinical symptoms of strep throat.

Laboratory tests

The specimen is streaked onto blood agar plates. Beta-hemolytic colonies that are gram-positive streptococci and also show sensitivity to bacitracin indicate *Streptococcus pyogenes*. Rapid enzyme-linked immunosorbent assays are also used and provide fast results.

Treatment

Streptococcal pharyngitis is self-limiting and usually lasts only 5 to 7 days without therapy. Sensitive strains are treated with a β-lactam antibiotic, such as penicillin. Erythromycin is used if the patient is allergic to penicillin. Drugs are given orally for a period of 10 days to avoid relapse due to regrowth of antibiotic-resistant bacteria and to prevent the development of rheumatic fever.

Prevention

- There is no vaccine for the prevention of group A streptococcus infections. Tonsillectomies have been suggested but have not been proven successful.

- Good personal hygiene habits, such as covering the mouth when sneezing or coughing and washing the hands after wiping or blowing the nose, coughing, or sneezing, help prevent infection.

- Prophylactic antibiotic therapy can be used to arrest the spread of *Streptococcus pyogenes* during epidemic outbreaks.

Tuberculosis

Worldwide, the prevalence of TB is about 2 billion persons. New cases number about 8 million yearly, and annual mortality worldwide is estimated at 3 million. This accounts for 7% of the total worldwide mortality and places tuberculosis as the number two cause of death by infectious disease (after pneumonia). Approximately 1 in 10 new cases of TB is caused by a resistant strain, and 1 in 100 is multidrug resistant. TB is fatal for up to 50% of untreated patients, and multidrug-resistant TB cases have a reported fatality rate of more than 70%

Cause of the disease

Mycobacterium tuberculosis, a bacterial pathogen, is an acid-fast, rod-shaped streptobacillus. It is aerobic and grows very slowly. The waxy, acid-fast cell wall restricts the diffusion of many chemicals, making the pathogen resistant to disinfectants and many antibiotics.

Transmission

Reservoir

Infected humans are the reservoir for *M. tuberculosis*.

Mode of transmission

The pathogen is transmitted by the airborne and droplet modes. The bacterium is resistant to temperature change and drying and survives as suspended particles in the air for several hours.

Pathogenesis

Entry

Airborne particles or respiratory droplets containing *M. tuberculosis* are inhaled.

Attachment

The organism attaches to alveolar macrophages after entering the lungs.

Avoiding host defenses

The organism is engulfed by alveolar macrophages but avoids fusion with lysosomes, resulting in the pathogen being protected within the host cell.

Damage

Replication within the macrophage results in cell lysis. Other macrophages are drawn to the site of infection and layer around the infected cells, forming tubercles or small granulomas. The tubercles can block alveoli and bronchioles. If the immune system cannot contain the mycobacteria in the tubercles, the pathogen spreads to other organs.

Clinical features

Approximately 10% of infected people go on to develop active TB. The lungs are the most commonly affected organ.

Clinical signs and symptoms of pulmonary TB include a bad cough that produces bloody sputum, chest pain, chronic fever, weakness or fatigue, chills, night sweats, weight loss, and loss of appetite.

Diagnosis

Clinical

Diagnosis of a person with suspected TB is made by using a Mantoux tuberculin skin test. A Mantoux skin test is performed by injecting a small amount of purified protein derivative or tuberculin intradermally in the skin of the forearm. The test is read 48 to 72 hours later; if the site of injection shows an area of swelling and redness larger than 15 millimeters in a healthy person, the test is considered positive. A positive skin test is followed up with a chest radiograph. Inactive cases will have granulomas, showing successful walling off of the pathogen.

Laboratory

Specimen: A sputum sample is taken.

Test: The test is acid-fast staining to detect acid-fast bacilli or polymerase chain reaction to detect *Mycobacterium tuberculosis*-specific DNA.

A positive culture for *M. tuberculosis* can be used to confirm the diagnosis, although diagnosis may also be made based simply on the clinical presentation of the patient.

Treatment

Because the pathogen grows so slowly and has a waxy coating covering its cell wall, long-term therapy is required with antibiotics that can penetrate into the mycobacterium.

Treatment with isoniazid for 6 to 12 months is commonly used for people diagnosed with *M. tuberculosis* infection to prevent the development of tuberculosis.

Active tuberculosis is typically treated with a combination of four drugs—isoniazid, rifampin, pyrazinamide, and either ethambutol or streptomycin—for anywhere from 6 to 24 months. The combination of drugs is used to prevent *Mycobacterium tuberculosis* from becoming resistant to any single drug.

Prevention

- *Mycobacterium bovis* bacillus Calmette-Guérin (BCG) vaccine is used for prevention in countries with a high rate of TB.

- Health care workers and others who work where TB is common must be tested regularly to ensure that they are not infected.

- Those with active tuberculosis should be isolated so as not to spread the disease to others.

- Antibiotic prophylaxis with isoniazid can be used to prevent the development of active tuberculosis.

SECTION III

Outbreaks of Diseases of the Gastrointestinal Tract

We can't do anything. . . . They just die and die and die, and they keep coming and coming and coming.

FLORENCE PARENT, U.S. physician, commenting on a cholera epidemic among Rwandan refugees (*New York Times*, 22 July 1994)

The most common symptom resulting from infection by gastrointestinal (GI) tract pathogens is diarrhea. Although it is often not viewed as a serious disease, diarrhea is actually the third leading cause of death from infectious disease worldwide. Most of the nearly 3 million annual deaths are among children less than 5 years old in underdeveloped regions of the world, where basic technology and public infrastructure are lacking. About one-third of the world's population lacks treated water, and approximately one-sixth of the world's population lacks sewage treatment. As a result, fecally contaminated drinking water is common in many communities. The combination of diarrhea in undernourished and malnourished children and a lack of basic health care is a lethal mixture that much of the world struggles with on a daily basis.

In institutional settings, such as college campuses, where large numbers of people share dining and toilet facilities, GI tract pathogens can be spread by contaminated food or drinks or by contact with contaminated environmental surfaces. Frequent hand washing, disinfection of toilet facilities, and proper cooking and preparation of food reduce the risk of spreading diarrheal pathogens.

The GI tract must defend against millions of microbes each day. To prevent infection and disease, the GI tract uses chemical and physical methods of defense. Chemical defenses include the low pH of gastric juice. HCl is secreted by parietal cells of the gastric mucosa. The acid conditions lead to denaturation of microbial proteins while the food

83

is being processed in the stomach. There are also enzymes that digest and destroy microbes. Lysozyme, which is secreted in the mouth, digests peptidoglycan, the key component of bacterial cell walls. Without the protection of the cell wall, bacterial cells can be destroyed by osmotic lysis. The pancreas produces a host of enzymes that hydrolyze proteins, carbohydrates, and nucleic acids. Bile from the liver solubilizes lipids, which can then be digested by pancreatic lipases. As a result, most microbes are digested for nutrients in the same way as the food we eat. The mucus layer that coats the GI tract acts as a physical barrier that inhibits the attachment of microbes. If microbes are unable to attach to the epithelium of the mucosa, they are eliminated with the feces.

Both the mouth and the large intestine have abundant normal floras, microbes that are permanent residents in and on us and that help to keep us healthy. These organisms act as microbial antagonists to inhibit pathogenic microbes by effectively consuming nutrients and utilizing the available microenvironments. As a result of the long-term adaptations of the members of the normal flora to their human hosts, it is difficult for pathogens to outcompete them.

Even with these defenses, the GI tract is a common site of infection. Successful microbes must attach to host tissues, survive the acidity of the stomach, not be destroyed by digestive enzymes, and outcompete the normal flora. *Streptococcus mutans*, which initiates dental caries formation, utilizes sucrose to synthesize a sticky capsule that enables it to attach to the pellicle of a tooth. Some pathogenic *Escherichia coli* and *Salmonella* strains have pili that enable them to adhere to specific parts of the intestines. Flagella help them penetrate the mucus coating. Although some microbes are resistant to acid denaturation, bile, or enzymatic digestion, others can survive by being contained in a layer of food that acts as protection. Rotavirus is not easily denatured by an acid environment. As a result, ingestion of only a small number of virus particles is sufficient to cause disease. Diarrhea-causing protozoa, such as *Entamoeba histolytica*, *Giardia lamblia*, and *Cryptosporidium parvum*, produce cysts that protect the microbe from host defenses until they reach the intestines, where they begin to reproduce and cause disease. Although the normal flora inhibits the growth of microbial pathogens, it can be unbalanced by antibiotic therapy or diarrhea, allowing pathogens to compete more easily for nutrients and microenvironments.

The outbreaks presented in this section emphasize that even in countries with excellent health care and well developed infrastructures for water and sewage treatment, GI tract pathogens are still a major source of illness and death. Gastrointestinal diseases can be spread to large numbers of people through common vehicles—food, drinking water, and contaminated recreational waters. Solutions to prevent future outbreaks require careful and complete compliance with accepted practices that prevent microbial growth or contamination.

Where natural disasters or war destroy sewage and water treatment facilities or displace populations into primitive areas, GI tract pathogens abound and can rapidly spread to cause thousands of deaths. At times, coordinated efforts by more developed countries are needed to quickly intervene to avoid significant loss of life.

Table III.1 Selected outbreak-causing gastrointestinal-tract pathogens

Organism	Key physical properties	Disease characteristics
Bacteria		
Campylobacter spp.	Microaerophilic, curved, gram-negative bacilli	Diarrhea
Clostridium botulinum	Anaerobic, gram-positive, endospore-forming bacillus that produces a potent neurotoxin which causes muscle paralysis	Botulism, flaccid paralysis
Enterohemorrhagic *Escherichia coli*	Non-sorbitol-fermenting gram-negative bacillus (*E. coli* O157:H7)	Bloody diarrhea, hemolytic-uremic syndrome
Enterotoxigenic *Escherichia coli*	Lactose-fermenting, gram-negative bacillus	Watery diarrhea
Listeria monocytogenes	Gram-positive, catalase-positive coccobacillus	Adults can have a range of illnesses from a mild flu-like illness to meningitis; can be transmitted vertically and cause fetal damage or death
Salmonella spp.	Non-lactose-fermenting, motile, gram-negative bacillus; produces H_2S from protein catabolism	Invasive diarrhea, typhoid fever
Shigella spp.	Non-lactose-fermenting, nonmotile, gram-negative bacillus	Bloody diarrhea, severe dysentery
Staphylococcus aureus	Gram-positive coccus that produces a heat-stable enterotoxin	Food poisoning, causing vomiting
Vibrio spp.	Gram-negative, curved bacillus with a monopolar flagellum	Cholera, massive watery diarrhea
Protozoa		
Cryptosporidium parvum	Forms acid-fast, chlorine-resistant round cysts	Self-limiting diarrhea (chronic in AIDS)
Entamoeba histolytica	Forms round cysts and amoebae	Diarrhea, amebic dysentery, liver abscess
Giardia lamblia	Forms oval cysts and flagellated trophozoites	Diarrhea with foul-smelling stools
Viruses		
Hepatitis A virus	Nonenveloped polyhedral capsid with single-stranded RNA	Self-limited hepatitis
Noroviruses (Norwalk agents)	Nonenveloped polyhedral capsid with single-stranded RNA	Diarrhea and vomiting
Rotavirus	Nonenveloped wheel-like capsid with double-stranded RNA	Diarrhea and projectile vomiting, primarily in young children

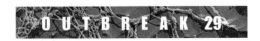

A *Salmonella enterica* Serovar Enteritidis Outbreak from Eating Eggs

MULTISTATE, 1997

Los Angeles County, California

In August 1997, the Los Angeles County Department of Health Services received reports of gastrointestinal illness in members of a Girl Scout troop and some of their parents. The ill persons had eaten food prepared in a private residence by the scouts. Stool cultures taken from 12 ill persons all yielded *Salmonella* (Fig. 29.1 and 29.2).

An investigation by the Los Angeles County Department of Health Services found that of 17 persons at the dinner, 13 had gastrointestinal illness. Cheesecake served at the dinner was associated with illness; all 13 ill persons and two well persons ate the cheesecake. The cheesecake contained raw egg whites and egg yolks that were cooked in a double boiler until slightly thickened. The California Department of Health Services and Department of Food and Agriculture investigated the farm that supplied the eggs. Of 476 environmental cultures taken from manure, feed, and water, 21 (4.4%) yielded the pathogen. All positive cultures were from manure. The pathogen was also isolated from 1 (0.5%) of 200 pooled egg samples obtained at the farm.

Washington, D.C.

In October 1997, the District of Columbia Bureau of Epidemiology and Disease Control received reports of gastroenteritis among 75 attendees at seven events (a workshop dinner, a nursing home luncheon, and five meals in private residences) at which lasagna from the same commercial manufacturer was served. Stool cultures from nine patients yielded *Salmonella*. Three patients were hospitalized; none died.

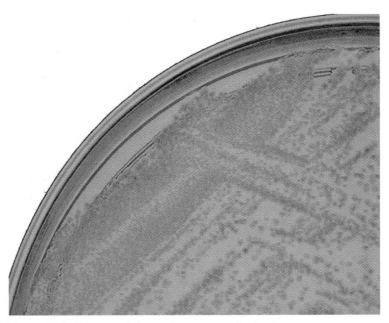

Figure 29.1 Growth of the pathogen on MacConkey agar.

The District of Columbia Bureau of Epidemiology and Disease Control interviewed 48 of the 75 attendees. Of the 47 persons who ate lasagna at the events, 39 became ill; the only person who did not eat lasagna did not become ill. Lasagna was the only food item common to all events. Cultures of two leftover lasagnas and one lasagna made on the same day but not eaten yielded the diarrhea-causing pathogen. The lasagnas were prepared commercially by a company in Gaithersburg, Maryland, using fully cooked meat or spinach sauce and a mixture of raw eggs, ricotta and mozzarella cheeses, and spices. Although the lasagnas were not labeled with a manufacture date, investigators determined that most, if not all, of the lasagnas implicated were made on the same day from a single batch of the egg-cheese mixture. The product was then frozen (except for one event, in which the lasagnas were kept refrigerated as a special order) and held without further cooking until they were purchased. For at least four of the six events for which lasagnas were purchased frozen, the lasagna was not thawed before being reheated.

A trace-back investigation led to two egg processors. Sampling of the farms that supplied eggs to these processors showed that 5 of 13 poultry houses had environmental samples positive for *Salmonella*.

Clark County, Nevada

In November 1997, 91 persons who ate either of two meals served 2 weeks apart at a hotel restaurant in Las Vegas, Nevada, developed gastroenteritis. Fifteen patients were hospitalized; none died. Stool cultures taken from ill persons yielded *Salmonella*.

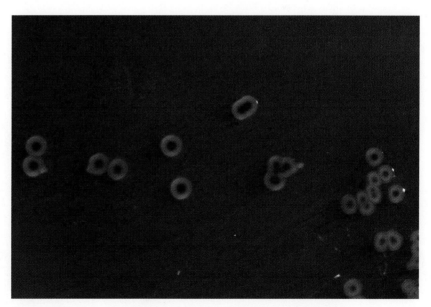

Figure 29.2 Growth of the pathogen on Hektoen enteric agar.

An investigation by the Clark County Health District found 28 culture-confirmed and 63 probable cases. Two separate case-control studies implicated broccoli with hollandaise sauce. Broccoli with hollandaise sauce was offered on a special menu that rotated biweekly. The hollandaise sauce was prepared from pooled eggs, cooked to a temperature inadequate to kill bacteria, and kept at room temperature for several hours until it was served.

Samples taken from those infected were cultured. Tests indicated that the pathogen was a facultatively anaerobic gram-negative motile rod that did not ferment lactose and produced H_2S (Fig. 29.1 and 29.2).

QUESTIONS

1. Besides *Salmonella*, what other pathogens might have accounted for the outbreak?

2. Why is *Salmonella* infection often associated with eating raw or undercooked eggs?

3. Describe the pathogenesis of *Salmonella*.

4. How would you have treated those affected by the disease?

5. How could future outbreaks of this pathogen be prevented?

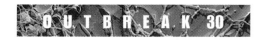

A *Cryptosporidium* Outbreak Associated with Swimming Pool Use

OHIO, 2000

In July 2000, the Delaware City/County Health Department (DCCHD) learned of several laboratory-confirmed cases of diarrhea potentially linked to a private swim club. To determine associated exposures, a descriptive study and two telephone-based case-control studies were conducted: a community-based study to examine potential sources of the outbreak and a swim club-based study to identify club-related risk factors. People were asked about sources of drinking water, recent travel, visits to pools and lakes, swimming behaviors, contact with ill persons or young animals, and day care attendance.

All case patients were in central Ohio from 17 June to 18 August. The DCCHD identified 700 clinical cases among residents of Delaware County and three neighboring counties. The outbreak began in late June. Of 268 stool samples submitted to the DCCHD, 186 (70%) tested positive for the pathogen. The median age of these case patients was 6 years (range, 1 to 46 years). The median duration of illness was 7 days (range, 1 to 36 days). Symptoms included diarrhea (91%), loss of appetite (87%), abdominal cramps (83%), and vomiting (35%).

Swimming at the private club was strongly associated with illness in the community case-control study. Activities that increased the risk for pool water getting in the mouth (e.g., standing under a pool sprinkler) increased the risk for illness. At least five fecal accidents, one of which was diarrheal, were observed in the pool.

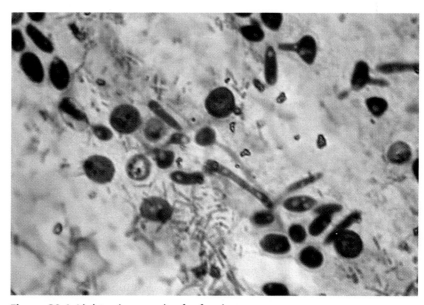

Figure 30.1 Light micrograph of a fecal smear.

Antigen tests for viral pathogens were negative. Laboratory cultures were negative for bacterial pathogens. Microscopic analysis did not reveal any trophozoites or nucleated cysts (different stages of the protozoal pathogens). However, small, acid-fast cysts were observed (Fig. 30.1), indicating *Cryptosporidium* as the cause of the outbreak. Cysts are protozoal reproductive structures. An acid-fast cyst has a waxy protective coating surrounding it.

QUESTIONS

1. How is *Cryptosporidium* transmitted? What is its natural reservoir?

2. How does *Cryptosporidium* infection cause diarrhea?

3. Explain why individuals suffering from diarrhea were asked about their sources of drinking water, recent travels, visits to pools and lakes, swimming behaviors, contact with ill persons or young animals, and day care attendance.

4. Explain how you would have managed this outbreak and prevented further outbreaks caused by the same pathogen.

Diarrhea among Attendees of the Washington County Fair

NEW YORK, 1999

The Washington County Fair was held from 23 to 29 August 1999. Approximately 110,000 people attended the fair. On 3 September, the New York State Department of Health (NYSDOH) received reports that at least 10 children who had attended the fair had been hospitalized with bloody diarrhea. Because these patients may have represented early cases of a developing outbreak with serious health consequences, the NYSDOH initiated an investigation to identify additional fair attendees with diarrhea. To do so, the NYSDOH issued press releases, conducted daily press briefings, and contacted emergency departments, laboratories, and infection control practitioners by fax and telephone. Laboratories were asked to culture all diarrheal stool specimens.

The investigation identified 921 persons who reported diarrhea after attending the fair. Analysis of these 921 cases demonstrated that there were two separate pathogens causing diarrhea. Those people with uncomplicated cases of diarrhea were found to have *Campylobacter jejuni* infections. For those with bloody diarrhea, stool cultures yielded pathogenic gram-negative rods (Fig. 31.1) that fermented lactose but did not ferment sorbitol (Fig. 31.2). The pathogen was motile and a facultative anaerobe (it could grow with or without oxygen), produced several toxins, and had peritrichous flagella (flagella that surrounded the cell).

Since both pathogens are usually transmitted through fecally contaminated food or water, the investigation began with an analysis of the water supplied to the fairgrounds. Although most of the grounds were supplied with chlorinated water, in one area, a shallow well supplied unchlorinated water to several food vendors, who used the water to make beverages and ice. The well was located near the barn that housed dairy cattle.

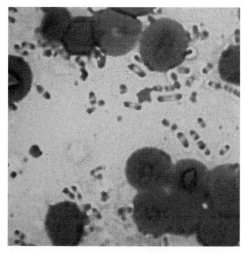

Figure 31.1 Gram stain of the pathogen.

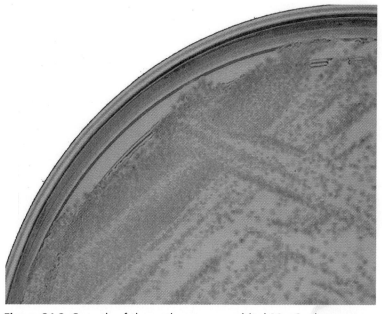

Figure 31.2 Growth of the pathogen on sorbitol-MacConkey agar.

To confirm that this water source may have been the source of the outbreak, a case-control study was conducted. The case patients were residents of Washington County who developed diarrhea after attending the fair and whose stool cultures yielded the pathogen. The controls were residents of Washington County randomly selected from the telephone directory who had attended the fair and who were matched by age group. Thirty-two case patients and 57 controls were compared. The results are shown below.

| Activity at fair | No. participating in the activity | |
	Case patients (*n* = 32)	Control patients (*n* = 57)
Drinking water from suspect well	16	3
Drinking beverages from vendors supplied by suspect well	10	6
Physical contact with animals	6	5
Eating food at the fair	30	52

QUESTIONS

1. What is the reservoir for *Campylobacter*? How is it usually spread?

2. What pathogen most likely caused the bloody diarrhea? Explain your reasoning.

3. Explain why each activity in the table was investigated, and give the most likely sources of most of the infections.

4. Explain how the pathogen causes serious, life-threatening complications.

5. You have been recruited as an advisor to the NYSDOH to help them manage their present resources. Your goal is to minimize any further illness and deaths and reduce the risk of spread of the infection.

   a. What would be your first priority? Explain.

   b. What would be your second priority? Explain.

An Amebiasis Outbreak

GEORGIA, 1998

On 27 August 1998, the regional office of the World Health Organization for Europe asked the Istituto Superiore di Sanità (the National Health Institute of Italy) for an immediate assessment of an increase in the incidence of intestinal disease (diarrhea and its complications) in Georgia's capital city, Tbilisi (population, 1.7 million), which had been reported by the Georgian Minister of Health. The collapse of the previous economic system and the civil war in 1993 seriously impaired the social and health situations in Georgia. In 1996, over 65% of the population was estimated to be below the poverty level. Health services were free of charge only for emergency situations; otherwise, drug treatment and hospital care had to be paid for by the patient.

In July 1998, more than 10 cases of liver abscesses were caused by complications of amebiasis. The patients were admitted to hospitals in Tbilisi. An emergency committee was set up by the Ministry of Health and arranged for diagnosis and treatment to be offered free of charge. The Georgian National Center for Disease Control asked hospital doctors and microbiologists to notify it of all suspected cases of amebiasis, giving the age, sex, address, workplace, and profession of patients and the symptoms, their dates of onset, date of hospital admission, laboratory results, and treatment of the disease. In order to detect additional cases, active case ascertainment was carried out by the local health authorities at the end of July by conducting doorstep interviews in the neighborhood where cases had already been identified. By 10 August, television broadcasts were advising the public to go to the hospital if they were suffering from bloody or mucous diarrhea or had symptoms that could indicate liver abscess (for example, fever with upper abdominal pain).

Laboratory tests were used to confirm infection by *Entamoeba histolytica*. Fecal smears showed the presence of round protozoal cysts.

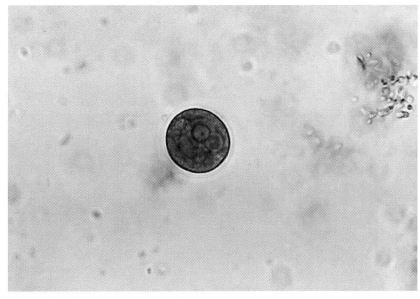

Figure 32.1 Light micrograph of a fecal smear.

One hundred seventy-seven cases of intestinal disease were reported to the National Center for Disease Control between 26 May and 3 September 1998, comprising 71 cases of intestinal disease and 106 probable cases of liver abscess. Four patients with liver abscess died.

Ninety-one percent of the patients lived on the left side of the River Kura, and patients who did not live there worked on that side of the river. The highest attack rates were close to a water filtration system that used surface water from a large lake. All districts with high attack rates were fed by this source. At this water treatment works, the filters were of poor quality, and routine maintenance was not documented. Districts with lower attack rates were fed by ground water. In Tbilisi as a whole, between 600 and 700 breakdowns of the water supply and sewage system were reported between April and September 1998, but the routine *Escherichia coli* index in drinking water, investigated by two different laboratories, was never reported to be significantly increased. No previous problems with the water treatment works had been reported.

QUESTIONS

1. How is *Entamoeba histolytica* transmitted?

2. How would you have treated those affected by uncomplicated cases of diarrhea caused by this pathogen?

3. How would you have controlled the outbreak?

4. Since your resources are significantly limited, propose a low-cost solution to prevent continued outbreaks caused by this pathogen.

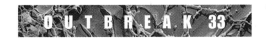

A Typhoid Fever Outbreak Linked with a Frozen Fruit Drink

FLORIDA, 2002

Typhoid fever is spread by food and water contaminated by the feces or urine of infected persons, with between 2 and 5% of those infected becoming asymptomatic carriers. Although about 17 million people around the world are infected each year and 600,000 die, clean water and safe sewage management have greatly reduced the risk in the United States. For more than 20 years, the annual U.S. incidence has been less than 1 case per 100,000 population, and almost all of the 400 or so cases seen each year have been in people who traveled to areas where the disease is endemic.

In 2002, in an outbreak in Florida, at least 16 people were infected over a relatively short time. These patients were not acquainted with one another, lived in several different counties, received drinking water from at least four different water systems, shared no common recreational or social activities, did not use the same grocery stores or restaurants, and with one exception had not recently been out of the country. Laboratory tests (Fig. 33.1) identified *Salmonella enterica* serovar Typhi in all cases, and deoxyribonucleic acid (DNA) analysis confirmed all pathogen isolates to be identical with each other.

Three patients mentioned that they had consumed fruit shakes made with a tropical fruit called mamey. This fruit, also called zapote, is commonly used in fruit shakes called batidos, where it is mixed with milk, ice, and sometimes sugar. When 11 other patients were asked open-ended questions about fruit and beverage use in a matched case-control analysis, 10 said they had drunk mamey batidos.

Food testing and tracebacks to manufacturers showed that mamey shakes consumed by the patients were made with commercially packaged frozen fruit from two manufacturing plants in Guatemala and one in Honduras. None of the samples obtained from 49 supermarkets and 12 distributors showed *Salmonella enterica* serovar Typhi, but all contained fecal coliforms and *Escherichia coli*.

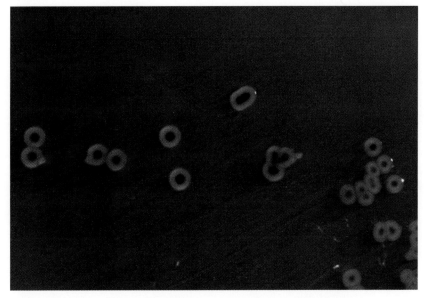

Figure 33.1 Growth of the pathogen on Hektoen enteric agar.

95

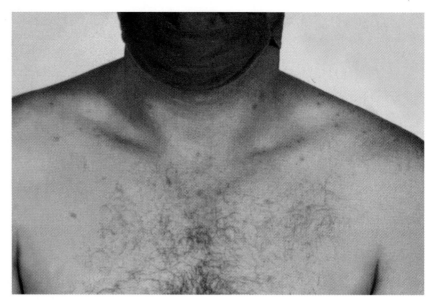

Figure 33.2 Rose spot rash.

QUESTIONS

1. Why was the discovery of fecal coliforms in the packaged frozen fruit important in identifying it as the most likely source of the typhoid fever pathogen?

2. What are the clinical features of typhoid fever?

3. What features of *Salmonella enterica* serovar Typhi enable it to cause systemic disease rather than just diarrhea?

4. How would you have treated those with typhoid fever?

5. How would you have stopped this outbreak and prevented future occurrences?

OUTBREAK 34

A *Giardia* Outbreak in a Day Care Nursery

JUNEAU, ALASKA, 1982

A nonprofit day care center-nursery cared for about 30 children, both infants and toddlers. The day care center cared for children over 2.5 years of age who were toilet trained, while the nursery accepted children 3 years old and under who were not yet toilet trained. The day care center was situated in an old building in downtown Juneau.

For the previous 5 years, there had been annual outbreaks of diarrhea in the nursery. Morbidity had been documented among children and their family members. Although numerous control measures were recommended in past years, they were poorly implemented, and outbreaks continued to occur. The day care center did not consistently prohibit accepting for care children who were ill or strictly enforce hand-washing procedures among staff.

In late August 1982, five cases of diarrhea were identified when a nursery employee submitted stool samples from children with chronic diarrhea to the Southeastern Regional Laboratory, Division of Public Health. As part of the epidemiologic investigation, the Juneau Health Center, in cooperation with the nursery, discovered an additional eight cases of diarrhea caused by the same pathogen from the total nursery population of 24. Nine of 10 (90%) infants less than 16 months old were affected, and 4 of 24 (17%) toddlers (aged 16 months through 3 years) were affected. Two cases of diarrhea caused by the pathogen were identified among siblings of positive children. Both had attended the nursery during July and were enrolled in the day care center.

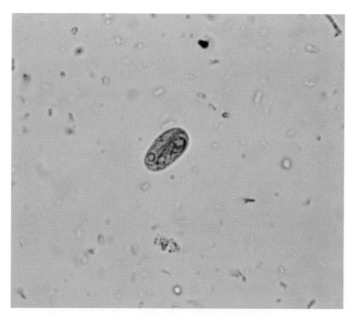

Figure 34.1 Light micrograph of a fecal smear.

Clinical signs and symptoms of the infected children showed that 52% had suffered foamy diarrhea for more than 1 week during the summer, with bloating and loss of appetite in half of them. Forty-eight percent of the infected children were asymptomatic.

The pathogen was identified by microscopically examining fecal smears. Oval cysts were observed, indicating infection by *Giardia lamblia*.

QUESTIONS

1. Besides *Giardia*, list four pathogens that could have caused the diarrhea.

2. How would you have treated those infected by the pathogen?

3. Describe an appropriate way to have managed the outbreak.

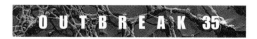

A Food-Borne Outbreak of Bloody Diarrhea

MULTISTATE, 2000

A multistate outbreak of bloody diarrhea with at least 30 culture-confirmed cases in California, Oregon, and Washington was linked to eating a nationally distributed five-layer dip. The onset of symptoms occurred between 10 and 23 January 2000. The implicated product was manufactured by Señor Felix's Mexican Foods (Baldwin Park, California) and distributed under the brand names Señor Felix's 5-Layer Party Dip (sold in 16-ounce, 20-ounce, and 41-ounce containers), Delicioso 5-Layer Party Dip (33-ounce containers), and Trader Joe's 5-Layer Party Dip (20-ounce containers). The dip consisted of layers of beans, salsa, guacamole, nacho cheese, and sour cream. The dip was made without the addition of food preservatives.

The clinical features of the infection included abdominal cramps, fever, and bloody diarrhea. Symptoms usually developed 1 to 3 days after the party dip was eaten.

Samples taken from those infected were cultured on selective and differential media (Fig. 35.1). Further tests indicated that the pathogen was a gram-negative nonmotile rod. Fecal samples showed abundant erythrocytes and leukocytes (Fig. 35.2).

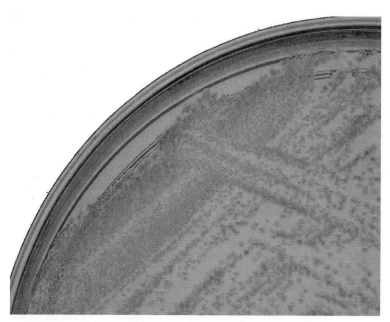

Figure 35.1 Growth of the pathogen on MacConkey agar.

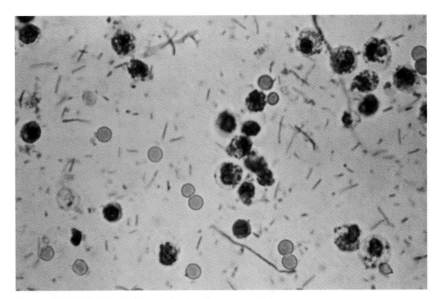

Figure 35.2 Light micrograph of a feces sample.

QUESTIONS

1. On the basis of the laboratory results, diagnose the disease and describe the pathogenic agent.

2. Given this pathogen, would you expect secondary outbreaks of bloody diarrhea?

3. Describe how this pathogen is typically transmitted.

4. How would you have stopped this outbreak and prevented further outbreaks like this from occurring?

A Multistate Outbreak of Listeriosis

NORTHEASTERN UNITED STATES, 2002

A multistate outbreak of *Listeria monocytogenes* infection caused 46 culture-confirmed cases and seven deaths in eight states. The infection was linked to eating sliced turkey delicatessen meat. Cases were reported from Pennsylvania (14 cases), New York (11 in New York City and 7 in other locations), New Jersey (5), Delaware (4), Maryland (2), Connecticut (1), Massachusetts (1), and Michigan (1).

Eating food contaminated with *Listeria* can be fatal. The majority of cases occur among pregnant women, the elderly, and persons with weakened immune systems. The illness typically begins with influenza-like symptoms and sometimes with diarrhea, which usually occur within 1 week after eating contaminated food. In serious cases the disease progresses to include high fever, severe headache, and neck stiffness.

Listeria was isolated from the blood of those most severely affected. The pathogen was identified in a Gram stain of a blood sample (Fig. 36.1). Growth on blood agar revealed hemolytic colonies.

QUESTIONS

1. For what complications are untreated and/or pregnant patients at increased risk?

2. Why is this pathogen often associated with processed meat?

3. How would you have treated those affected by the disease?

4. How would you have managed this outbreak?

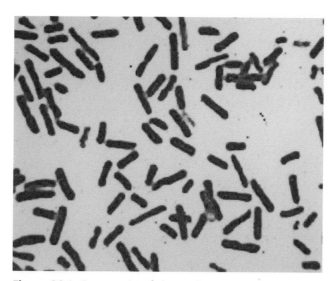

Figure 36.1 Gram stain of the pathogen.

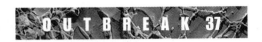

Food-Borne Paralysis from Eating Home-Pickled Eggs

ILLINOIS, 1997

On 23 November 1997, a previously healthy 68-year-old man became nauseated, vomited, and complained of abdominal pain. During the next 2 days, he developed diplopia (double vision), dysarthria (difficulty speaking), and respiratory impairment. Physical examination confirmed multiple cranial-nerve abnormalities, including muscle weakness around the eyes (extraocular motor palsy) and diffuse flaccid paralysis. A food history revealed no exposures to home-canned products; however, the patient had eaten pickled eggs that he had prepared 7 days before the onset of illness; gastrointestinal symptoms began 12 hours after ingestion of the eggs.

The pickled eggs were prepared using a recipe that consisted of hard-boiled eggs, commercially prepared beets, hot peppers, and vinegar. The intact hard-boiled eggs were peeled and punctured with toothpicks and then combined with the other ingredients in a glass jar that was closed with a metal screw-on lid. The mixture was stored at room temperature and was occasionally exposed to sunlight.

Bacteria were cultured from the pickling liquid, beets, and egg yolk. Bacteria grew only under anaerobic conditions. The Gram and endospore staining results are shown in Fig. 37.1 and 37.2. Cultures of the peppers did not yield any bacteria. Beets from the original commercial containers were not available. The pH of the pickling liquid was 3.5. However, the pH of the egg yolk was estimated to be 6.8.

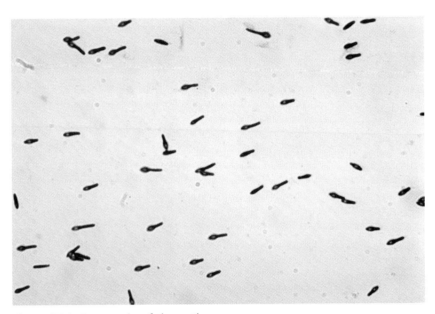

Figure 37.1 Gram stain of the pathogen.

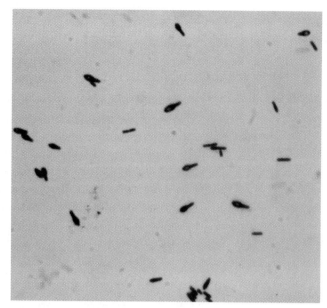

Figure 37.2 Endospore stain of the pathogen.

QUESTIONS

1. What disease did the man have, and what pathogen caused it?

2. Describe the physical characteristics of the pathogen.

3. What food preparation procedures could be changed to prevent this disease?

4. Describe the pathogenesis of the disease.

5. What other uses are there for the paralysis-causing toxin?

6. Describe an appropriate way to have treated the man's disease.

7. What is the pathogen's reservoir?

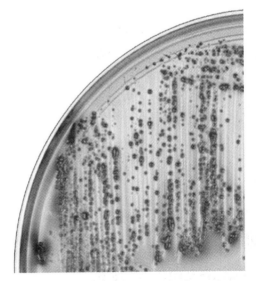

Bloody Diarrhea Associated with Eating Ground Beef

UNITED STATES, 2002

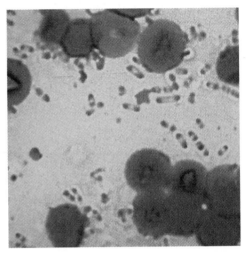

Figure 38.1 Gram stain of the pathogen.

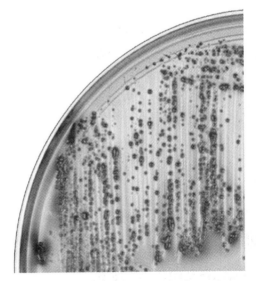

Figure 38.2 Growth on MacConkey agar.

During July 2002, the Colorado Department of Public Health and Environment identified an outbreak of bloody diarrhea infections among Colorado residents that was linked to eating contaminated ground beef products produced by a commercial beef-packing plant. Initial investigation identified 28 cases of illness in Colorado and six other states. Seven patients were hospitalized; five developed hemolytic-uremic syndrome (HUS). The median age of the patients was 15 years (range, 1 to 72 years). The dates of symptom onset ranged from 13 June to 7 July.

Symptoms of the disease included bloody and nonbloody diarrhea, vomiting, and abdominal cramps. The illness typically resolved within 7 to 10 days. A subset of patients, particularly the young and the elderly, developed HUS, characterized by hemolytic anemia (anemia resulting from lysis of erythrocytes), thrombocytopenia (a decrease in platelets that causes blood to fail to clot), and renal failure.

Interviews with 16 patients with confirmed infections revealed that all had eaten ground beef during the 7 days before illness. Furthermore, in every case, the ground beef had been purchased at grocery chain A between 10 and 24 June. The pathogen was cultured from an opened package of ground beef collected from a patient's home. A trace back by the Colorado Department of Public Health and Environment of ground beef collected from a patient's home indicated that it was reground by grocery chain A with meat produced on 31 May by a single commercial beef-packing plant. The extent to which the meat was repackaged and distributed under other labels was unclear.

Independent of the outbreak investigation, the beef packing plant identified the pathogen during routine microbiologic testing conducted by the U.S. Department of Agriculture (Fig. 38.1 and 38.2). Antigen tests were used to specifically identify the pathogenic nature of the isolated bacteria by testing for the types of H (flagellar) and O (lipopolysaccharide) antigens.

The commercial beef-packing plant produced 18.6 million pounds of fresh and frozen ground beef and beef trimmings between 12 April and 11 July.

QUESTIONS

1. What is the pathogen most likely to have caused the outbreak of bloody diarrhea?

2. How does this pathogen cause HUS?

3. Describe how you would have treated those affected by the pathogen.

4. How would you have managed the outbreak?

5. How would you prevent yourself from getting this disease?

A Hepatitis Outbreak Associated with Restaurant Onions

PENNSYLVANIA, 2003

The Pennsylvania Department of Health and the Centers for Disease Control and Prevention (CDC) investigated an outbreak of hepatitis among patrons of a restaurant (restaurant A) in Monaca, Pennsylvania. As of 20 November 2003, approximately 555 people infected with the liver pathogen were identified, including at least 13 restaurant A food service workers and 75 residents of six other states who dined at restaurant A. Three persons died.

Approximately 9,000 people ate food at restaurant A during the 2 to 6 weeks before the outbreak or had exposures to ill people involved in the outbreak. One hundred eighty-one people reported eating at restaurant A from 3 to 6 October. All infected restaurant A food service workers became ill after 26 October, suggesting that a food service worker could not have been the source of the outbreak. However, these ill food service workers were working in restaurant A during late October and early November, when they could have been infectious.

This form of hepatitis is characterized by a 2- to 6-week incubation period followed by nausea, vomiting, loss of appetite, fatigue, dark urine, and jaundice (yellowing of the skin and of the sclera of the eye). Those who died suffered from hemorrhagic complications.

Blood tests were used to detect the presence of antibodies to viruses that caused the disease. An indirect enzyme-linked immunosorbent assay (ELISA) was used to identify a viral pathogen. The virus was a positive-sense, single-stranded ribonucleic acid (RNA) virus with a polyhedral capsid and no envelope.

A case-control study was conducted to identify a menu item(s) or ingredient(s) associated with illness. A case patient was defined as a person who had onset of illness between 14 October and 12 November, had

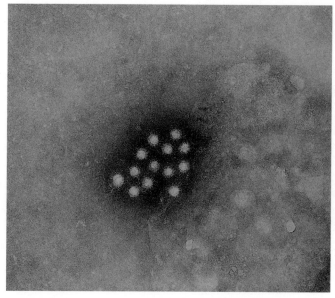

Figure 39.1 Transmission electron micrograph of the viral pathogen.

laboratory confirmation of the infection, reported eating food prepared at restaurant A between 3 and 6 October, and had eaten only once at restaurant A during the 2 to 6 weeks before the onset of illness. Controls included persons without the infection who either had dined with case patients at restaurant A or were identified through credit card receipts as having dined at restaurant A between 3 and 6 October. Enrolled case patients and controls were asked about restaurant A food that they had eaten. Of 133 menu items, only chili con queso and mild salsa were significantly associated with illness. Mild salsa was eaten by 94% of case patients compared with 39% of controls. Chili con queso was eaten by 15% of case patients compared with 3% of controls. Both menu items associated with illness contained uncooked or minimally heated fresh green onions. Among 11 case patients who reported not eating mild salsa, 7 ate at least one of the other 52 menu items that contained green onions. Eating a menu item containing green onions was reported by 98% of case patients compared with 69% of controls.

During interviews conducted at restaurant A, food service workers described green onion storage, washing, and preparation practices. Green onions were shipped in 8.5-pound boxes containing multiple small bundles (six to eight green onions per bundle). Each box was unpacked, and the bundles were stored upright (root side down) and refrigerated in a bucket with ice included in the shipment. The green onions were stored for ≤5 days before being processed, which consisted of rinsing intact onion bundles, cutting the roots off, and removing the rubber bands. Green onions from each box were chopped by machine to yield approximately 8 quarts. The chopped green onions were refrigerated for approximately 2 days. Periodically (i.e., every 1 to 3 days), salsas were prepared in batches of 40 to 80 quarts. Mild salsa included chopped fresh green onions; hot salsa did not. Salsas were refrigerated in 8-quart containers with a shelf life of 3 days. Mild and hot salsas were ladled into bowls and provided free with tortilla chips upon seating at restaurant A. Preliminary trace-back information indicated that the green onions supplied to restaurant A were grown in Mexico.

QUESTIONS

1. Identify the pathogen causing the outbreak.

2. How was the pathogen probably transmitted?

3. How would you have treated those who were ill from the pathogen?

4. How would you have contained this outbreak and prevented future outbreaks?

5. Suggest possible sources of contamination either in the field or during shipping of the green onions.

A Rotavirus Outbreak among College Students

WASHINGTON, D.C., 2000

On 31 March 2000, student health services at a university in Washington, D.C., notified the city health department that a number of students had become ill with acute gastroenteritis beginning on 29 March. Some ill students reported eating tuna or chicken salad sandwiches from dining hall A on campus.

The health department initiated an outbreak investigation. Telephone interviews were conducted with students who reported illness to student health services, with additional ill students who were identified during the interviews, and with healthy controls selected randomly from the university registry of students residing on campus. Controls and case patients whose illness onset occurred between 27 and 31 March were questioned about their food histories, residence and dining halls, sources of water, use of a public-access computer or sports equipment at the university gym, and attendance at social or athletic events.

A total of 108 students had gastrointestinal symptoms between 26 March and 11 April. The attack rate among students residing on campus was 5%, with no significant differences in attack rates by gender, occupancy of residence hall, or grade level. Among the 83 case patients for whom a complete lists of symptoms were reported, 77 (93%) had diarrhea, 75 (90%) had abdominal pain or discomfort, 69 (83%) had loss of appetite, 67 (81%) had nausea, 64 (77%) had fatigue, 56 (67%) had vomiting, 49 (59%) had headache, 48 (58%) had chills, 48 (58%) had subjective or low-grade fever, and 42 (51%) had muscle pain (myalgia). Sore throat, cough, and/or congestion were reported by six case patients with onsets on or after 2 April. The median duration of illness was 4 days.

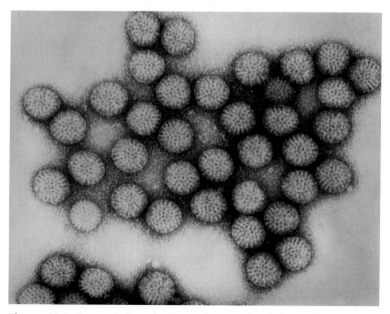

Figure 40.1 Transmission electron micrograph of the pathogen.

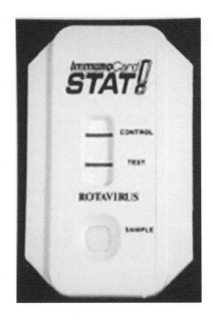

Figure 40.2 Rapid test for rotavirus.

Of those who completed the telephone interview, 40 (91%) of 44 case patients and 27 (68%) of 40 controls ate at least one delicatessen sandwich from campus dining hall A between 27 and 30 March.

Laboratory tests for bacteria, protozoa, and noroviruses (Norwalk-like viruses) were negative. Using electron microscopy, enzyme immunoassay (Fig. 40.2), and reverse transcriptase polymerase chain reactions, specimens that contained rotavirus were identified. Positive stool specimens from students and employees were identified. Two of the three positive employees were line cooks who reported having symptoms of gastroenteritis on 27 March and 2 April, respectively.

QUESTIONS

1. Besides rotavirus, list several possible causes of this outbreak and briefly describe the physical characteristics of each pathogen.

2. How could rotavirus have been transmitted in this outbreak?

3. Why is it unusual for a population of this age group to be infected with this pathogen?

4. How would you have treated those affected by the pathogen?

5. How would you have stopped this outbreak and prevented further outbreaks like this from occurring?

A Cholera Outbreak in a Refugee Camp

ZAIRE, 1994

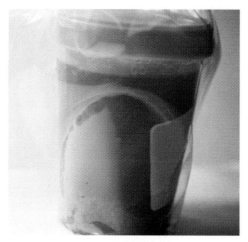

Figure 41.1 Stool sample.

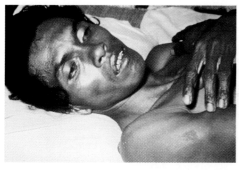

Figure 41.2 Dehydration caused by cholera.

In the spring of 1994, civil war broke out in Rwanda. In a 3-month period, 500,000 people were killed and 3.9 million were displaced as they fled the areas of fighting. In 1 week in July, 1,000,000 refugees fled to Goma, Zaire. In the days that followed, all of the trees in the town were used by refugees to build fires for warmth and cooking. The refugee camp surrounded a lake, the only source of water in the area. The land in the region consists of a thin layer of topsoil over hard volcanic rock. Most of the refugees were undernourished.

Newspaper accounts of the disaster that beset the refugees indicated that deaths due to infectious disease occurred extremely rapidly. Because it takes time to mobilize governments and resources to deal with a problem of this magnitude, the number of deaths due to disease was extremely high. The Rwandan refugee tragedy did, however, emphasize that microbes are still a major threat to human health.

19 July 1994: CARE, an international humanitarian organization, estimated that to provide adequate food to feed the people for the next month, 100 trucks carrying 40 tons each of rice, beans, and cooking oil must arrive every hour for 24 hours. The terrain and fighting made this nearly impossible. Most refugees had no shelter. The camp was dotted with makeshift tents made of plastic sheeting and blankets for those lucky enough to have carried them or found them as they fled the fighting. The chief concern of Joelle Tanguy, head of Doctors without Borders USA, was not food and shelter but infectious disease. One day, she confirmed one case of cholera in the refugee camp. The patient had profuse watery diarrhea that was milky colored (Fig. 41.1). He was extremely dehydrated (Fig. 41.2) and losing massive amounts of water. Bacteriological analysis of a stool sample indicated *Vibrio cholerae,* a gram-negative, curved, rod-shaped bacterium (Fig. 41.3).

20 July 1994: Dr. Tanguy reported the first death from cholera. An additional 120 cases were confirmed.

21 July 1994: Officially, 250 people had died from the cholera epidemic; however, several doctors reported counting 800 dead on the side of a 5-mile stretch of the road leading to Goma. After 5 miles, they decided to stop counting.

25 July 1994: One week after the first confirmed case, official counts were 14,000 people dead and 90,000 infected. Bulldozers were used to dig through the rock to make mass graves. At the grave sites, traffic jams built up as trucks waited to unload the corpses. Trucks that could carry only 40 bodies were running 24 hours a day. In the camp, refugees wore handkerchiefs, scarves, and surgical masks in the streets to try to cope with the stench of rotting bodies and stinging fumes from fires. The refugee count was estimated at 2.4 million.

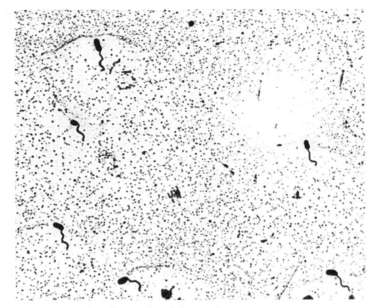

Figure 41.3 Flagellar stain of the pathogen.

The nearest airport to Goma was too small to land large aircraft. The nearest airport which could handle large aircraft had been damaged by war in Rwanda, and roads joining this airport to Goma were blocked by continued fighting.

26 July 1994: Officially, the death toll stood at 18,000; however, privately, United Nations officials estimated the death count at 50,000, with 1,800 dying each day. Bodies now lay side by side for 100 yards along the road to Goma. They were piled two and three high in rows three and four deep. United Nations Undersecretary General Peter Hansen said, "We are facing nothing short of a catastrophe." Andrew Middleton, an aid worker, was more to the point: "It's a. . . nightmare."

QUESTIONS

President Clinton ordered the U.S. military to participate in humanitarian relief for the area. If you were to advise the president, how would you answer the following questions.

1. How is this pathogen being transmitted?

2. Describe how the pathogen causes the lethal diarrhea and an appropriate treatment.

3. After an airport and a road for transportation into the area are secured, what should be the military's first priority in order to minimize deaths due to this illness? Explain why.

4. What should be the second priority? Explain why.

Amebiasis

Ten percent of all the people in the world are infected by *Entamoeba histolytica*, the causative agent of amebiasis. The highest prevalence occurs in developing countries with the lowest levels of sanitation. Only a small percentage of those infected develop clinical disease.

Cause of the disease

Entamoeba histolytica, a eukaryotic pathogen, belongs to the ameba group, since it moves using pseudopodia and obtains its nutrition by phagocytosis. *E. histolytica* is found in both trophozoite and cyst forms.

Transmission

Reservoir

Fecally contaminated food or water is the reservoir for *E. histolytica*.

Mode of transmission

The mode of transmission is via the oral-fecal route.

Pathogenesis

Entry

E. histolytica enters through the mouth after a person has ingested fecally contaminated food or drink or has touched a contaminated specimen and brought the hands into contact with the mouth.

Attachment

E. histolytica attaches to the lumen of the large intestine and invades the intestinal mucosa.

Avoiding host defenses

An acid-resistant cyst allows *E. histolytica* to evade destruction by digestive acids in the stomach.

Damage

The parasite burrows a path into the submucosa, causing an ulcer. From the large intestine, the protozoan can spread to other parts of the body. The disease may invade the liver, causing an abscess to form.

Exit

The pathogen exits through the feces.

Clinical features

Infections can cause severe dysentery or may be asymptomatic. Symptoms of the disease generally include abdominal pains, stomach cramps, and bloody diarrhea.

Diagnosis

Sample

A fecal swab, feces samples, or aspirations of intestinal lesions following endoscopy are obtained.

Test

Light microscopy of an iodine-stained feces sample shows round cysts.

Treatment

Common antiprotozoals used to treat *Entamoeba histolytica* infection include metronidazole and tinidazole for those suffering from symptoms of amebiasis.

Prevention

- The hands should be washed thoroughly after using the toilet and before handling food.
- Treating known carriers would also be expected to reduce outbreaks of the disease.

Botulism

Food-borne botulism occurs at a rate of about 1,000 cases annually worldwide. European cases are most commonly associated with contamination of home-processed meats, while Alaskan, Canadian, and Japanese outbreaks often involve preserved seafood. Chinese cases are related to home-processed bean products. Home-processed foods are responsible for most (94%) outbreaks in the continental United States.

Cause of the disease

Clostridium botulinum, a bacterial pathogen, is a gram-positive, rod-shaped bacterium commonly found in soil and sediments. It forms endospores that allow the obligate anaerobe to survive in an oxygen-rich environment. The endospores are also heat resistant, allowing the pathogen to survive during improper food processing. *Clostridium botulinum* produces a potent neurotoxin.

Transmission

Reservoir

Clostridium botulinum is commonly found in the soil and in anaerobic sediments of aquatic environments.

Mode of transmission

Botulism is caused by ingestion of food contaminated with the toxin (adult or food-borne botulism), when an infant without a completely developed intestinal flora ingests *Clostridium*-contaminated food (infant botulism), or when a wound with poor circulation is infected with botulism endospores (wound botulism).

Pathogenesis

Entry

The pathogen or toxin enters by ingestion or through wounds.

Attachment

The toxin attaches to cells at the neuromuscular junctions. The bacteria, if they are ingested, may attach to the large intestine.

Avoiding host defenses

The toxin is acid stable and survives passage through the stomach. It also avoids defenses, because it is able to cause disease at a concentration that is too low to be immunogenic. The bacteria normally cannot outcompete the flora of the large intestine for an anaerobic microenvironment. However, infants are susceptible to *Clostridium botulinum* infection, since the normal flora are incompletely developed.

Damage

The bacteria produce the botulinum toxin, which blocks neurotransmitter release at the neuromuscular junction, causing paralysis.

Exit

The disease is noncommunicable (it is not spread from person to person).

Clinical features

Symptoms usually occur within 12 to 36 hours after intoxication. Symptoms include general weakness, dizziness, double vision, trouble speaking or swallowing, difficulty breathing, weakness of other muscles, abdominal distention, and constipation. These may progress to respiratory failure, complete paralysis, and death.

Diagnosis

Botulism is diagnosed by demonstrating the presence of the toxin in the serum or feces of the patient or in the food which the patient consumed. The toxin is detected by using a mouse bioassay.

Treatment

Botulinum antitoxin injections can be helpful in preventing the condition from getting worse if given soon after symptoms begin. The antitoxin is derived from horse serum and is available through the Centers for Disease Control and Prevention. Intensive supportive treatment is required, and a respirator may be necessary. Intravenous fluids and nutrition may be necessary during hospitalization because of difficulty swallowing.

Prevention

- Infant botulism is often associated with children under 1 year old eating unpasteurized honey. Avoiding feeding raw honey to infants can reduce the risk of botulism.

- Most outbreaks of food-borne botulism result from spores contaminating improperly prepared home-canned vegetables, sausages, meats, and seafood products. The endospores can only be killed through a sterilization process. Pressure cooking of home-canned foods for an appropriate time and at appropriate temperature and pressure effectively kills the endospores. Improper canning provides an ideal anaerobic environment loaded with nutrients in which the spores can germinate and the bacteria can produce toxin. If a can is bulging, or the contents have a peculiar color, odor, or cotton-like mold growth, the food should not be eaten.

- Jams and jellies have a high sugar concentration and thus plasmolyze (remove water through osmosis) *Clostridium botulinum*.

- Properly pickled foods have an acidic pH, which inhibits endospore germination.

- Wound botulism is prevented by prompt disinfection, treatment, and care of puncture wounds and deep lacerations.

- Heating food for 30 minutes at 80°C destroys the toxin.

Campylobacteriosis

Campylobacteriosis is the most commonly identified food-borne bacterial infection in the world. An estimated 2 million cases of *Campylobacter* enteritis occur in the United States annually, accounting for 5 to 7% of cases of gastroenteritis. A large animal reservoir is present, with up to 100% of poultry, including chickens, turkeys, and waterfowl, having asymptomatic infections in their intestinal tracts.

Cause of the disease

Campylobacter jejuni, a bacterial pathogen, is a microaerophilic, gram-negative, slender, curved rod with monopolar or bipolar flagella.

Transmission

Reservoir

C. jejuni is found in the GI tracts of cattle, sheep, and birds, especially poultry.

Mode of transmission

The pathogen is primarily acquired from fecally contaminated water, unpasteurized milk, or undercooked poultry and meats.

Pathogenesis

Entry

Ingestion of bacteria introduces the pathogen into the GI tract.

Attachment

The pathogen attaches to the jejunum, ileum, or colon, where it replicates.

Avoiding host defenses

The pathogen initially infects only epithelial tissue and avoids circulating antibodies and cells of the immune system.

Damage

Localized destruction of intestinal mucosa and tissue caused by endotoxin release causes an inflammatory response. Tissue destruction and fluid loss from inflammation cause diarrhea.

Clinical features

Infection can be asymptomatic or cause serious bloody diarrhea with ulcerations of the intestinal mucosa. The most common clinical symptoms of *Campylobacter* infection include diarrhea, malaise, headache, fever, nausea or vomiting, and abdominal pain. Clinical features usually last less than 10 days.

Diagnosis

Specimen

A fecal swab or feces sample is obtained.

Test

Transparent colonies grow on blood agar at 42°C in a microaerophilic environment. Colonies are catalase positive and oxidase positive and produce H_2S.

Treatment

Patients should drink plenty of fluids as long as the diarrhea lasts. In severe cases, antibiotics, such as erythromycin, are typically given.

Prevention

- Cook all poultry products thoroughly.
- Wash hands with soap before and after handling raw foods of animal origin.
- Avoid cross-contamination of utensils and food preparation areas.
- Wash hands with soap after having contact with pet feces.
- Avoid consuming unpasteurized milk and untreated surface water.
- Make sure that persons with diarrhea, especially children, wash their hands carefully and frequently with soap to reduce the risk of spreading the infection.
- *Campylobacter* can spread through a chicken flock via their drinking water. Providing clean, chlorinated water sources for the chickens might prevent *Campylobacter* infections in poultry flocks and thereby decrease the amount of contaminated meat reaching the marketplace.

Cholera

Epidemics of cholera occur after natural disasters and wars that leave large numbers of people without adequate water and sewage treatment.

Cause of the disease

Vibrio cholerae, a bacterial pathogen, is a comma-shaped, gram-negative bacterium that is motile by a unipolar flagellum. The pathogen is facultatively anaerobic (it can grow with or without oxygen) and can be a free-living inhabitant of fresh water.

Transmission

Reservoir

Fecally contaminated water and shellfish grown in fecally polluted waters are reservoirs of the pathogen.

Mode of transmission

The pathogen is transmitted via the oral-fecal route from contaminated food, such as shellfish, or water. *V. cholerae* is not usually transmitted person to person.

Pathogenesis

Entry

Since the pathogen is acid sensitive, infection requires the ingestion of large numbers of *V. cholerae* bacteria.

Attachment

The pathogen attaches to the epithelium of the large intestine.

Avoiding host defenses

Infection is restricted to the surface epithelium, so the pathogen is not initially exposed to circulating antibodies or cells of the immune system.

Damage

V. cholerae releases cholera toxin, which activates an enzyme of the intestinal mucosa. Enzyme activation leads to a series of metabolic changes that cause the ion pumps in the large intestine to reverse the osmolarity gradient. As a result, water is not absorbed by the large intestine but is actively secreted, causing massive diarrhea.

Exit

The pathogen exits through the feces.

Clinical features

A 2- to 5-day incubation period is followed by the abrupt onset of vomiting and profuse watery diarrhea with flecks of mucus. The stools quickly lose solid material. The liquid is white and opalescent and is known as rice water stool.

Cholera victims can lose up to 20 liters of fluid a day. The serious dehydration leads to hypotension, an increased pulse rate, an increased respiratory rate, sunken eyes and cheeks, etc.

Hypovolemic shock (a life-threatening drop in blood pressure due to low blood volume) and metabolic acidosis can cause death within a few hours of onset, especially in children. In untreated cases, mortality is as high as 60%.

Diagnosis

Clinical signs and symptoms are used to diagnose cholera. Organisms can be identified by dark-field microscopy showing large numbers of comma-shaped organisms.

Treatment

Treatment consists of rapid replacement of fluids and electrolytes using oral or intravenous rehydration solution.

Antimicrobial agents reduce the volume of cholera stool purged by half and shorten the duration of symptoms. Common antibiotics include doxycycline and trimethoprim-sulfamethoxazole.

Prevention

- There is a vaccine available, but it offers brief and incomplete immunity.
- If water treatment or sewage treatment facilities are damaged by natural or man-made disasters, people

should drink boiled or treated water, cook food thoroughly, avoid undercooked or raw fish, and eat cooked vegetables.

Cryptosporidiosis

Cryptosporidium parvum causes a self-limited diarrheal illness in healthy individuals, mostly children. Only recently has cryptosporidiosis been recognized as a cause of self-limited diarrhea in persons with a normal immune system and severe prolonged diarrhea in patients with acquired immune deficiency syndrome (AIDS).

Cause of the disease

C. parvum, a eukaryotic protozoal pathogen, has a complex life cycle that includes the formation of sporozoa and thick-walled oocysts that are acid-fast during staining.

Transmission

Reservoir

The pathogen can be carried by humans and a wide range of animals, including cattle, cats, deer, and horses.

Mode of transmission

The pathogen is spread by the oral-fecal route through contaminated drinking water, recreational water, or food that has been contaminated.

Pathogenesis

Entry

Ingestion of approximately 100 infected oocysts in fecally contaminated material is sufficient for infection.

Attachment

The pathogen attaches to the epithelial cells of intestinal villi.

Avoiding host defenses

Oocysts have an acid-resistant capsule that allows them to pass through the low pH of the stomach without damage and to proceed into the intestines. The cysts develop into sporozoites, which attach to the intestinal epithelium.

Damage

After ingestion of oocysts, asexual release of sporozoites is initiated. Sporozoites attach to and penetrate the intestinal mucosa, where they mature into other forms of the parasite and rupture the infected cells. Damaged tissue and inflammation prevent water absorption, causing diarrhea.

Exit

Infective thick-walled oocysts are excreted through feces.

Clinical features

Symptoms may last about 1 to 3 weeks and appear 2 to 10 days after the initial infection. They include loose, watery diarrhea; stomach cramps; and slight fever. In immunocompromised patients, *Cryptosporidium* infection leads to chronic watery diarrhea with severe cramps, weight loss, a low-grade fever, and severe dehydration.

Diagnosis

Sample

A fecal sample is taken.

Tests

Modified acid-fast staining and detection of acid-fast oocysts by microscopic examination of a stool specimen are performed.

Treatment

Those with a healthy immune system will recover in 1 to 3 weeks without treatment. Oral fluids and electrolytes help to prevent dehydration from diarrhea.

In immunocompromised patients, such as AIDS patients, nitrazoxanide or paromomycin is often used to inhibit growth of the pathogen. Although paromomycin inhibits eukaryotic protein synthesis, it is not absorbed by the GI tract, so oral administration preferentially inhibits *Cryptosporidium* in the GI tract.

Prevention

- Practice good hygiene.
- Wash hands thoroughly with soap and water (after using the toilet, changing diapers, handling animals, or cleaning up feces; before eating or preparing food; and after handling anything contaminated with fecal matter).
- Avoid drinking untreated water from lakes, streams, pools, hot tubs, or other water sources. Thick-walled oocysts can survive extreme environments, including high levels of chlorination.
- Rinse and peel fruits or vegetables to be eaten raw to prevent ingestion of food that may be contaminated with feces.
- Drink bottled water without ice when traveling to places with poor sanitation.
- Boil contaminated water for at least 10 minutes or filter the water to remove any bacterial, protozoan, or viral pathogens.

Enterohemorrhagic *Escherichia coli*

Even though *E. coli* is a normal resident of the large intestine, where the bacterium does not cause disease, some strains are among the most frequent causes of some of the many common bacterial infections, including urinary tract infections and diarrhea, and other clinical infections, such as neonatal meningitis and pneumonia. The urinary tract is the most common site of infection by *E. coli*, which accounts for more than 90% of all uncomplicated urinary tract infections. The O157:H7 and O111 variants of *E. coli* are enterohemorragic and cause bloody diarrhea that can be complicated by hemolytic-uremic syndrome.

Cause of the disease

E. coli O157:H7 or O111 is a gram-negative bacterial pathogen. *E. coli* is part of the normal flora of all healthy individuals. However, mutant strains like *E. coli* O157:H7, which carries the H7 antigen on its flagella and the O157 antigen on the O oligosaccharide of the lipopolysaccharide of the outer membrane, cause hemorrhagic diarrhea.

Like nonpathogenic *E. coli*, the pathogen is a facultative anaerobe with peritrichous flagella and ferments lactose. However, the O157:H7 variant does not ferment sorbitol, as does the usual nonpathogenic strain.

Transmission

Reservoir

Cattle can carry *E. coli* O157:H7 in their intestines and appear healthy.

Mode of transmission

Transmission is via the oral-fecal route through ingestion of contaminated meat. Also, anything contaminated with cow feces, including unpasteurized cider, and petting zoos in fairs can be sources of infection.

Pathogenesis

Entry

During the slaughter of cattle, the bacteria can be mixed into the meat. Eating inadequately cooked beef can transmit *E. coli* O157:H7. It can also be found on cow's udders and can be transmitted by drinking unpasteurized milk.

Attachment

The pathogen adheres to mucous surfaces in the gut via fimbriae.

Avoiding host defenses

Initial infection is restricted to the epithelium of the intestine, so the pathogen is not initially exposed to circulating antibodies and cells of the immune system.

Damage

The pathogen produces Shiga-like toxins, which cause cell death along the intestinal mucosa, and an endotoxin, which leads indirectly to capillary damage. Vascular damage in the colon by the Shiga-like toxins allows inflammatory mediators into the circulation. The mediators then initiate HUS.

Exit

The pathogen exits in the feces.

Clinical features

Clinical features include severe bloody diarrhea, abdominal cramps, and potentially HUS, a serious complication in which red blood cells are destroyed and the kidneys fail. HUS has a 50% mortality rate in children under 5 years of age.

Diagnosis

Specimen

A fecal swab or stool sample is obtained.

Tests

Diagnostic tests are isolation of *E. coli* that does not ferment sorbitol on sorbitol MacConkey agar and detection of O157 and H7 antigens by an ELISA.

Treatment

Most people recover in 5 to 10 days without any antibiotic or other treatment. For serious infections, antibiotics are given after testing for antibiotic-resistant properties of the pathogen. HUS is treated with blood transfusions and kidney dialysis.

Antidiarrheal agents may make the symptoms worse, because preventing bowel movements allows the pathogen to grow to high concentrations within the GI tract, potentially causing more damage and increasing the risk of serious complications.

Prevention

- Cook all meat thoroughly.
- Consume only pasteurized milk and juices.
- Wash hands carefully and frequently to reduce risk.

Giardiasis

Giardia infects infants in the developing world early in life and has peak prevalence rates of 15 to 20%. In the United States, *Giardia* is primarily found among children in day care centers, in institutions, and on Native American reservations.

Cause of the disease

Giardiasis is caused by *Giardia intestinalis* (also known as *Giardia lamblia*), a eukaryotic protozoan pathogen that uses flagella for motility (flagellate).

Transmission

Reservoir

During the past 2 decades, *Giardia* infection has become recognized as one of the most common causes of waterborne disease (it is found in both drinking and recreational water) in humans in the United States. The pathogen lives in the intestines of both humans and other animals and survives in the environment for long periods as a cyst.

Mode of transmission

Transmission is via the oral-fecal route. The organism is often ingested by accidentally swallowing fecally contaminated recreational water or eating uncooked food. It can also be spread through fomites, such as diaper-changing tables or toys contaminated with feces from an infected person.

Pathogenesis

Entry

The route of entry is the oral-fecal route. The cyst is found in fecally contaminated soil, food, or water or on surfaces.

Attachment

The motile trophozoite stage of the pathogen attaches firmly to the epithelial tissue of the duodenum using its adhesive disk.

Avoiding host defenses

Infection by trophozoites is limited to the epithelial surface, so they initially avoid circulating antibodies and cells of the immune system. The cysts that are produced have a thick protective wall that resists bile and digestive enzymes.

Damage

The pathogen damages the villi of the intestinal tract, causing malabsorption of nutrients and diarrhea.

Exit

Cysts are excreted with the feces.

Clinical features

Infection can be asymptomatic or cause diarrhea; gas, or flatulence; greasy and foul-smelling stools that tend to float; stomach cramps; and nausea. Symptoms of giardiasis normally begin 1 week after infection and may last 2 to 6 weeks.

Diagnosis

Sample
A stool sample is obtained.

Test
Light microscopy is used to find oval cysts in feces.

Treatment
Fluid and electrolyte replacement prevents dehydration. Otherwise-healthy adults are often treated with metronidazole. Metronidazole is activated to cause DNA damage leading to cell death by a protozoan-specific pathway and in the reducing environment caused by the *Giardia* infection.

Prevention
- Wash hands with soap and water after using the toilet or changing diapers and before eating or preparing food.
- If a person has had an infection with *Giardia* recently, he or she should not swim in recreational water (pools, hot tubs, lakes or rivers, the ocean, etc.), since *Giardia* can be shed for at least 2 weeks after diarrhea stops. The pathogen can be passed on while swimming and can contaminate water for several weeks, resulting in outbreaks of *Giardia* infection among recreational water users.
- Avoid fecal exposure during sexual activity.
- Do not swallow recreational water.
- Do not drink untreated water from shallow wells, lakes, rivers, springs, ponds, and streams.
- Do not use untreated ice or drinking water when traveling in countries where the water supply might be unsafe.

Hepatitis A Virus Infections
Hepatitis A virus (HAV) has a worldwide distribution. The areas with the highest fraction of the population infected with HAV include urban Africa, Asia, and South America, where evidence of past infection is nearly universal among the people living there. Acquisition in early childhood is the norm in these regions and is usually asymptomatic. Factors predisposing humans to early acquisition include overcrowded conditions, poor sanitation, and lack of a reliable and clean water resource.

In the United States, persons aged 5 to 14 years are most likely to acquire acute HAV infection. Over the last 40 years, the average age of infected persons has steadily increased as a result of improved sanitation and hygiene measures. Currently, high-risk populations account for most cases, including contacts of recently infected individuals, foreign travelers (particularly those traveling to developing nations), male homosexuals, child care workers, institutionalized individuals, and those living in poverty.

Food handlers at the point of preparation are an infrequent source of outbreaks in the United States, although cases have been documented. Virtually any food can be contaminated with HAV.

Cause of the disease
HAV is a very small nonenveloped virus with a polyhedral capsid and single-stranded RNA for genetic information.

Transmission

Reservoir
Infected humans are the reservoir for HAV.

Mode of transmission
HAV is transmitted via the oral-fecal route through contaminated food, water, or fomites.

Pathogenesis

Entry
The pathogen is ingested with fecally contaminated food or water.

Attachment
The virus attaches to cells of the intestinal epithelium; replication damages the tissue, allowing entry into the blood and spread to the liver.

Avoiding host defenses
The virus is an intracellular pathogen that initially avoids circulating antibodies and immune system cells.

Damage
HAV probably enters the bloodstream after intestinal infection and then infects liver cells. Liver damage is probably caused indirectly by cellular immune responses to the infection and includes necrosis (tissue death) and inflammation of liver tissues. The damage decreases the liver's ability to process bilirubin, a breakdown product of hemoglobin from damaged red blood cells. As a result, bilirubin accumulates in the blood, causing jaundice.

Exit
The pathogen exits in the feces.

Clinical features

The incubation stage is anywhere from 15 to 40 days. For symptomatic infections, hepatitis A symptoms include fever, anorexia or unwillingness to eat, nausea, vomiting, jaundice, dark-yellow urine, and light-colored stools.

Diagnosis

Specimen

A blood sample is taken.

Tests

Indirect ELISA is used to look for a rising concentration of anti-HAV antibodies, or PCR analysis of serum, food, or environmental samples is performed.

Treatment

Most people infected with HAV recover without intervention after a few weeks. Recovery is aided by plenty of bed rest. In some cases, immunoglobulin can be administered.

Prevention

- The hepatitis A vaccine is effective in preventing the contraction of hepatitis A.

- Since the pathogen is spread from fecally contaminated material, proper sanitation and hygiene are most important to prevent the spread of HAV. Thoroughly washing the hands after using the toilet or preparing food is important.

- When traveling to countries where water sanitation may not be adequate, drink water only if it is treated or boiled, and eat only hot cooked foods or fruits that you peel yourself.

Listeriosis

Listeriosis is a rare food-borne disease, with approximately 2,000 cases reported per year in the United States. Even though it is rare, it is of significant concern to women who are pregnant. The pathogen can infect the developing fetus, causing neonatal listeriosis, a disease with a 20 to 30% mortality rate.

Cause of the disease

Listeria monocytogenes, a bacterial pathogen, is a gram-positive, pleomorphic (variably shaped) bacillus. It uses a flagellum for locomotion.

Transmission

The bacterium is very resistant to common food preservation agents, such as heat, salt, nitrite, and acids. It survives on cold surfaces and can also multiply at refrigerator temperatures.

Reservoir

The pathogen can contaminate foods of animal origin, such as meats and dairy products, and can contaminate raw foods during processing.

Mode of transmission

Horizontal: Transmission can occur through eating fecally contaminated food.

Vertical: The pathogen can cross the maternal-placental barrier and infect the fetus.

Pathogenesis

Entry

Consumption of contaminated food is the route of entry.

Attachment

The pathogen is engulfed by monocytes, macrophages, or polymorphonuclear leukocytes.

Avoiding host defenses

The pathogen can survive and multiply in leukocytes. A toxin that it produces ruptures the phagocytic vacuole and the lysosomal membranes, releasing the bacteria to multiply inside the leukocyte.

Damage

Infected leukocytes seed the pathogen in the liver, spleen, and lungs. When pregnant women are infected, the pathogen localizes in the central nervous system of the fetus. The pathogen produces several toxins that cause damage, including beta-hemolysin, which lyses erythrocytes, and an endotoxin-like cell wall component that can damage tissues.

Clinical features

Infection produces flu-like symptoms, such as fever, chills, and upset stomach, and gastrointestinal symptoms, such as nausea, vomiting, and diarrhea. If the pathogen crosses the blood-brain barrier, it may cause meningitis symptoms—headache, stiff neck, confusion, loss of balance, and convulsions.

Infected pregnant women may experience only a mild, flu-like illness; however, infection during pregnancy can lead to premature delivery, infection of the newborn, or stillbirth. In infections during pregnancy, the mother usually survives while the child has a mortality rate of 80%.

Diagnosis

Specimen

Blood, cerebrospinal fluid, amniotic fluid, or placenta is used as a specimen.

Test

L. monocytogenes forms small beta-hemolytic colonies on blood agar. The pathogen can also grow at 4°C, is catalase positive (dissociates H_2O_2), and does not hydrolyze hippurate.

Treatment

When infection occurs during pregnancy, antibiotics given promptly to the pregnant woman can often prevent infection of the fetus or newborn. Penicillin, ampicillin, garamycin, and sulfamethoxazole-trimethoprim have all been used successfully for listeriosis treatment.

Prevention

- Wash hands frequently and thoroughly with hot soapy water.
- Avoid cross-contamination of ready-to-eat foods and preparation areas with raw meat, poultry, and seafood.
- Cook food at safe temperatures, and reheat lunch meats, cold cuts, and other delicatessen-style meats until they are steaming hot.
- Refrigerate or freeze perishables, including ready-to-eat foods, within 2 hours.
- Pregnant women should avoid soft cheeses, like feta and Brie.
- Do not use unpasteurized dairy products.

Salmonellosis

Salmonellosis is one of the most common bacterial infections in the United States. It is estimated that more than 2 million cases occur each year. The incidence of *Salmonella* infection is greatest among children, with outbreaks also common among individuals who are institutionalized and residents of nursing homes. Nations with an adequate public health infrastructure report frequencies of gastroenteritis similar to those in the United States. Gastroenteritis is far more common in areas where sanitation is inadequate.

Cause of the disease

Salmonellosis is caused by *Salmonella*, a bacterial pathogen. The genus *Salmonella* is divided into more than 2,000 serotypes on the basis of differences in cell wall and flagellar antigens. These serotypes are divided into several different serovars (different strains within a serovar grouping), including *Salmonella enterica* serovar Typhi (which causes typhoid fever) and *S. enterica* serovar Enteritidis (a diverse group of bacteria with over 2,000 serotypes that cause diarrhea).

The pathogen is a gram-negative, facultatively anaerobic bacillus. It produces H_2S from the metabolism of proteins and is motile, using peritrichous flagella.

Transmission

Reservoir

The GI tracts of humans and other animals are reservoirs of the pathogen.

Mode of transmission

Transmission is via the oral-fecal route, i.e., eating contaminated food.

Pathogenesis

Entry

The pathogen's route of entry is via ingestion of fecally contaminated food, often undercooked beef, poultry, eggs, or dairy products, or contact with pet reptiles.

Attachment

The pathogen attaches to the mucosal epithelium of the small intestine.

Avoiding host defenses

Initially, the infection is restricted to the epithelial tissue, so the pathogen is not exposed to circulating antibodies or cells of the immune system. When *Salmonella* cells bind to the intestinal epithelium, they signal the host cell membrane to engulf the bacteria.

Damage

Salmonella disrupts the epithelial tissue and invades the lamina propria of the small intestine, where it causes an inflammatory response, resulting in fluid loss and causing diarrhea.

Exit

The pathogen exits through feces.

Clinical features

The disease has an incubation period of 18 to 24 hours, followed by diarrhea, abdominal cramps, and fever.

Diagnosis

Specimen

A feces sample from an infected person serves as a specimen.

Tests

Cultural: The test is growth on selective agar, such as salmonella-shigella agar. *Salmonella* turns the agar black as a result of H_2S production.

Noncultural: Widal agglutination testing identifies O and H antigens.

Treatment

Many cases are self-resolving and last only 5 to 7 days with no extensive treatment needed. In cases of severe dehydration (especially in infants and the elderly), fluid and electrolyte replacement may be necessary.

Antibiotics are given if the disease spreads from the intestinal tract, resulting in a systemic infection. Typical antibiotics include amoxicillin and trimethoprim-sulfamethoxazole.

Prevention

- Public water and sewage treatment prevents infection.
- Thoroughly wash produce, meat, and poultry. Completely cook beef, poultry, and eggs before eating them.
- Wash hands before and after handling food and after using the restroom.
- Avoid cross-contamination of clean food and utensils with raw meats.
- Do not drink unpasteurized milk.
- Children, especially under 1 year of age, should avoid contact with pet reptiles.

Shigellosis

Approximately 20,000 to 30,000 cases of shigellosis are reported annually in the United States. Shigellosis occurs worldwide, most frequently in areas with unhygienic living conditions or in overcrowded areas with poor sanitation. It is also commonly found wherever war or natural disasters disrupt the public health infrastructure. Bacteremia occurs primarily in malnourished children and carries a mortality rate of 20% as a result of renal failure, hemolysis, thrombocytopenia, gastrointestinal hemorrhage, and shock. Hemolytic-uremic syndrome may complicate infections with *Shigella* species (spp.) and *Escherichia coli*, and this complication carries a mortality rate higher than 50%.

Cause of the disease

Shigella spp. include *Shigella dysenteriae* (which causes the most severe form of shigellosis) and *Shigella sonnei* (the most common species causing shigellosis in the United States).

Shigella is a slender gram-negative, rod-shaped bacterial pathogen. It is facultatively anaerobic and produces H_2S from protein metabolism.

Transmission

Reservoir

The GI tract of humans is the reservoir of *Shigella*.

Mode of transmission

Infection occurs via person-to-person transmission by the oral-fecal route or from contaminated fomites and/or contaminated food.

Pathogenesis

Entry

The pathogen is most commonly transmitted from fecally contaminated water and by unsanitary handling of food by food handlers. A small inoculum (10 to 200 organisms) is sufficient to cause infection.

Attachment

The bacteria attach to and penetrate the epithelial cells of the intestinal mucosa.

Avoiding host defenses

The bacteria infect epithelial cells and are not initially exposed to circulating antibodies or cells of the immune system.

Damage

After invasion, the bacteria multiply intracellularly. With this multiplication come local inflammation, fluid loss, and epithelial cell dysfunction, which result in tissue destruction. The pathogen can also release an exotoxin that causes local tissue destruction.

Exit

The pathogen exits in the feces.

Clinical features

The illness usually begins 1 to 4 days after the bacteria are swallowed and can last up to 7 days. Symptoms include watery or bloody diarrhea and an acute fever resulting from local inflammation associated with tissue destruction; acute abdominal cramps and/or pains caused by tissue destruction; nausea or vomiting; and blood, mucus, or pus in the stools from the infected tissue.

Shigellosis can have serious complications, including severe dehydration due to excess fluid loss as a result of diarrhea, convulsions in young children, mucosal ulcerations, rectal bleeding, and hemolytic-uremic syndrome that results from damage to the kidneys by exotoxin release.

Diagnosis

Specimen

A fecal sample is obtained.

Test

A test for growth on Hektoen enteric agar is performed. *Shigella* colonies appear green without a black center, because they do not produce H_2S like *Salmonella*.

Treatment

Patients with mild symptoms tend to recover on their own. For more serious cases, a physician may prescribe an antibiotic to speed up the recovery process. Antibiotics are usually chosen after the pathogen is screened for antibiotic resistance. Treatment with a drug that *Shigella* is resistant to kills only normal flora, allowing *Shigella* to utilize the nutrients and microenvironments previously occupied by the normal flora and leading to a more serious *Shigella* infection. Properly chosen antibiotics will help kill the bacteria and shorten the duration of the illness.

In order to prevent dehydration, the patient should drink plenty of liquids to replace those lost from diarrhea and vomiting.

The use of antidiarrheal agents can make the illness worse.

Prevention

- There is no vaccine to prevent shigellosis.
- Proper sanitation and hygiene are most important to prevent the spread of *Shigella*. Thoroughly washing the hands after using the toilet or preparing food is important.
- When traveling to other countries where water sanitation may not be adequate, drink only treated or boiled water and eat only hot cooked foods or fruits that you have peeled yourself.

Typhoid Fever

An estimated 12 million to 33 million cases of typhoid fever occur globally each year. The disease is always present (endemic) in many developing countries of the Indian subcontinent, South and Central America, and Africa. Outbreaks of typhoid fever have also occurred amid the recent social upheaval in Eastern Europe.

Cause of the disease

Salmonella enterica serovar Typhi, a bacterial pathogen, is a facultatively anaerobic, gram-negative rod with O antigens 9 and 12. The pathogen is mobile with peritrichous flagella and has a polysaccharide capsule.

Transmission

Reservoir

Salmonella enterica serovar Typhi is a human-only pathogen that can be found contaminating a number of foods exposed to human fecal material: shellfish taken from beds contaminated with fecal waste; vegetables fertilized with fecal material or watered with sewage-containing H_2O; and fecally contaminated food, water, or milk.

Mode of transmission

Infection is by the oral-fecal route of transmission or from person to person.

Some persons can be asymptomatic carriers for months to years, providing a continuous source from which others can be infected (about 3% of untreated individuals will become chronic carriers, because the pathogen survives in the gall bladder).

Pathogenesis

Entry

The route of entry is ingestion of bacteria from shellfish grown in water contaminated with human feces or of water, milk, or other food.

Attachment

The pathogen attaches to the surface of the mucosa of the small intestine.

Avoiding host defenses

The Vi antigen, a protein on the surface of *Salmonella*, blocks binding of certain classes of antibodies. *Salmonella enterica* serovar Typhi is also highly resistant to bile. The pathogen is phagocytized by macrophages; however, it is not destroyed but multiplies in the protected intracellular environment.

Damage

On secondary entry into the intestine after replicating in the lymphoid tissue, the large number of bacteria causes necrosis of the Peyer's patches, which may lead to abscess formation or septicemia.

Exit

The pathogen is excreted in the feces.

Clinical features

There are two broad features of the disease: gastroenteritis and fever.

Symptoms include diarrhea in children and either constipation or diarrhea in adults and high fever, muscle aches (myalgia), weakness, stomach pains, headache, loss of appetite, flu-like symptoms, and cough. In 30% of cases, a rash of flat rose-colored spots that blanch with applied pressure is experienced on the trunk.

Diagnosis

Specimen
Blood or feces are used as a specimen.

Tests
Testing for growth of black-centered colonies on salmonella-shigella agar or agglutination testing to identify O and H antigens is performed.

Treatment
The drug inhibits DNA replication by inhibition of DNA gyrase. Ampicillin can be used to eliminate the postinfective carrier state. For severe cases of typhoid fever, chloramphenicol is used. It is used only in severe cases because it has rare but very serious side effects.

In addition to antibacterial agents, fluids and electrolytes should be used to replace those lost through diarrhea.

With proper treatment, patients with typhoid fever usually recover within 2 to 4 weeks, although relapses may occur if the treatment has not fully eradicated the infection.

Prevention
- There is an oral vaccine for patients 2 years of age and older.
- Wash hands properly and frequently.
- In areas where typhoid fever is common, drink only boiled or bottled water.
- Eat thoroughly cooked food that is served hot.
- Avoid unwashed fruit.

Viral Gastroenteritis
Rotavirus is the most common cause of severe diarrhea among children, resulting in the hospitalization of approximately 55,000 children each year in the United States and the death of over 600,000 children annually worldwide. Another common cause of gastroenteritis is a group of viruses known as noroviruses. The CDC estimates that 23 million cases of acute gastroenteritis are due to norovirus infection, and it is now thought that at least 50% of all food-borne outbreaks of gastroenteritis can be attributed to noroviruses. Among the 232 outbreaks of norovirus illness reported to the CDC from July 1997 to June 2000, 57% were food borne, 16% were due to person-to-person spread, and 3% were waterborne; in 23% of the outbreaks, the cause of transmission was not determined. In the study, common settings for outbreaks included restaurants and catered meals (36%), nursing homes (23%), schools (13%), and vacation settings or cruise ships (10%).

Cause of the disease
Several viral pathogens cause acute gastroenteritis in humans. Common pathogens include rotavirus and noroviruses.

Rotavirus has a unique wheel-like appearance (hence its name). It is a nonenveloped virus with an icosohedral capsid (20 sides to its polyhedral shape) and has 11 segments of double-stranded RNA.

Noroviruses are a group of small, polyhedral, nonenveloped viruses using single-stranded RNA as genetic information.

Transmission

Reservoir
Infected humans are the reservoir for noroviruses.

Mode of transmission
Transmission occurs via the oral-fecal route or through contaminated fomites.

Pathogenesis

Entry
The viral pathogen is ingested with contaminated food or water or through contact with contaminated surfaces.

Attachment
One of the outer capsid proteins binds to receptors on the surface of the epithelium of the small intestine.

Avoiding host defenses
The viruses are acid resistant, allowing them to survive the acidity of the stomach. They are also intracellular pathogens that infect the epithelial layer, allowing the initial infection to avoid circulating antibodies or cells of the immune system.

Damage
Damage is direct as a result of the lytic cycle of the virus destroying infected cells. The tissue damage also induces an inflammatory response. Diarrhea is caused by the tissue damage inhibiting the ability of the villi to absorb fluids and by the fluid released due to the inflammation.

Exit
The viral pathogen exits in the feces.

Clinical features
The disease is often called the "stomach flu," although it is not caused by any of the influenza viruses. The

main symptoms of viral gastroenteritis are watery diarrhea and vomiting. Infants infected with rotavirus often experience projectile vomiting. The affected person may also have headache, fever, and abdominal cramps (stomach ache). In general, the symptoms begin 1 to 2 days following infection with a virus that causes gastroenteritis and may last for 1 to 10 days, depending on which virus causes the illness.

Diagnosis

Specimen

A stool sample is obtained.

Tests

Viral gastroenteritis caused by rotavirus can be diagnosed by rapid antigen detection. Noroviruses are diagnosed by a reverse transcriptase polymerase chain reaction.

Treatment

Normally, the disease is self-limiting, requiring only oral rehydration therapy to prevent dehydration. However, about 1 in 40 children with rotavirus gastroenteritis requires hospitalization for intravenous fluids. The CDC recommends that families with infants and young children keep a supply of oral rehydration solution (ORS) at home at all times and use the solution when diarrhea first occurs in the child. ORS is available at pharmacies without a prescription. Parents should follow the written directions on the ORS package and use clean or boiled water.

Prevention

- An effective vaccine was approved for rotavirus in 1998. However, it is no longer recommended for infants in the United States because of data that indicated a strong association between the vaccine and intussusceptions (bowel obstructions) among some infants during the first 1 to 2 weeks following vaccination.

- Wash hands with soap and water after using the toilet or changing diapers and before eating or preparing food.

Outbreaks of Sexually Transmitted Diseases

AIDS was . . . an illness in stages, a very long flight of steps that led assuredly to death, but whose every step represented a unique apprenticeship. It was a disease that gave death time to live and its victims time to die, time to discover time, and in the end to discover life.

HERVÉ GUIBERT, *To the Friend Who Did Not Save My Life* (1991)

Pathogens that cause sexually transmitted diseases (STDs) are sensitive to temperature changes and drying. Consequently, the pathogens require direct intimate contact for successful transmission. Although sexually transmitted pathogens are not as easily spread as respiratory pathogens, STDs are still widespread and common.

The genitourinary tract has a number of significant defenses to prevent the attachment and growth of microbial pathogens. Physical defenses include urination and vaginal secretions; pathogens that do not attach to host tissues are simply washed away before causing disease. A mucus coating lines much of the genitourinary tract, inhibiting the attachment of pathogens to host cell receptors. Chemical defenses also inhibit pathogen growth. Urine tends to have an acidic pH, which is not optimum for the growth of many bacteria. In the vagina, organisms in the normal flora, like *Lactobacillus*, break down glycogen to glucose and ferment the glucose to lactic acid. This drops the pH to approximately 5, which inhibits the growth of the pathogenic form of *Candida albicans*, the pathogen responsible for vaginal yeast infections.

Microbial pathogens bypass these defenses in several ways. *Escherichia coli*, the most common pathogen causing urinary tract infections, has flagella that allow it to swim up the urethra into the bladder, where it can lodge and lead to infection. *Neisseria gonorrhoeae* has adhesins on its pili that attach to the urogenital epithelium. This prevents the pathogen from being washed away. Other pathogens, such as *Haemophilus ducreyi* and *Treponema pallidum*, take advantage of microscopic breaks in the mucosa or skin surface to bypass normal defenses.

College students are among the highest-risk groups for sexually transmitted diseases. For example, in a 3-year study of college age females, 43% became infected with human papillomavirus (HPV). The majority of these infections were by serotypes of HPV associated with a high risk for developing cervical cancer. Among all sexually active women, greater than 50% were infected, 15% had active infections, and 1% had genital warts.

This chapter emphasizes the widespread and cross-cultural nature of STDs and the difficulties of prevention. In theory, the prevention of STDs appears simple. However, determining effective strategies for changing sexual behavior and the politics of providing treatment and prevention resources make the real world of STD management both challenging and interesting.

Table IV.1 Selected outbreak-causing sexually transmitted pathogens

Organism	Key physical properties	Disease characteristics
Bacteria		
Chlamydia trachomatis	Obligate intracellular pathogen; very small	Nongonococcal urethritis, lymphogranuloma venereum, PID
Haemophilus ducreyi	Fastidious pleiomorphic gram-negative bacillus	Chancroid (genital ulcers)
Neisseria gonorrhoeae	Gram-negative intracellular diplococcus	Gonorrhea, PID
Treponema pallidum	Gram-negative spirochete	Primary syphilis (chancre), secondary syphilis (rash and systemic symptoms), tertiary syphilis (neurological, cardiovascular, and tissue degeneration), neonatal syphilis (birth defects)
Protozoa		
Trichomonas vaginalis	Flagellated protozoan	Vaginitis
Viruses		
Herpes simplex virus types 1 and 2	Enveloped polyhedral capsid with double-stranded DNA	Recurrent genital ulcers, fetal/neonatal infections
Human immunodeficiency virus (HIV) types 1 and 2	Enveloped polyhedral capsid with single-stranded RNA: retrovirus	AIDS, neonatal infection
Human papillomaviruses	Nonenveloped double-stranded DNA virus	Genital warts, cervical cancer

OUTBREAK 42

An Outbreak of Sexually Transmitted Disease among Teenagers

GEORGIA, 1996

In 1996, an unusual outbreak of an ulcerative STD was documented in a group of teenagers in a middle-size town in Georgia. The pathogen was initially diagnosed in six white female subjects, two white male subjects, and two African-American male subjects. Four of the female subjects were younger than 16 years old.

An investigation of the outbreak by the Georgia Division of Public Health indicated a large network of sexual contacts that potentially exposed more than 200 teenagers and young adults to the pathogen. At least 1 year before the outbreak was detected, a group of 18 young white girls began meeting with two different groups of young men: one set of white males aged 17 to 21 and a set of less affluent African-American males of similar ages. Meetings took place while the girls' parents were gone for the evening. The groups met for drug and alcohol use and sexual activities. Injectable drugs were not used. Sexual activities were usually public (in a car or in a hidden public place) and involved sequential and simultaneous sex partners. Several of the girls who were part of the outbreak were pregnant at the time of disease diagnosis. Thirteen other girls became pregnant after completion of their treatment. During interviews, the adolescent women indicated that most parents had not taken action in response to the outbreak nor increased levels of communication at home about sexual activity or drug use.

Dark-field microscopy was used to analyze the pathogen from scrapings of the ulcers. The pathogen could not be cultured in the laboratory.

QUESTIONS

1. List several STDs that could cause this type of outbreak, and briefly describe several physical characteristics of each pathogen.

2. Based on the laboratory results, diagnose the disease and describe the pathogenic agent.

3. Describe the pathogenesis of the microbe.

4. How would you have managed this outbreak?

5. For what complications are untreated and/or pregnant individuals at increased risk?

Figure 42.1 Dark-field microscopy of the pathogen.

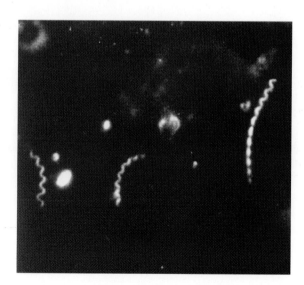

A Chancroid Outbreak among Hispanic Men

CALIFORNIA, 1981

From 1 May 1981 to 19 March 1982, 389 patients with chancroid ulcers on their genitals were seen in the Orange County (California) Special Diseases Clinic. Ninety-five percent of the cases were in men with genital ulcers (ranging from 0.3 to 2.5 centimeters in diameter) and/or enlarged inguinal nodes. The lesions were single or multiple, superficial or deep, and often with ragged edges and a purulent (pus-filled) base. Tender unilateral or bilateral inguinal nodes were present in 32% of patients, and in some patients, they progressed to the formation of buboes.

Dark-field and serologic tests for syphilis, cultures for herpes simplex virus, and serologic tests for lymphogranuloma venereum-causing chlamydiae (bacteria that cause extensive swelling of the lymph nodes in the groin) were negative in nearly all instances. The pathogen that was isolated was fastidious and grew only on chocolate agar. A Gram stain of pus from the lesion indicated a gram-negative rod-shaped pathogen.

Ninety-one percent of the patients were Hispanic men, many of whom were recent immigrants from Mexico living in central Orange County in crowded apartments (5 to 15 occupants per single housing unit). At least 77% of these men had had recent sexual contact with prostitutes. Physical examination of two prostitutes from that area, who presumably had multiple contacts with male patients who had the disease, showed no lesions. However, the pathogen was identified when cultures of the cervix, urethra, and vagina were done.

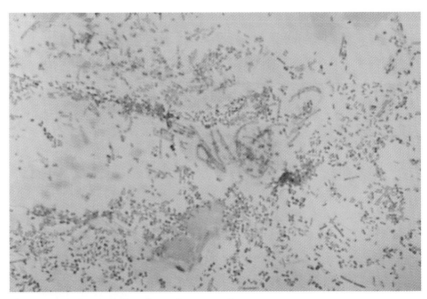

Figure 43.1 Gram stain of an ulcer scraping.

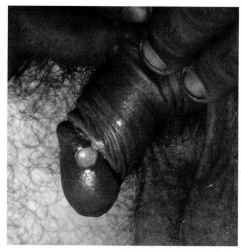

Figure 43.2 Ulcer resulting from the pathogen.

Antimicrobial susceptibility tests performed at the Centers for Disease Control and Prevention (CDC) on 29 isolates of the pathogen from this outbreak showed resistance to sulfamethoxazole and tetracycline.

QUESTIONS

1. Why were laboratory tests done for syphilis, herpes simplex virus, and lymphogranuloma venereum?

2. Identify the pathogen that was spread in this cluster of sexual contacts.

3. What other STDs does chancroid increase the risk of acquiring?

4. How would you have treated the affected individuals?

5. Describe how you would have prevented this epidemic from spreading.

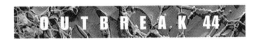

An Outbreak of Sexually Transmitted Disease in the Pornography Industry

CALIFORNIA, 2004

The adult film industry in Southern California produces about 4,000 films and videos a year. Although the San Fernando Valley pornography industry is believed to generate up to $9 billion a year, most of its productions are turned out by just a few dozen companies and producers. In that relatively closed environment, sexual contacts often overlap among many pornographic-film performers.

The STD infection rate in the performing population of adult pornographic films was "getting out of hand" in mid-July 2004, according to Adult Industry Medical Care Foundation cofounder Sharon Mitchell. Her foundation tests 1,200 adult film performers monthly for STDs.

In April 2004, the primary case patient, a pornographic-film actor who was uninfected in March, tested positive for an enveloped retrovirus with a polyhedral capsid and single-stranded ribonucleic acid (RNA). Mitchell and her staff from the Adult Industry Medical Care Foundation used their database of video productions to find 13 primary sexual contacts (two of whom tested positive for the STD) and about 65 secondary sexual contacts who had had intercourse with the primary contacts.

A director and producer of pornographic films who had worked with the primary case patient several times said the actor's infection was "just catastrophic" and called him "a total gentleman." The director estimated that he had filmed 40,000 sex scenes in the last 5 years. He stated that his wife, who had performed in more than 1,000 adult films, was so careful that she had never been infected with a sexually transmitted disease.

The Los Angeles County Health Department issued subpoenas for the records relating to the STD scare from the Adult Industry

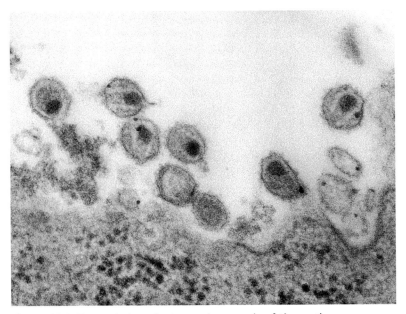

Figure 44.1 Transmission electron micrograph of the pathogen.

Medical Care Foundation. Adult industry lawyers tried to prevent the information from being released. "We have a moral and legal obligation to protect our population of patients from any type of intrusion and confusion at this point," said Sharon Mitchell. "They realize this is an occupational hazard." Sharon Mitchell is herself a former adult film actress who earned a master's degree in public health and a Ph.D. in human sexuality before cofounding the medical foundation. Although some production companies require actors to use condoms, she said, most do not. "Films are picked up for distribution faster if the actors are not wearing condoms, and the talent earns more money for not wearing condoms," Mitchell said.

QUESTIONS

1. What STDs are commercial sex workers at high risk for contracting?

2. Identify the pathogen and the STD that were spread in this cluster of sexual contacts.

3. To what opportunistic pathogens will those infected with this STD eventually become susceptible?

4. How would you have treated the affected individuals?

5. Describe how you would have prevented this epidemic from spreading.

6. How does the legal system in your state determine when public safety issues regarding the spread of infectious disease outweigh issues of confidentiality of medical records?

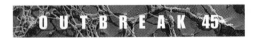

An Outbreak of Azithromycin-Resistant Gonorrhea

KANSAS CITY, MISSOURI, 1999

In the United States, an estimated 700,000 to 800,000 people are infected with *Neisseria gonorrhoeae* each year. This STD pathogen was once easily treated with penicillins before penicillinase-producing *Neisseria gonorrhoeae* developed. Penicillinase is an enzyme produced by most bacteria that are resistant to penicillins. The enzyme degrades penicillin so that it will not harm the cell. During the 1980s, resistance to penicillin and tetracycline among gonococcal isolates became widespread; as a result, the CDC recommended that other antimicrobial agents be used to treat gonorrhea. Since 1993, the CDC has recommended the use of fluoroquinolones for gonorrhea treatment. Fluoroquinolone therapy is used frequently because it is an inexpensive, oral, and single-dose therapy. However, because of the increased prevalence of fluoroquinolone-resistant *N. gonorrhoeae* in Asia, the Pacific Islands (including Hawaii), Massachusetts, New York City, and California, fluoroquinolones are no longer recommended for treating gonorrhea acquired in those locations.

Between March and December 1999, the Gonococcal Isolate Surveillance Project identified a cluster of 12 men with gonorrhea that had decreased susceptibility to the macrolide azithromycin. The patients were seen at the Kansas City, Missouri, STD clinic. The medical records of the 12 patients indicated that their median age was 33 years and that 10 were black. Six reported sex with a commercial sex worker, and all 12 denied sexual contact with other men. Two were infected with human immunodeficiency virus (HIV). Two reported antimicrobial use during the 30 days before diagnosis.

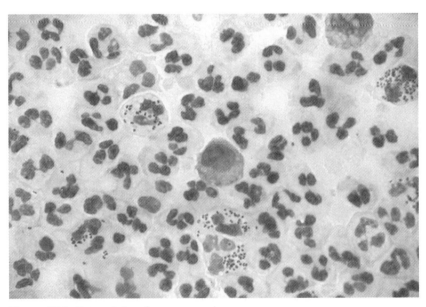

Figure 45.1 Gram stain of a pus sample.

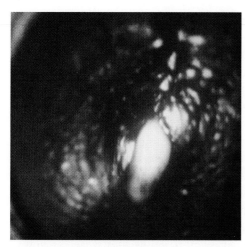

Figure 45.2 Pus discharge.

Preliminary laboratory data suggested that the gonococcal strains among the 12 patients were identical. All isolates were susceptible to ceftriaxone, cefixime, spectinomycin, ciprofloxacin, and penicillin but showed resistance to tetracycline.

QUESTIONS

1. What risk factors did the men have for acquiring a drug-resistant strain of *Neisseria gonorrhoeae*?

2. What complications can be caused by gonorrhea?

3. Describe the pathogenesis of *Neisseria gonorrhoeae*.

4. Why is *Neisseria gonorrhoeae* becoming resistant to the drugs that are used to treat it?

5. Why is it often important to know where an STD was contracted?

6. What actions should be taken to decrease the development of drug resistance in *Neisseria gonorrhoeae* in the United States?

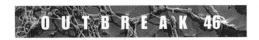

Invasive Cervical Cancer among Women

UNITED STATES, 1992 TO 1999

Approximately 13,000 new cases of invasive cervical cancer occur annually, and over 4,000 women die of the disease, about twice as many as die of AIDS. To characterize the incidence of invasive cervical cancer, the CDC analyzed incidence data for Hispanic and non-Hispanic women from 1992 to 1999. Microscopically confirmed invasive cervical cancer cases were selected, and the numbers of incidences per 100,000 women were calculated (Fig. 46.1 and 46.2).

From 1992 to 1999, a total of 14,759 invasive cervical cancer cases were diagnosed (53% localized, 40% advanced, and 7% unstaged). Twenty-two percent were among Hispanic women, and 78% were among non-Hispanic women. Invasive disease confined to the cervix was categorized as localized; cancers that had spread beyond the cervix to regional nodes or metastasized to other sites were categorized as advanced. The incidence of invasive cervical cancer was 16.9 per 100,000 for Hispanic women and 8.9 for non-Hispanic women. Among women aged >30 years, the cervical cancer incidence for Hispanic women was approximately twice that for non-Hispanic women. Regardless of the stage of disease at diagnosis, incidences for Hispanic women were approximately twice those for non-Hispanic women in each year from 1992 to 1999.

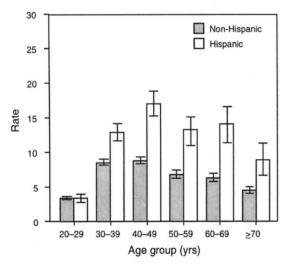

* Per 100,000 women.
† Localized-stage cancer is confined to the cervix.

Figure 46.1 Incidence of localized invasive cervical cancer among Hispanic and non-Hispanic women, by age group.

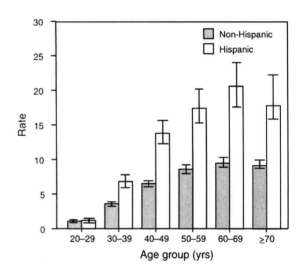

* Per 100,000 women.
† Advanced-stage cancer (includes regional and distant) requires direct extension to corpus uteri or any site beyond the cervix, lymph node involvement, or metastasis.

Figure 46.2 Incidence of advanced invasive cervical cancer among Hispanic and non-Hispanic women by age group.

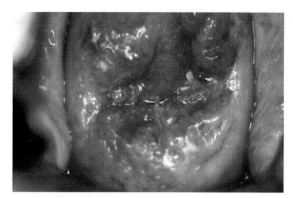

Figure 46.3 Cervical cancer.

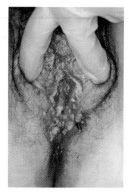

Figure 46.4 Genital warts.

Human papillomavirus (HPV) is a tumor-causing virus which can cause benign tumors (genital warts) or malignant tumors (cervical cancer). Several strains of HPV are responsible for 93% of cervical cancers. Cervical cancer screening (Pap smears) identifies precancerous lesions and prompts early treatment to prevent advanced-stage cancer and death.

QUESTIONS

1. Why is invasive cervical cancer generally at a low level in the population until women are >30 years old?

2. What are the main risk factors for cervical cancer?

3. Describe the pathogenesis of cervical cancer.

4. Does condom use prevent the sexual transmission of the pathogen that causes cervical cancer?

5. What other STD is caused by other serotypes of the HPV pathogen?

6. How would you decrease the spread of cervical cancer in the United States?

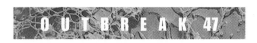

An Outbreak of Lymphogranuloma Venereum in Homosexual Men

THE NETHERLANDS, 2003

In mid-December 2003, a cluster of an ulcerative STD that causes enlargement of the lymph nodes in the groin was detected in men who have sex with men and was reported to the Municipal Health Service in Rotterdam, The Netherlands, by the Erasmus Medisch Centrum sexually transmitted infection outpatient clinic. A majority of these men were HIV infected. Consequently, there were concerns that the outbreak might extend through a large part of Western Europe.

In February 2003, the first case, involving a white, HIV-infected, bisexual man, was diagnosed at the sexually transmitted infection clinic as proctitis (inflammation of the colon due to infection). Two HIV-infected homosexual men presented with proctitis at the outpatient clinic in Rotterdam in April 2003. Although there was apparently no link to the first patient, laboratory results showed that they were infected with the same pathogen. A cluster of cases of the same infection was found through contact tracing, and two other cases, not connected to this cluster, presented themselves. Most patients presented with proctitis and some with constipation. Infections of the rectum by this pathogen result in much more severe inflammation than other STD infections.

All of the patients were white and between 26 and 48 years old. Thirteen of them were HIV positive (and already aware of their HIV status), and eight also had another sexually transmitted infection along with HIV infection. One of the patients had very recently been diagnosed as infected with hepatitis C virus, and sexual transmission was thought to be the only possible route of his infection. All of the men reported unprotected sexual contact. Many sexual contacts were

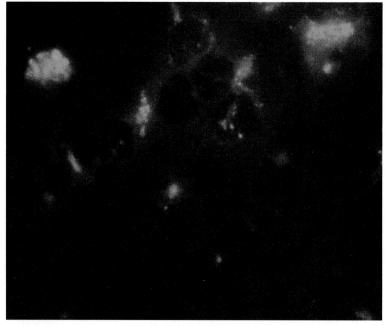

Figure 47.1 Direct fluorescent-antibody assay for *Chlamydia trachomatis.*

anonymous, hampering individual contact tracing. Sexual contacts among these men were reported in Germany, Belgium, the United Kingdom, and France.

The pathogen, a very small intracellular, gram-negative bacterium, was identified by PCR and by direct fluorescent-antibody assays.

QUESTIONS

1. Identify the pathogen that was spread in this cluster of sexual contacts.

2. How would you have treated the affected individuals?

3. Assume you have been sent by the World Health Organization to review grant applications to combat the outbreak. Your primary goal is to minimize the number of illnesses caused by the pathogen. Which two grants from those listed below would receive your highest recommendation? Explain why.

   a. The U.S. National Institutes of Health Emerging Pathogens Group has requested funds for a new vaccine development study.

   b. An international research consortium has requested funds to determine how the pathogen avoids immune recognition.

   c. A regional hospital near a locality where the disease is common has requested additional funds to pay for a study to best determine how to prevent the disease.

   d. The Health Department has requested funds to test and treat those affected at free clinics.

   e. A local health care clinic in a locality where the disease is common has requested funds to take blood samples from anyone who requests it for the purpose of identifying whether they are carrying the pathogen.

   f. An individual university microbiologist has requested funds to determine differences in pathogenesis between homosexual men and heterosexuals affected by the same pathogen.

A Syphilis Outbreak Connected with a Cybersex Chat Room

SAN FRANCISCO, CALIFORNIA, 2000

One-third of adult Internet visits are directed to sexually oriented web sites. Consequently, it is not surprising that the Internet is often used to seek sexual partners. Chat rooms where individuals initially meet to arrange participation in high-risk sexual activities are now being used to help trace sexually transmitted diseases. Identification of the sexual contacts of those infected could help reduce the spread of sexually transmitted pathogens.

The city of Denver provides health care at a public health clinic where HIV counseling and testing is provided. During an 8-month period, Mary McFarlane and CDC coworkers interviewed 856 people who visited the clinic. Their results indicated that those who sought sex partners over the Internet were at high risk for acquiring STDs. First, those who found sexual partners in Internet chat rooms tended to have high-risk sex. Second, people who had sex with partners who had been identified in online chat rooms were more likely to be homosexual and male. These individuals were more likely than the general population to have had more sex partners, more anal sex, and more sex with men who have sex with men and were more likely to have sex with a partner known to be HIV positive.

In San Francisco, an outbreak of an ulcerative STD was identified in two gay men who reported meeting most of their sex partners on the Internet. The disease was characterized by a painless ulcer on the penises of the men. Laboratory tests from the ulcer identified the pathogen by using dark-field microscopy and silver staining of infected tissue. An investigation of the chat room participants indi-

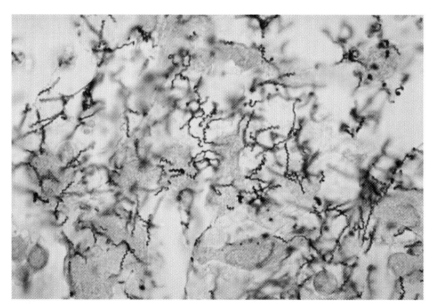

Figure 48.1 Light micrograph of silver-stained infected tissue.

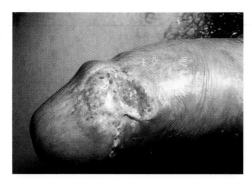

Figure 48.2 Lesion on the penis.

cated they had an average of six sex partners. Users of the chat room identified themselves only by screen names. Contact tracing by the Health Department was hindered because the Internet service provider refused to provide the Health Department with identifying information about chat room members without a federal subpoena.

QUESTIONS

1. Name the pathogen that infected the two men.

2. How would you have treated the affected men?

3. What potential complications were the men at risk for if they were not treated?

4. Describe how you would have prevented an epidemic from occurring in the sexual partners of these men.

5. Do you think the Public Health Service (PHS) should have had access to the real names of visitors to the cybersex chat room for the purpose of preventing the spread of syphilis or other STDs?

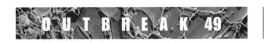

The Impact of AIDS Worsens Famine

SOUTHERN AFRICA, 2002 TO PRESENT

The HIV/acquired immune deficiency syndrome (AIDS) epidemic is fueling a widening and increasingly deadly famine in southern Africa. The African famine is an example of how the impact of HIV/AIDS reaches beyond the loss of life and health care costs traditionally associated with disease.

There are 42 million people living with HIV/AIDS worldwide. Of those infected, 38.6 million are adults, 19.2 million are women, and 3.2 million are children under the age of 15. Five million new infections with HIV occurred in 2002; of these, 4.2 million were in adults (2 million of whom were women). A total of 3.1 million people died of HIV/AIDS-related causes in 2002.

Sub-Saharan Africa has the highest number of HIV-positive individuals (29.4 million people living with HIV/AIDS). In sub-Saharan Africa, the epidemic continues to expand. An estimated 3.5 million new infections occurred in 2002, and 2.4 million Africans died of the disease.

In the predominantly agricultural societies in South Africa, Lesotho, Malawi, Mozambique, Swaziland, Zambia, and Zimbabwe, the populations are battling serious AIDS epidemics, with more than 5 million adults currently living with HIV/AIDS in these countries out of a total adult population of some 26 million. These six countries also have a total of 600,000 children under 15 living with HIV infection.

AIDS is combining with other factors—including droughts, floods, and in some cases short-sighted national and international policies—to cause a steady fall in agricultural production and to cut deeply into household income. AIDS-related deaths in farm households

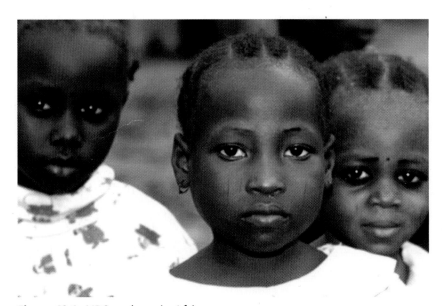

Figure 49.1 AIDS orphans in Africa.

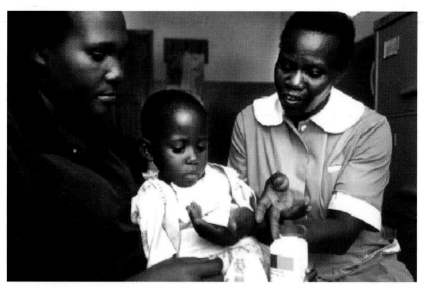
Figure 49.2 A child receives treatment for AIDS.

cause crop output to plummet—often by up to 60%. A 2002 study in central Malawi, for example, showed that about 70% of surveyed households had suffered labor losses due to sickness. Household incomes also have decreased, leaving people with less money to buy food. Seven million agricultural workers in 25 African countries have died of AIDS since 1985. In 2001 alone, AIDS killed nearly 500,000 people in the six predominantly agricultural countries threatened with famine, most of whom were in their productive prime. As a result, more than 14 million people are now at risk of starvation.

QUESTIONS

1. Describe the epidemiology of HIV in sub-Saharan Africa.

2. Why is the observed incidence of HIV/AIDS higher in Africa than in other areas of the world?

3. In order to minimize the number of deaths in the six agricultural countries significantly affected by AIDS-related deaths, what would be your first priority among the activities listed below? Assume you have the financial resources to complete only one objective. Explain the rationale for your choice.

    a. Provide antiretroviral therapy to those showing signs of AIDS.

    b. Educate the public on the importance of consistent and correct condom use.

    c. Set up a research center designed to develop an HIV vaccine.

    d. Provide food to those who are currently starving.

    e. Educate the surviving populace about how to develop a sustainable agricultural system.

4. What would be your second priority? Explain the rational for your choice.

AIDS

AIDS is now the number one cause of death in sub-Saharan Africa, surpassing malaria. It is estimated that 29.4 million people are currently living with HIV/AIDS in sub-Saharan Africa—that is two-thirds of the HIV/AIDS cases reported globally. According to the Joint United Nations Program on HIV/AIDS, an estimated 3.5 million adults and children in sub-Saharan Africa became infected with HIV in 2002 and 2.4 million people died of AIDS-related illness in Africa. What sets AIDS apart, however, is that it kills so many adults in the prime of their working and parenting lives, decimating the workforce. The epidemic has impoverished families, orphaned millions, and shredded the fabric of communities. Of the 13 million children orphaned by AIDS worldwide, 10 million live in sub-Saharan Africa.

In at least 10 African countries, prevalence rates among adults exceed 10%. In several of the countries with the highest adult infection rates, life expectancy has now dropped to less than 40 years, with a child born today having over a 50% chance of dying of AIDS.

Cause of the disease

HIV is an enveloped virus with a polyhedral capsid and single-stranded RNA as its genetic information. HIV is called a retrovirus because it has an enzyme, reverse transcriptase, that catalyzes the synthesis of single-stranded RNA to double-stranded deoxyribonucleic acid (DNA).

Transmission

Reservoir
Humans are the only reservoir of HIV.

Mode of transmission
Horizontal: The virus is spread by direct intimate contact as an STD or as a blood-borne pathogen via the parenteral route.

Vertical: The virus can be spread to newborn children during birth, when there is a potential for maternal and placental blood exchange to occur. Infants can also acquire HIV through a mother's breast milk.

Pathogenesis

Entry
Entry of the virus requires blood-to-blood or blood-to-semen exchange.

Attachment
The protein on the outside of the HIV envelope (gp160) binds to lymphocytes, neurons, and macrophages, which carry the $CD4^+$ receptor protein.

Avoiding host defenses
The virus is an intracellular pathogen, so it can avoid circulating antibodies. In addition, HIV can form a provirus, in which the viral DNA has been incorporated into the chromosome of its host cell. In a proviral state, the virus can be dormant for long periods until it is stimulated to complete its normal replication cycle.

Overcoming defenses
As a result of the infection, CD4 lymphocytes are destroyed. CD4 lymphocytes normally activate both the humoral immune system (B cells and antibodies) and the cell-mediated immune system (T cells and cytotoxic T cells). Also, the virus is very error prone. Many mutations occur as the virus synthesizes its genetic information using an error-prone enzyme, reverse transcriptase. This produces a heterogeneous mix of mutant viruses, allowing it to quickly adapt to changing defenses and antiviral agents.

Damage
Damage is direct, as infected cells lose their functions and die. Indirect damage results from loss of immune functions, resulting in a person with AIDS acquiring a number of opportunistic infections (infections that are easily defeated by a person with a healthy immune system).

Exit
HIV exits through the blood or semen of infected individuals.

Clinical features

After the primary infection by HIV, a person will experience a mononucleosis-like illness. After recovery, there is a long period (about 10 years) during which the virus continues to replicate and cause damage to the organs and cells of the immune system, but there is little clinical expression of the disease. Following the asymptomatic (no-symptom) period, those with HIV infections begin to experience chronic systemic problems, including weight loss, persistent fever, persistent lymphadenopathy (swollen lymph nodes), persistent diarrhea, and night sweats. AIDS is characterized as an HIV infection where the patient has a CD4 lymphocyte count of less than 200 cells/milliliter and experiences the chronic systemic signs and symptoms plus an opportunistic infection. *Pneumocystis carinii* is the most common cause of death among people with AIDS. It is a fungal pathogen that causes pneumonia in people whose immune systems function poorly (immunocompromised people).

Diagnosis

Specimen
A blood sample is obtained.

Test
Initially, an enzyme-linked immunosorbent assay is used to screen for antibodies to HIV. If the first test is positive, the infection is confirmed through a second sample using a Western blotting technique to identify HIV-specific proteins or by polymerase chain reaction (PCR) analysis to identify HIV-specific DNA sequences.

Treatment
HIV infection is treated with a "triple cocktail" composed of two inhibitors of the reverse transcriptase enzyme and one inhibitor of the HIV protease. Both enzymes are unique to HIV-infected cells. The reverse transcriptase inhibitors are nucleoside analogs that have a high affinity for reverse transcriptase. They lack the —OH group that normally links nucleotides together during DNA synthesis. The protease inhibitor has a unique structure that allows it to specifically bind to HIV protease and prevents it from cleaving a large polypeptide precursor, thus preventing virus assembly.

Prevention

Sexual transmission
- Abstinence and monogamy (one partner for life) prevent the transmission of all STDs.
- Consistent and correct latex condom use is an effective way to prevent the spread of HIV.
- General risk can be decreased by limiting the number of different sexual partners and not having intercourse with individuals who are at high risk for acquiring STDs, e.g., commercial sex workers (CSWs).
- Public education may also work to induce changes in high-risk sexual behavior.
- The spread of HIV can be reduced in a community by screening high-risk groups and providing easy and free treatment programs.

Blood-to-blood transmission
- Pregnant women should take anti-HIV medications to prevent spread to the newborn infant.
- Intravenous drug users should not share needles.
- The blood supply must be screened to eliminate HIV-contaminated blood.
- Contact tracing of HIV-positive blood donors should take place.
- Hemophiliacs should be supplied with recombinant blood-clotting factors.
- Health care workers should always employ universal precautions: wearing gloves and masks and using needle disposal devices.

Chancroid

Chancroid is uncommon in industrialized nations; however, it is a frequent cause of genital-ulcer disease in developing countries. The ulceration of genital tissues also greatly increases the risk for HIV transmission. In the United States and Europe, most cases are part of localized outbreaks, and they generally have involved traditional STD core populations, such as drug users or prostitutes and their clients.

Cause of the disease
Haemophilus ducreyi, a bacterial pathogen, is a gram-negative, irregularly rod-shaped bacterium that is typically seen as short rods or chains. It is mostly found in tropical and subtropical regions of the world and is usually associated with poor socioeconomic and hygiene conditions.

Transmission

Reservoir
Infected humans are the reservoir of this pathogen.

Mode of transmission
The disease is transmitted via direct sexual contact.

Pathogenesis

Entry
The pathogen is spread to the reproductive tract or external genitalia by direct contact with an infected lesion. It enters the tissue through small skin abrasions.

Attachment
The pathogen attaches to the epithelium of the reproductive tract.

Avoiding host defenses

The pathogen restricts its initial infection to the epithelial surface and avoids defenses of the immune system.

Damage

The pathogen produces a cytotoxin that causes local tissue destruction and an inflammatory response with swelling and pus formation.

Exit

The pathogen exits in pus from a lesion.

Clinical features

The incubation period between contact and the initial appearance of skin ulcers ranges from 4 to 10 days. The disease is most commonly seen in men, especially those who are uncircumcised. After exposure, one or more sores or raised bumps arise on the genital organs, surrounded by a narrow red border filled with pus. This lesion ruptures, leaving a painful open sore. If left untreated, the lymph glands in the groin can become infected, resulting in severe pain and enlargement and ulceration of the nodes. In females, an infection is typically characterized by painful urination or bowel movements, painful intercourse, rectal bleeding, or vaginal discharge.

Diagnosis

Specimen

A swab of fluid or pus from a lesion is obtained.

Test

Noncultural: Microscopic detection of gram-negative rods in short chains that often appear similar to a school of fish is the diagnostic test.

Treatment

Chancroid is commonly treated with macrolide antibiotics, such as azithromycin. Erythromycin stimulates the dissociation of peptidyl-transfer RNA (tRNA) from bacterial ribosomes, preventing complete translation of proteins.

Prevention

- Abstinence and monogamy prevent the transmission of all STDs.

- Consistent and correct latex condom use is an effective way to prevent the spread of *Haemophilus ducreyi*.

- General risk can be decreased by limiting the number of different sexual partners and not having intercourse with individuals who are at high risk for obtaining STDs, e.g., CSWs.

- Public education may also work to induce changes in high-risk sexual behavior.

Chlamydial Nongonococcal Urethritis

Approximately 4 million cases of chlamydial infection are reported per year in the United States, with an overall prevalence of 5%. At-risk groups (e.g., sexually active adolescent girls) have a higher prevalence, with an incidence of 10%. Fifteen- to 24-year-old women represent about 80% of infections, with the highest rates among economically disadvantaged young women. Up to 40% of women with untreated *Chlamydia* infection will develop pelvic inflammatory disease (PID). Of those with PID, 20% will become infertile; 18% will experience debilitating, chronic pelvic pain; and 9% will have a potentially life-threatening tubal pregnancy.

Cause of the disease

Chlamydia trachomatis, a bacterial pathogen, is an obligate intracellular bacterium that has two different forms: an elementary body that is transmitted between hosts and a reticulate body that replicates inside the host cells. It is a very small (0.20-micrometer) gram-negative bacillus.

Transmission

Reservoir

Symptomatic and asymptomatic humans are the reservoir.

Mode of transmission

Horizontal: Direct intimate contact is required to transmit the pathogen, since it is sensitive to changes in temperature and to drying.

Vertical: Newborn infants can develop conjunctivitis after being exposed to *Chlamydia* during birth.

Pathogenesis

Entry

The pathogen enters the reproductive tract via sexual contact.

Attachment

The elementary body has adhesins that bind to receptors on the urogenital epithelium, preventing the pathogen from being washed away by urine or vaginal discharges.

Avoiding host defenses

The pathogen survives inside host cells of the reproductive epithelium, which are initially protected from circulating antibodies and cells of the immune system.

Damage

Direct damage is caused by *Chlamydia* lysing its host cell to release elementary bodies. The tissue damage causes an inflammatory response, resulting in swelling, pain, and pus formation.

Exit

The pathogen exits in pus.

Clinical features

Approximately 75% of women and 50% of men are asymptomatic carriers of the pathogen.

For symptomatic females, there is a 14-day incubation period followed by an increased or abnormal, foul-smelling vaginal discharge. They may also experience painful urination, unusual vaginal bleeding, or bleeding after sexual intercourse. Lower abdominal pain may also result as the cervix becomes inflamed.

For symptomatic males, the disease presents as pain during urination and a pus discharge from the penis and possibly pain and swelling in the testicles.

Diagnosis

Specimen

Males: A urine sample is obtained.
Females: A sample of cervical mucus is obtained.

Tests

Tests include PCR using *Chlamydia trachomatis*-specific primers and a direct fluorescent-antibody test using a *Chlamydia*-specific monoclonal antibody conjugated to a fluorescent dye. The chlamydiae are visualized under an immunofluorescence microscope.

Treatment

Chlamydia infections are commonly treated with tetracycline or macrolide antibiotics. Doxycycline effectively inhibits bacterial growth by preventing binding of aminoacyl-tRNA to 70S ribosomes. Like all tetracyclines, it is not used in pregnant women (it can harm fetal development) or children less than 8 years old (it stains the teeth a permanent brown color). The macrolide erythromycin stimulates the dissociation of peptidyl-tRNA from bacterial ribosomes, preventing completion of protein formation.

Prevention

- Abstinence and monogamy prevent the transmission of all STDs.
- Consistent and correct latex condom use is an effective way to prevent the spread of *Chlamydia trachomatis*.
- General risk can be decreased by limiting the number of sexual partners and not having intercourse with individuals who are at high risk for acquiring STDs, e.g., CSWs.
- Physicians are required to notify the Public Health Service when *Chlamydia* is identified in one of their patients. The PHS does contact tracing, in which they follow up with infected individuals to identify and recommend treatment for previous sexual partners. In this way, asymptomatic carriers can be identified and treated before they experience complications or spread the pathogen to other sexual partners.
- The spread of *Chlamydia* can also be reduced in a community by screening high-risk groups and providing easy and free treatment programs.
- Public education may also work to induce changes in high-risk sexual behavior.

Cervical Cancer and Genital Warts

The cost of the health care burden for cervical cancer and genital warts is second only to that of AIDS among STDs, with an annual cost of $1.6 billion to $6.0 billion. There are 5.5 million infections per year in males and females. Among all sexually active women, over 50% have been infected by more than one type of HPV. Fortunately, the majority have only asymptomatic infections; only about 1% of those infected develop clinical disease. In the United States, there are 14,000 cases of cervical cancer per year, causing 5,000 deaths—twice as many deaths in the female population as are caused by AIDS.

Cause of the disease

HPV has a polyhedral capsid and double-stranded DNA as genetic information. It does not possess an envelope. HPV is a tumor-causing virus. Benign tumors form warts, and malignant tumors cause cancer. There are about 100 different serotypes of HPV, with about 30 causing infections of the genital mucosa. About a dozen of these cause high-risk infections that can progress to invasive cancer. Evidence of HPV infection is found in 93% of cases of cervical cancer.

Transmission

Reservoir

Humans are the only reservoir. The pathogen can be carried by both symptomatic and asymptomatic carriers.

Mode of transmission

Horizontal: Transmission requires direct intimate contact.

Vertical: Transmission causes juvenile onset of recurrent respiratory papillomatosis.

Pathogenesis

Entry

Virus entry is via direct intimate contact with HPV-infected tissue. The infected tissue does not have to display clinical features for HPV to be passed to a new host.

Attachment

HPV attaches to the cervical epithelium and skin of the external genitalia.

Avoiding host defenses

The pathogen avoids circulating antibodies and cells of the immune system by replicating in a protected environment. HPV is an intracellular pathogen, and infection is restricted to the epithelial tissues. In addition, HPV can form a provirus, in which the viral DNA has been incorporated into the chromosome of the host cell. In a proviral state, the virus can be dormant for long periods until it is stimulated to complete its normal replication cycle.

Damage

Several of the viral proteins that are expressed early in the replication cycle bind to tumor suppressor proteins. As a result, the cell's normal division cycle is unregulated and the infected cells divide continuously.

Exit

HPV exits to enter a new host by direct contact.

Clinical features

For wart-causing HPV serotypes, infection is followed by a 1- to 6-month incubation period before warts form on the penis, vulva, and perianal region.

For cancer-causing HPV serotypes, there is an approximately 10-year period after infection before cervical-cell dysplasia and cervical cancer develop.

Diagnosis

Warts are diagnosed simply by the clinical presentation; 1.4 million persons in the United States have genital warts.

Abnormal cell growth in cervical tissue is diagnosed by histological examination of a Pap smear. About 50 million Pap smears are done per year; they identify 2.5 million low-grade abnormalities and 250,000 high-grade abnormalities.

Treatment

There are no systemic therapies to treat genital warts or cervical cancer. Treatment requires removing infected tissue using local destructive approaches, such as freezing tissue at and near the site of infection, laser oblation of infected tissue, and treatment with topical cytotoxic compounds. Since tissue that appears normal can still harbor the virus, there is a 10 to 20% recurrence for abnormal cervical tissue growth and a 20 to 50% recurrence for warts.

Prevention

- Unlike other STDs, the CDC has determined that latex condoms do not prevent the spread of HPV because the normal-appearing tissues around the genitals can be infected and spread the virus.
- Regular PAP smears detect cell abnormalities early, allowing affected tissue to be destroyed before cancer develops.
- Prevention requires either abstinence or monogamy.
- General risk can be decreased by limiting the number of different sexual partners and not having intercourse with individuals who are at high risk for acquiring STDs, e.g., CSWs.
- Public education may also work to induce changes in high-risk sexual behavior.

Gonorrhea

Worldwide, approximately 200 million new cases of gonorrhea occur each year. In developed countries, the incidence of gonorrhea is declining due to public health initiatives. In the United States, there are about 600,000 reported new infections per year, with many more estimated to occur but not be reported. The incidence of penicillinase-producing *N. gonorrhoeae* is rising and is expected to make the treatment of gonorrhea more difficult in the future.

Cause of the disease

Neisseria gonorrhoeae, a bacterial pathogen, is a gram-negative diplococcus that produces fimbriae.

Transmission
Reservoir
Symptomatic men and women and asymptomatic women are reservoirs.

Mode of transmission
Horizontal: Direct sexual contact is the mode of transmission. The pathogen is sensitive to drying and temperature changes and requires direct intimate contact.

Vertical: Newborn infants can develop conjunctivitis after being exposed to *Neisseria* during birth.

Pathogenesis
Entry
The pathogen enters the body via direct intimate contact.

Attachment
Adhesins on pili attach to tissues of the reproductive tract, the oral cavity, the conjunctiva of the eye, and the rectum. Although in women, the cervix usually is the initial site of infection, the disease can be carried on sperm cells and spread to and infect the uterus and fallopian tubes.

Avoiding host defenses
Attachment prevents the bacteria from being washed away by urine or vaginal discharges. In addition, the pathogen produces immunoglobulin A protease, which degrades the antibodies associated with mucosal immunity.

Damage
Growth of the pathogen causes direct tissue damage, which induces a large inflammatory response.

Exit
The pathogen exits through pus discharge.

Clinical features
Incubation
Incubation is for 2 to 10 days after sexual contact with an infected partner.

Females: Infection is asymptomatic in 50% of females. Symptomatic infections cause a painful or burning sensation when urinating and vaginal discharge that is yellow or bloody. Advanced infection can cause abdominal pain, bleeding between menstrual periods, vomiting, fever, and PID, a mixed infection of the upper reproductive tract that can lead to abscesses, chronic pain, ectopic pregnancy, or infertility.

Males: Symptoms include pus-containing discharge from the penis and a burning sensation during urination that may be severe.

Gonorrhea also increases the risk of HIV infection, so prevention and early treatment are critically important.

Diagnosis
Specimen
A cervical swab or pus sample is obtained.

Tests
Cultural: The pathogen grows on modified Thayer-Martin medium.

Noncultural: Testing may be done by PCR using *Neisseria gonorrhoeae*-specific primers or Gram stain of pus to detect gram-negative diplococci in leukocytes.

Treatment
Some strains of *Neisseria gonorrhoeae* produce β-lactamase, so penicillin-resistant cases of gonorrhea are increasing in incidence. A common treatment is a single intramuscular dose of ceftriaxone, a β-lactamase-resistant β-lactam. It is not unusual for gonorrhea to be complicated by a chlamydial infection; therefore, doctors usually prescribe a combination of antibiotics.

Prevention
- Abstinence and monogamy prevent the transmission of all STDs.

- Consistent and correct latex condom use is an effective way to prevent the spread of *N. gonorrhoeae*.

- General risk can be decreased by limiting the number of different sexual partners and not having intercourse with individuals who are at high risk for obtaining STDs, e.g., CSWs.

- Physicians are required to notify their state department of public health when gonorrhea is identified in one of their patients. The health department does contact tracing, in which they follow up with infected individuals to identify and recommend treatment for previous sexual partners. In this way, asymptomatic carriers can be identified and treated before they experience complications or spread the pathogen to other sexual partners.

- The spread of gonorrhea can also be reduced in a community by screening high-risk groups and providing easy and free treatment programs. Public education may also work to induce changes in high-risk sexual behavior.

- Antimicrobial agents are placed in the eyes of newborns to prevent infection by *Neisseria* (ophthalmia neonatorum).

Lymphogranuloma Venereum

Cause of the disease

Lymphogranuloma venereum is caused by *Chlamydia trachomatis* serotypes L1, L2, and L3, which are common in Africa, Asia, and South America. In Europe, Australia, and North America, these serotypes are found mostly among homosexual men. *Chlamydia trachomatis* is a gram-negative rod-shaped bacterium. It is very small and lives intracellularly.

Transmission

Reservoir
The reservoir for the pathogen is infected humans. Many infections, particularly in females, are asymptomatic.

Mode of transmission
The mode of transmission is direct contact as an STD.

Pathogenesis

Entry
The infectious form of *Chlamydia trachomatis*, the elementary body, enters the host tissues through minute abrasions in the mucosal surface.

Attachment
The elementary body attaches to specific receptors on the host cells and enters through endocytosis. Once inside the host cell, the elementary body differentiates into the metabolically active reticulate body, which divides to produce more elementary bodies.

Avoiding host defenses
Chlamydia trachomatis avoids host defenses because it is an intracellular pathogen and is not initially exposed to immune system antibodies and cells.

Damage
Elementary bodies are released from an infected cell through cell lysis. The cell destruction leads to an inflammatory response.

Exit
Pus and fluid from infected ulcers carry the pathogen to the new host.

Clinical

After a 1- to 4-week incubation, *Chlamydia trachomatis* serotypes L1, L2, and L3 cause an ulcerating papule as a primary lesion at the site of infection. The pathogen drains into the inguinal lymph nodes, causing the swelling characteristic of the disease. The illness is accompanied by high fever, headache, and myalgia (muscle aches) and may be complicated by abscesses that form in the lymph nodes. They typically rupture and discharge pus through the skin. Additional signs and symptoms in homosexual males include bloody proctitis with pus or mucous anal discharge and constipation.

Diagnosis

Chlamydia trachomatis can be detected directly by microscopy using a direct fluorescent-antibody test or by nucleic-acid-based tests using PCR.

Treatment

Lymphogranuloma venereum is treated with tetracycline or doxycycline. Erythromycin is used in pregnant women.

Prevention

- Abstinence and monogamy prevent the transmission of all STDs.

- Consistent and correct latex condom use is an effective way to prevent the spread of *Chlamydia trachomatis*.

- General risk can be decreased by limiting the number of different sexual partners and not having intercourse with individuals who are at high risk for acquiring STDs, e.g., CSWs.

- Physicians are required to notify the Public Health Service when *Chlamydia* is identified in one of their patients. The PHS does contact tracing, in which they follow up with infected individuals to identify and recommend treatment for previous sexual partners. In this way, asymptomatic carriers can be identified and treated before they experience complications or spread the pathogen to other sexual partners.

- The spread of *Chlamydia* can also be reduced in a community by screening high-risk groups and providing easy and free treatment programs.

- Public education may also work to induce changes in high-risk sexual behavior.

Syphilis

In the United States, syphilis is most prevalent among persons of minority race and ethnicity, with the highest incidence among African-Americans. Nationally, syphilis rates are approximately 60 times higher in African-Americans than in Caucasians, and more than 80% of all cases have been reported in the southern United States. Syphilis remains prevalent in many developing countries and regions, especially Eastern Europe and Siberia, where more than 1% of the population has the disease.

Cause of the disease

Treponema pallidum, a bacterial pathogen, is a gram-negative spirochete, a tightly coiled bacterium that moves by means of axial filaments.

Transmission

Reservoir
Infected humans are the reservoir.

Mode of transmission
Horizontal: Treponema pallidum is transmitted sexually and requires direct contact of skin or mucous membranes with infectious secretions of syphilis lesions.

Vertical: Transplacental transmission to the fetus from the infected mother causes significant developmental abnormalities.

Pathogenesis

Entry
The pathogen enters from an infected chancre when it comes into direct contact with a minute abrasion.

Attachment
The ends of bacteria attach to the hyaluronic-acid-containing extracellular matrix that joins capillary endothelial cells.

Avoiding host defenses
The cell surface of *Treponema pallidum* is rich in lipid and is antigenically nonreactive (only after the cell dies are antigens uncovered, followed by the host response).

Damage
Damage is caused by the body's inflammatory response at the sites of cell death. For primary syphilis, inflammation occurs at the site of initial infection; for secondary syphilis, inflammation occurs at various sites after systemic dissemination of the pathogen; and for tertiary syphilis, the inflammation is localized and leads to necrosis (tissue death) at many different sites.

Exit
The pathogen exits through pus from an infected chancre.

Clinical features

Primary syphilis
Symptoms include the development of an open, painless lesion called a chancre and enlarged inguinal lymph nodes. The chancre heals spontaneously.

Secondary syphilis
One to 3 months after primary syphilis, a flu-like illness occurs, characterized by muscle aches, headache, fever, swollen lymph glands, sore throat, patchy hair loss, weight loss, and fatigue. A pox-like rash also characterizes secondary syphilis. The rash consists of raised, pus-filled pox marks that are larger in size than chicken pox. (At one time, a syphilis rash was called the great pox to distinguish it from smallpox.) There is spontaneous resolution of secondary syphilis.

Tertiary syphilis
Three to 30 years later, when the immune system responds to the latent *Treponema* infection, large regions of tissue are damaged. Neurosyphilis is characterized by loss of feeling in the extremities, central nervous system damage, and insanity; cardiovascular syphilis causes aortic lesions leading to internal bleeding. Gummas are the most common form of tertiary syphilis. They are nodular lesions characterized by a granulomatous inflammation and can form in many places and cause organ failure at different locations.

Diagnosis

Specimen
For primary syphilis, a chancre scraping is used; for later stages, a blood sample is taken.

Tests
Chancre scrapings are examined under dark-field microscopy to observe spirochetes. Blood samples are analyzed by enzyme-linked immunosorbent assay to detect *Treponema*-specific antigens.

Treatment

Syphilis is commonly treated with a β-lactam class of antibiotics. Penicillin G is effective for treating primary and later stages of syphilis. If patients are allergic to penicillin, a tetracycline is often used.

Prevention

- Abstinence and monogamy prevent the transmission of all STDs.

- Consistent and correct latex condom use is an effective way to prevent the spread of *Treponema pallidum*.

- General risk can be decreased by limiting the number of different sexual partners and not having intercourse with individuals who are at high risk for acquiring STDs, e.g., CSWs.

- Physicians are required to notify the state department of health when syphilis is identified in one of their patients. The PHS does contact tracing, in which they follow up with infected individuals to identify and recommend treatment for previous sexual partners. In this way, asymptomatic carriers can be identified and treated before they experience complications or spread the pathogen to other sexual partners.

- The spread of syphilis can also be reduced in a community by screening high-risk groups and providing easy and free treatment programs.

- Public education may also work to induce changes in high-risk sexual behavior.

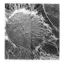 # Outbreaks of Diseases of the Skin, Eyes, and Deep Tissues

It takes a full five minutes of washing to flush out 99% of the most dangerous bacteria from your hands.
G. WILLIAMS, "Your Mother Was Right" (*Discover,* 1999)

The skin is an effective barrier to prevent microbes from infecting underlying tissues. It has little moisture and a relatively high salt concentration, which inhibits the growth of many potential pathogens. The normal flora of the skin also effectively consumes most available nutrients. In the process, oils are broken down to fatty acids, which lowers the pH of the skin's surface. Glands in the skin also produce lysozyme, which breaks down the peptidoglycan of bacterial cell walls.

The skin is composed of stratified squamous epithelium. The flattened cells are linked together by tight junctions, preventing microbes from passing between them. The epithelial cells of the skin are also filled with keratin, a waterproofing protein. These layers of cells are continually sloughed off but are replaced by rapidly growing cells at the base of the epidermal layer.

Microbes that infect the skin attach to the epithelium or to tissues in hair follicles or glands of the skin. To be successful as pathogens, they must outcompete the normal flora and overcome the chemical and physical defenses of the skin. Microbes that infect the underlying tissues must first penetrate the defenses of the skin. This is typically done by the parenteral route, through a cut, puncture wound, abrasion, or burn which breaks the skin. In outbreaks, the integrity of the skin is typically compromised by trauma or by medical procedures—surgery or needle sticks.

This section presents a variety of outbreaks of infection by viral and bacterial pathogens. Outbreaks in health care settings usually involve deviations from acceptable standards of practice. The challenges in prevention of future outbreaks lie in identifying the source of infection, revising procedures, and implementing appropriate quality assurance for compliance. Community-acquired infections of skin, blood, and connective tissue are common. Prevention and containment of local outbreaks require rapid identification of the reservoir and changing the conditions that promote transmission.

Table V.1 Selected outbreak-causing pathogens of skin, soft tissues, and blood

Organism	Key physical properties	Disease characteristics
Bacteria		
Bacillus anthracis	Gram-positive bacillus; aerobic; forms endospores; produces an antiphagocytic capsule and toxins	Naturally occurring; cutaneous lesions
Clostridium perfringens	Anaerobic; gram positive, endospore-forming bacillus	Gas gangrene
Group A streptococci (*Streptococcus pyogenes*)	Gram-positive streptococci; produce an antiphagocytic capsule; beta-hemolytic on blood agar	Impetigo, cellulitis, bacteremia, necrotizing fasciitis, strep throat
Pseudomonas aeruginosa	Non-lactose-fermenting, oxidase-positive, gram-negative bacillus; small porins make it resistant to antibiotics and disinfectants	Dermatitis, burn patient infections, community-acquired and nosocomial urinary tract infections, conjunctivitis
Staphylococcus aureus	Gram-positive staphylococcus; catalase positive; coagulase positive	Boils, abscesses, wound infections, cellulitis, bacteremia, endocarditis, pneumonia, food poisoning, conjunctivitis
Fungi		
Trichophyton spp.	Filamentous molds	Ringworm, athlete's foot, skin and nail infections
Viruses		
Hepatitis B virus	Enveloped polyhedral capsid with double-stranded DNA	Chronic hepatitis; seventh leading cause of death from infectious disease worldwide
Hepatitis C virus	Enveloped polyhedral capsid with single-stranded RNA	Chronic hepatitis
Herpes simplex virus types 1 and 2	Enveloped polyhedral capsid with double-stranded DNA	Cold sores, genital ulcers, neonatal infections
Human papilloma-viruses	Nonenveloped double-stranded DNA virus	Warts, genital warts, cervical cancer
Rubella virus	Enveloped polyhedral capsid with single-stranded RNA	German measles; can cause significant birth defects when pregnant women are infected
Rubeola virus	Enveloped helical capsid with single-stranded RNA	Measles; pneumonia and encephalitis complications
Varicella-zoster virus	Enveloped polyhedral capsid with double-stranded DNA	Chicken pox; shingles as a latent manifestation

An Outbreak of *Staphylococcus aureus* with Increased Vancomycin Resistance

ILLINOIS, 1999

Since 1996, *Staphylococcus aureus* with an intermediate level of vancomycin resistance (vancomycin-intermediate *Staphylococcus aureus* [VISA]) has been identified in Europe and Asia. The emergence of reduced vancomycin susceptibility in *S. aureus* increases the possibility that some strains will become fully resistant and that available antimicrobial agents will become ineffective for treating infections caused by such strains.

In April 1999, a 63-year-old woman with methicillin-resistant *Staphylococcus aureus* (MRSA) bacteremia was transferred from a long-term care facility to an Illinois hospital (hospital A). If a bacterium is resistant to methicillin, an antibiotic that is not degraded by bacterial penicillinases, then the bacterium has a mutation in a penicillin-binding protein so that it will not bind the penicillins. As a result, the bacterium is resistant to treatment by nearly all drugs of the penicillin group. The patient had a history of frequent hospitalizations for complications of hemodialysis-dependent end stage renal disease and multiple central-venous-catheter-associated infections. Thirteen days after hospital admission and 25 days after vancomycin therapy was initiated, a culture from her blood grew *S. aureus* with an intermediate level of vancomycin resistance. Three subsequent blood specimens drawn within the next 3 days confirmed the increased vancomycin resistance. The isolates were genetically identical and were resistant to penicillin, oxacillin, clindamycin, erythromycin, ciprofloxacin, and rifampin but susceptible to trimethoprim-sulfamethoxazole, tetracycline, and gentamicin and had intermediate susceptibility to chloramphenicol. No VISA strains were recovered from other body sites.

S. aureus can be transmitted by direct contact. It can also asymptomatically colonize the skin and nasal mucosa. As a result, both the facility's staff and members of the patient's family were potentially

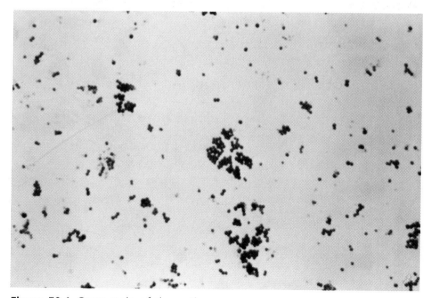

Figure 50.1 Gram stain of the pathogen.

exposed. Before her death, the woman was visited by friends in the long-term care facility and by her immediate family and grandchildren while in the hospital.

APPLICATION

Assume you are the head of the office in charge of public health activities for the state of Illinois. Your assignment is to minimize deaths and prevent future outbreaks of VISA infection. Although your resources are large, they are not infinite, and you must use the existing health care infrastructure (unless you can make a convincing case to the state legislature for additional funds). Consequently, you must prioritize your investment in manpower and resources to accomplish your task. How would you prioritize the expenditure of funds and resources? Focus your answers to address only one area of health care or research for each answer.

1. What would be your first priority? Why?

2. What would be your second priority? Why?

3. What would be your third priority? Why?

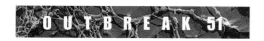

An Outbreak of *Pseudomonas* Dermatitis from a Hotel Pool and Hot Tub

COLORADO, 1999

In February 1999, the Colorado Department of Public Health and Environment was notified of approximately 15 people who had developed an infectious skin rash after they used a hotel pool and hot tub. The cases occurred among children and adults attending two birthday parties at the hotel and among community residents who entered the pool on a pay-to-swim basis.

Twenty-five community residents who used the pool and/or hot tub between 5 and 7 February were identified through discussions with area physicians, hotel management, and other swimmers. These community residents were interviewed by the Colorado Department of Public Health and Environment by using a telephone questionnaire. Case patients were defined as people who developed an infectious skin rash, with or without other symptoms, within 3 days of using either the pool or the hot tub at the hotel. Questionnaires were completed for 22 (88%) of the 25 people identified. Of the 20 people who had used the hot tub, 19 had developed a rash and met the case definition.

Analysis of the rash indicated the infection was primarily within hair follicles or in the dermis. Fourteen (74%) of the 19 case patients had more severe illnesses (a rash of ≥2 weeks duration or rash and one other symptom), some lasting more than 6 weeks.

Specimens collected from the hot tub filter and hand rail base during the environmental inspection in May were cultured. The pathogenic bacterium was motile using polar flagella and oxidase positive (it had a particular type of enzyme that many other gram-negative rods do not). Additional biochemical tests led to identification of the pathogen as *Pseudomonas aeruginosa*.

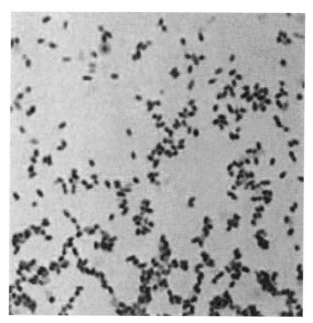

Figure 51.1 Gram stain of the pathogen.

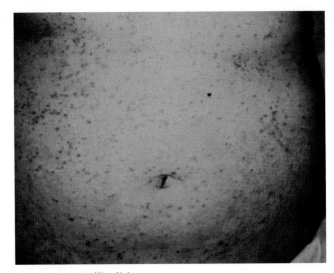

Figure 51.2 Folliculitis.

The pool and hot tub used separate filtration systems; each had an automated chlorination system that relied on an on-site probe to measure free-chlorine and pH levels and to deliver preset levels of chlorine using calcium hypochlorite tablets and muriatic acid for pH control. A printout of the hourly free-chlorine and pH levels in the pool and hot tub revealed that free-chlorine levels dropped below state-required levels (1 milligram/liter) on the evening of 4 February and remained below recommended levels for approximately 69 hours. The decline in pool chlorine levels was the result of a faulty chlorine pellet dispenser.

QUESTIONS

1. Besides *Pseudomonas*, list and describe three potential pathogens that could have caused the infectious skin rash.

2. What physical features make *Pseudomonas aeruginosa* a more likely pathogen than the others you listed?

3. How would you have treated the infection of the swimmers?

4. How would you have stopped the outbreak and prevented future outbreaks?

A Ringworm Outbreak in a Wrestling Team

ALASKA, 1993

Most of the members of the Wasilla High School wrestling team developed skin rashes during the winter of 1993. After notification of the outbreak by a local physician, the Alaska State Section of Epidemiology began an investigation. Of the 28 boys on the team who were examined, 79% reported having one or more skin lesions. The lesions lasted more than 5 days and were found on the upper body. None were found on the scalp or finger- or toenails. A total of 76 lesions were identified, with one wrestler having 28 lesions. The lesions were typically 1 to 3 centimeters in diameter and were scaly, round, and red.

An Anchorage dermatologist had evaluated three team members and identified eukaryotic filamentous cells on potassium hydroxide-treated skin scrapings from each boy. The Section of Epidemiology also obtained skin scrapings for examination and identified eukaryotic filamentous pathogens from 17 boys with suspicious lesions.

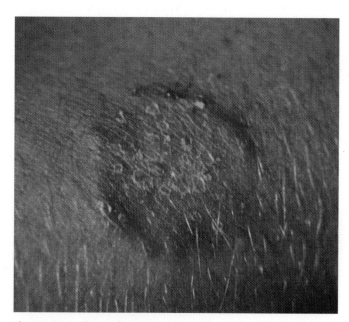

Figure 52.1 Skin infection.

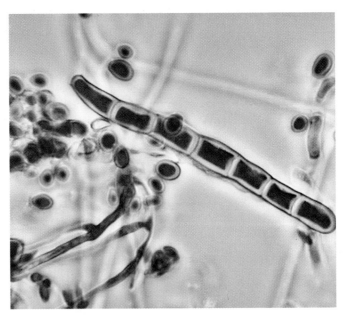

Figure 52.2 Light micrograph of the pathogen.

QUESTIONS

1. Name and describe the pathogen that caused the outbreak.

2. Describe how the pathogen is spread.

3. How would you have treated the lesions on the wrestlers?

4. How would you have stopped the outbreak and prevented future outbreaks?

An Outbreak of Conjunctivitis at an Elementary School

MAINE, 2002

On 18 October 2002, the nurse at an elementary school in Westbrook, Maine, notified the Maine Bureau of Health of an increase in the number of students with conjunctivitis. Between 23 September and 18 October, a total of 31 students in kindergarten and in first and second grades either were reported by parents to the nurse as having conjunctivitis or had conjunctivitis diagnosed by the nurse at school. Conjunctival swab cultures from some students grew an alpha-hemolytic, gram-positive streptococcus on blood agar.

School nurses and child care center managers were asked to report to the Maine Bureau of Health any child or staff member who had onset of conjunctivitis between 20 September and 6 December. Among 361 students, 28% had at least one episode of conjunctivitis. The attack rate was highest among first-grade students (51 of 136), followed by morning kindergarten. Conjunctivitis was also found among school staff, family members who did not attend school, and household contacts of infected students. School nurses and child care staff in the community reported an additional 77 students who had conjunctivitis.

The symptoms reported most commonly were red eyes; itchy, painful, or burning eyes; crusty eyes in the morning; grey or yellow discharge from the eyes; and swelling of the eyelids. Sixty-five students each missed an average of 2 days of school during their illnesses.

Isolates that were tested for antimicrobial susceptibility were resistant to erythromycin but were susceptible to penicillin and broad-spectrum cephalosporins.

QUESTIONS

1. Based on the laboratory results and clinical description, identify and describe the pathogenic agent.

2. How would you have treated those with conjunctivitis?

3. How does the pathogen cause tissue damage?

4. Why was the highest incidence of conjunctivitis in the first-grade and kindergarten classes?

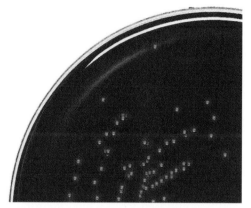

Figure 53.1 Colony morphology on blood agar.

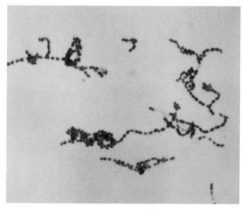

Figure 53.2 Gram stain of the pathogen.

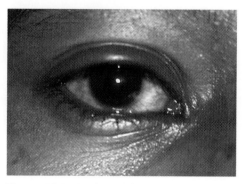

Figure 53.3 Conjunctivitis.

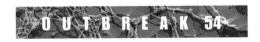

A Measles Outbreak among Internationally Adopted Children

UNITED STATES, 2001

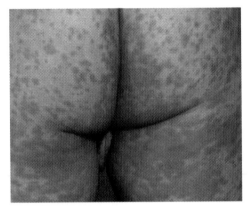

Figure 54.1 Macular rash.

On 16 February 2001, the Texas Department of Health was notified of a child, aged 10 months, adopted from orphanage A in China, who was taken to a Texas hospital with measles. The child had fever, conjunctivitis, Koplik's spots, and a macular rash. The ill adopted child (index case) had traveled with a fever on international (China-to-Los Angeles) and domestic (Los Angeles-to-Houston) flights on commercial airlines and had been part of a cohort of adopted children from China who had lived in orphanage A. These children and their adoptive families had spent 2 weeks or more together in China while the families were visiting the orphanage and completing the immigrant visa process.

The index case potentially exposed multiple people during the communicable period, including members of 63 families who had traveled to China to adopt children, representatives from 16 international adoption agencies who accompanied the families, staff at the local medical facility in China at which the patient was examined as a requirement for a U.S. immigrant visa, staff at the U.S. consulate, passengers and crew members of the international and domestic flights on which the patient traveled, and adoption agency representatives who met the returning family.

Investigation of other recently adopted children from China identified 10 children aged 9 to 12 months from seven states who were also infected. Analysis of the incubation period for the disease indicated the adopted children were probably infected in China. The Central China Adoption Agency and the Centers for Disease Control and Prevention were charged with developing a collaborative strategy to control and prevent further spread of this infectious disease.

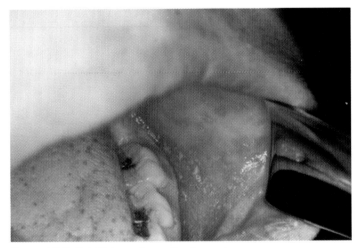

Figure 54.2 Koplik's spots on the buccal mucosa.

160

QUESTIONS

1. What pathogen caused the outbreak?

2. How was it transmitted?

3. Describe the serious complications that can result from the disease.

4. What is the risk group(s) primarily susceptible to serious complications from the disease?

5. What would have been your first priority for preventing the spread of this pathogen through the U.S. population?

6. What would have been your second priority?

7. How is the disease prevented?

8. Explain why the criteria for immunity to the disease are (i) having been born before 1957, (ii) a history of physician diagnosis of the disease, (iii) documentation of having received two doses of the vaccine, and (iv) serologic evidence of immunity.

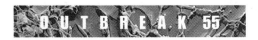

A Hepatitis Outbreak at a Pain Clinic

OKLAHOMA, 2002

In August 2002, the Oklahoma State Department of Health was informed of six patients with blood-borne infections who had received treatment from the same pain remediation clinic. Clinical features indicated the patients all had hepatitis: fatigue, anorexia, nausea, malaise, fever, jaundice, vomiting, dark-colored urine, white stools, and abdominal pain. A preliminary investigation by the Oklahoma State Department of Health found that a certified registered nurse anesthetist reused needles and syringes routinely during clinic sessions. A single needle and syringe were used to administer each of three different sedation medications to up to 24 sequentially treated patients at each clinic session. These medications were administered through intravenous tubes.

On the basis of these findings, an investigation was initiated. Serologic testing for blood-borne pathogens was completed for 793 (87%) of the 908 patients attending the clinic. A total of 100 infections that probably were acquired in the clinic were identified.

Several pathogens were identified through direct and indirect enzyme-linked immunosorbent assays (ELISAs). Sixty-nine patients were infected with a virus having a positive-sense single-stranded ribonucleic acid (RNA), a polyhedral capsid, and an envelope. Thirty-one were infected with a double-stranded deoxyribonucleic acid (DNA) virus with a double-shelled capsid.

QUESTIONS

1. Name three different viruses that cause hepatitis.

2. Which two viruses were transmitted at the clinic?

3. How would you have treated the individuals affected by the disease?

4. How would you have stopped the outbreak and prevented similar outbreaks in the future?

5. What actions should be taken with regard to the nurse and the clinic administration?

An Outbreak of Flesh-Eating Bacteria

SAINT JOHN, CANADA, 2004

In late April 2004, a 37-year-old woman died of necrotizing fasciitis (massive death of connective tissues) after routine day surgery at St. Joseph's Hospital in Saint John, Canada. Another man who was at the same hospital was also infected with the virulent strain but survived. The two patients confirmed to have the disease were both patients at the same day surgery unit at St. Joseph's Hospital in Saint John. Five other patients, who also had surgery on the same day as those diagnosed with necrotizing fasciitis, were tested for the pathogen—three were infected. In the 16 months preceding the cases described above, 12 people were also diagnosed with the infection and survived. In the 3 years before that, there was only one case per year in the Saint John region. Health officials said they had not found the source of the disease.

The health officials said it was difficult to pinpoint the source because the bacterium that caused the infection is common and comes in many forms. In its invasive form, it causes severe tissue damage that needs to be removed surgically. This can result in the amputation of the affected limb. Some people are transient carriers; others are chronic carriers. A transient carrier is a person who picks up the bacteria temporarily and can pass them on. A chronic carrier has the bacteria indefinitely. None of the staff who were screened were shown to be chronic carriers.

Laboratory results of tests on blood isolated from individuals infected by the pathogen indicated the pathogen was a beta-hemolytic, bacitracin-sensitive, gram-positive coccus arranged in chains.

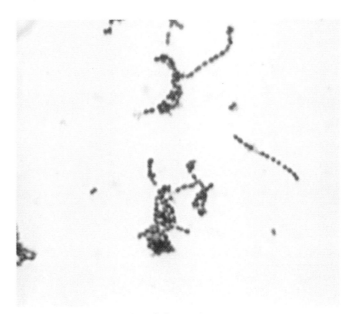

Figure 56.1 Gram stain of the pathogen.

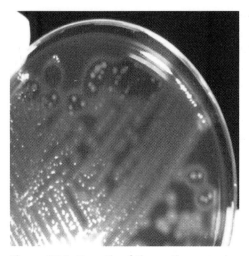

Figure 56.2 Growth of the pathogen on blood agar.

QUESTIONS

1. What is the name of the pathogen that caused the necrotizing fasciitis?

2. What characteristics of the pathogen enabled it to invade tissues and cause massive damage?

3. How was the pathogen transmitted?

4. What type of investigation would you have performed to discover the source of the pathogen?

An Outbreak of Invasive Group A *Streptococcus* at a Child Care Center

BOSTON, MASSACHUSETTS, 1997

On 2 February 1997, a previously healthy 4-year-old girl (patient 1) who had had onset of chicken pox on 30 January was taken to a local hospital because of swelling, tenderness, warmth, and redness over her left upper arm and shoulder. Pus-filled skin lesions were not present, and a blood culture did not grow any bacteria. The patient was admitted to the hospital and received intravenous clindamycin, but her symptoms did not improve. She underwent surgical exploration and subsequently received a total fasciotomy (removal of the connective tissue surrounding the muscle) of her left arm. Cultures of tissue specimens obtained at surgery grew a beta-hemolytic bacterium on blood agar plates. The hemolytic colonies were Gram stained to reveal gram-positive streptococci. Other clinical tests indicated the pathogen had group A antigen on its surface.

On 6 February, 7 days after the onset of chicken pox infection, an abscess was diagnosed in a 3-year-old child who went to the same day care center as patient 1. No obviously infected lesions were located over or near the abscess, and a blood culture was negative. The abscess was incised and drained, and the contents also grew group A streptococci.

A total of 39 children aged 1 to 4 years were enrolled in the child care center. Of the 14 classmates of patients 1 and 2, 3 had pharyngitis (sore throat) caused by the pathogen and 2 carried the pathogen asymptomatically in their pharynxes. Two additional possible cases of infection were identified, one with an infected chicken pox lesion and the other with leg cellulitis. Of the 25 children in other classrooms, 1 had scarlet fever. Of the 92 household contacts, 3 had pharyngitis, and the bacterium was carried by 2 healthy individuals. Of the 13 child care center workers, 1 carried the bacterium.

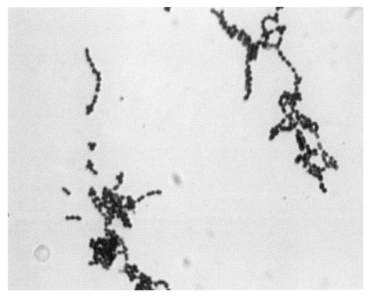

Figure 57.1 Gram stain of the pathogen.

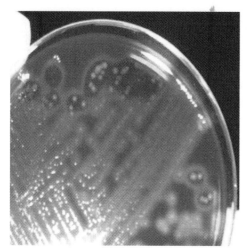

Figure 57.2 Growth of the pathogen on blood agar.

The first case of chicken pox occurred on 15 January; of the other 11 children susceptible to chicken pox, 10 had onset of chicken pox between 29 January and 1 February. Of these, seven were identified with the bacterial infection. Of 112 environmental surfaces cultured to assess the possible role of fomites (nonliving intermediates that can carry pathogens to a new host), six plastic food utensils were positive for the pathogen.

Children who spent more than 30 hours per week at the child care center were significantly more likely to be infected with the pathogen than children who spent 30 hours or less per week there.

QUESTIONS

1. What pathogen caused this outbreak?

2. Describe how the chicken pox outbreak contributed to the spread of the pathogen.

3. How would you have treated those with purulent lesions? Cellulitis? Pharyngitis? Scarlet fever? Asymptomatic carriers?

4. What characteristics of the pathogen enable it to cause invasive infections?

5. How would you have managed this outbreak?

A Skin Infection Outbreak at a High School

HOUSTON, TEXAS, 2002

Since the second week of school, faculty and students at Sam Rayburn High School in Houston, Texas, had to cope with an outbreak of boils and skin infections. The outbreak affected many on the football team and dance team and then spread to other students and schools, resulting in about 50 cases.

One mother had two children who contracted the bacterial infection. She said they were infected at Sam Rayburn High School, where they both attended class. The mother stated that her son, who was on the football team, had to make 20 trips to the doctor and had missed about 13 days of school because of the boils on his skin. The mother claimed the school district was not responding to the outbreak.

Laboratory tests were used to identify the pathogen. The pathogen was catalase positive (it had an enzyme that breaks down H_2O_2), coagulase positive (it had an enzyme that causes blood to clot), and was resistant to β-lactams, including ampicillin/clavulanate and methicillin.

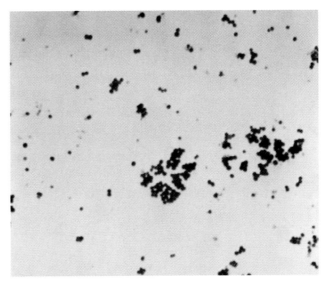

Figure 58.1 Gram stain of the pathogen.

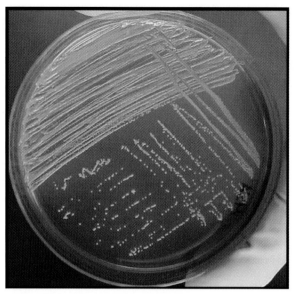

Figure 58.2 Growth of the pathogen on mannitol salt agar.

QUESTIONS

1. What pathogen caused this outbreak?

2. What type of mutation causes resistance to β-lactams and methicillin? How does this differ from the changes that cause resistance to many β-lactams but not methicillin?

3. Describe the mode of transmission of the pathogen and explain why it appeared to primarily affect the football and dance teams.

4. What was the reservoir for the pathogen?

5. Describe the pathogenesis for boils.

6. How would you have treated those affected?

7. How would you have managed this outbreak and prevented future outbreaks?

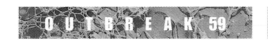

A Gas Gangrene Outbreak after a Tsunami

PAPUA NEW GUINEA, 1998

A tsunami hit the coastal town of Aitape, Papua New Guinea. In response to the disaster, a United Nations Disaster Assessment and Coordination team conducted an aerial survey of the devastated area. The scene as seen from the air was one of near-total devastation, with trees, vegetation, and buildings mostly destroyed. Twelve days after the giant wave struck, seven evacuation centers were established in isolated inland areas. Most had no road access, and relief items and personnel had to be flown in by helicopter. The evacuation centers had about 9,000 people who needed daily food, water, and shelter. Twenty-eight people were missing, and over 2,100 were dead.

Attending to the severely injured and the sick was the top priority during the emergency phase. The opening of the Australia-New Zealand army field hospital in Vanimo allowed surgery to be performed locally. The Australian military field hospital at Vanimo was successful in its relief efforts until one evening, when 13 patients with gas gangrene arrived. The infection affected patients who had previously been injured with deep wounds. The pathogen quickly caused a massive life-threatening infection. As a result, already exhausted doctors and nurses were faced with another 12-hour stretch of emergency surgery to try to save lives and limbs.

One of those brought in was an 8-year-old boy from Malol village. His left leg was too far gone to save and was amputated below the knee. The head of the Australian medical team, Major Paul Taylor, said the pathogen had been identified as an anaerobic soilborne bacterium that produced gas and a toxin that seriously damaged tissue. When a large infection is found deep in the lower limb, there is almost no way to successfully clear the infection.

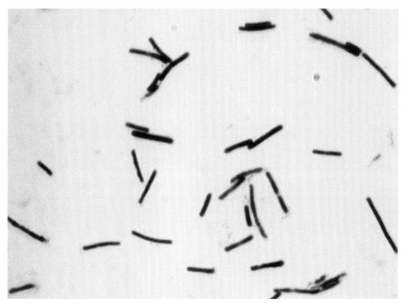

Figure 59.1 Gram stain of the pathogen.

QUESTIONS

1. What pathogen causes gas gangrene?
2. Why does the pathogen affect those with traumatic injuries?
3. How does the infection cause massive tissue damage?
4. How would you have treated those affected by the pathogen?
5. How would you have stopped the outbreak?

Bacterial Conjunctivitis

Conjunctivitis is considered extremely common worldwide. In the United States, conjunctivitis is responsible for approximately 30% of all eye complaints from people seeking treatment in the emergency department. Conjunctivitis can be caused by allergies, viruses, and bacteria.

Cause of the disease

Streptococcus pneumoniae is a common cause of bacterial conjunctivitis. It is a gram-positive, lancet-shaped bacterium usually found in pairs or short chains. The pathogen produces a toxin causing alpha-hemolysis of erythrocytes (it damages red blood cells so that they release a green pigment); it is nonmotile and facultatively anaerobic (it grows with or without oxygen). The pathogen has a polysaccharide capsule that offers protection from phagocytosis

Transmission

Reservoir

The pathogen is commonly found in the upper respiratory tract, especially the nasopharynx.

Mode of transmission

The pathogen is spread by droplets or through direct contact or by indirect contact via fomites contaminated with the pathogen.

Pathogenesis

Entry

The pathogen is commonly introduced from the environment by individuals rubbing their eyes. Pathogen-containing droplets can be introduced into the eye by coughing or sneezing.

Attachment

Streptococcus pneumoniae attaches to cell surface glycolipids on the host cell.

Avoiding host defenses

The pathogen has an antiphagocytic capsule.

Damage

The pathogen produces many tissue-damaging enzymes and toxins, including neuraminidase (which contributes to invasiveness), proteases (which suppress host cell immunity and facilitate colonization), and pneumolysin O (which inhibits phagocytic attack). In addition, *S. pneumoniae* produces teichoic acids and peptidoglycans that cause an inflammatory response leading to red eyes, tissue swelling, and pus production.

Exit

The pathogen can exit through pus discharge from the eye.

Clinical features

Conjunctivitis, also called pinkeye, normally presents as red, swollen eyes with pus discharge. Unlike allergic conjunctivitis, bacterial conjunctivitis often is not accompanied by ocular itching. An inflamed membrane and a velvety, beefy-red conjunctiva suggest bacterial conjunctivitis. People experience morning crusting and difficulty opening the eyelids. Furthermore, bacterial pinkeye is usually not seasonal.

Diagnosis

Specimen

A pus sample is obtained.

Tests

Growth of alpha-hemolytic colonies on blood agar and identification of gram-positive streptococci by microscopy are the diagnostic tests.

Treatment

Treatment for bacterial conjunctivitis typically involves several different classes of antibiotics, which inhibit a broad spectrum of pathogens. Eye drops commonly have neomycin, polymyxin B, and dexamethasone, an anti-inflammatory agent. Neomycin inhibits gram-negative pathogens by blocking formation of the 30S initiation complex during protein synthesis. Polymyxin B inhibits gram-positive pathogens by damaging bacterial cytoplasmic membranes by binding to phospholipids, thus altering permeability and causing general damage.

Prevention

- Wash hands frequently and thoroughly.
- Avoid touching and rubbing the eye.
- Replace eye cosmetics regularly, and do not share eye cosmetics with others.
- Do not share towels or handkerchiefs.
- Properly use and care for contact lenses.

Gas Gangrene

Gas gangrene cases are relatively rare, with only several thousand cases reported annually in the United States. Most cases are the result of trauma from motorcycle accidents. Worldwide, gas gangrene has the highest incidence in areas with poor access to proper wound care. Although rare, the infection is life threatening, with a mortality rate of 25% even when treated. The mortality rate can be much higher if treatment is delayed.

Cause of the disease

Clostridium perfringens, a bacterial pathogen, is a gram-positive, rod-shaped bacterium that can form endospores, specialized cells that are resistant to drying, temperature changes, O_2, antibiotics, disinfectants, and heat. The pathogen is an obligate anaerobic organism that does not tolerate O_2. When an endospore from soil or feces is introduced into a suitable anaerobic environment, such as a puncture wound, it germinates and produces reproducing vegetative cells. The vegetative cells use fermentative metabolism and produce CO_2 as a by-product.

Transmission

Reservoir

The pathogen is found in soil and the intestinal tracts of animals.

Mode of transmission

The pathogen is transmitted via the parenteral route by entering traumatic wounds. Gangrene is a noncommunicable disease; it cannot be spread person to person. An infection causing gangrene is acquired by contamination of a wound with soil or feces.

Pathogenesis

Entry

Entry is via dirt- or feces-contaminated wounds with significant vascular damage that prevents oxygenated blood delivery to the site of injury.

Attachment

Penetrating traumatic injury makes it difficult to remove the pathogen from the damaged tissues.

Avoiding host defenses

Traumatic injury to a tissue reduces blood supply to the muscle. This results in lactic acid fermentation in the muscle tissue, causing a drop in pH. The lowered pH and lack of O_2 provide a suitable environment for clostridial growth. With reduced blood supply, normal host defenses are impaired.

Damage

The pathogen produces alpha-toxin, which is the primary cause of damage, and at least 20 other, different toxins. Many are hemolytic (they lyse erythrocytes) and dermonecrotic (they kill cells of soft tissues). Some enzymes digest connective tissues, which allows the pathogen to invade deeper tissues. As the surrounding tissue is destroyed, gas from fermentation is produced in the muscle bundles, increasing the pressure and restricting blood flow. Thus, the pathogen creates an anaerobic environment and can spread into the damaged tissue.

Clinical features

The typical incubation period for gas gangrene is less than 24 hours. Local swelling and pain are followed by the skin turning a bronze color and then progressing to a blue-black color with hemorrhagic swellings. Local effects include necrosis of muscle and subcutaneous fat and clotting of blood vessels. Marked swelling also restricts further blood supply to the region, making it easier for the anaerobic *Clostridium perfringens* to spread. Fermentation of glucose probably is the main mechanism of gas production in gas gangrene. The production of gas breaks apart the muscle bundles and facilitates rapid spread of the infection. Destruction of erythrocytes and fluid loss can cause renal failure and shock, leading to death. Gas gangrene is lethal in 25% of cases, but this can approach 100% when treatment is delayed.

Diagnosis

Clinical

Clinical diagnosis is based on the presence of necrotic tissue plus a radiograph of the infected area showing the typical feathering pattern of gas in soft tissue.

Laboratory

A Gram stain of pus or infected tissues reveals large gram-positive bacilli.

Treatment

The combination of aggressive surgical debridement (removal of dead tissues) and effective antibiotic therapy is the determining factor for successful treatment of this life-threatening infection. Using a hyperbaric chamber to increase the O_2 concentration in the damaged tissue may help reduce further damage.

Currently, a combination of penicillin and clindamycin is widely used. Penicillin blocks cell wall formation, killing the pathogen. Clindamycin is a macrolide that inhibits protein synthesis by stimulating the dissociation of peptidyl-transfer RNA (tRNA), thereby preventing completion of proteins. By blocking protein synthesis, clindamycin prevents synthesis of the tissue-damaging toxins.

Patients with gas gangrene frequently have multiple serious conditions as a result of the infection and require intensive supportive care.

Prevention

- Gas gangrene is most often a complication of traumatic injury. As a result, it is prevalent following wars and natural disasters, when aid for injuries may be unavailable or delayed. Rapid cleaning and treatment of injuries are the keys to prevention.

Group A Streptococcus Infections

Group A streptococci (GAS) can infect a variety of tissues. Erysipelas is an acute infection of the skin associated with lymphatic involvement. Cellulitis (infection of the tissue under the skin) is inflammation of the skin and subcutaneous tissues and is associated with local pain, tenderness, swelling, and redness, along with systemic symptoms, including fever, chills, and malaise. Necrotizing fasciitis (destruction and death of connective tissue due to infection) is a rapidly invasive infection with GAS that may arise following minor trauma or from the spread of GAS from the throat to the site of blunt trauma or muscle strain. Any of these conditions can lead to the spread of GAS to the blood. GAS bacteremia is a serious infection with a mortality rate of 25 to 48%.

Cause of the disease

Necrotizing fasciitis and other invasive skin infections are often caused by invasive forms of *Streptococcus pyogenes*, a bacterial pathogen.

Streptococcus pyogenes is a gram-positive streptococcus. It has the group A antigen on its surface. The M protein on the cell wall is antiphagocytic. Invasive *Streptococcus pyogenes* also produces a number of enzymes that enable it to digest connective tissues and lyse erythrocytes.

Transmission

Reservoir

The reservoir for *Streptococcus pyogenes* is the skin and upper respiratory tract mucous membranes.

Mode of transmission

Streptococcus pyogenes enters the human body through the respiratory tract, skin, superficial membranes, or traumatized tissues. It is transmitted through direct contact or respiratory droplets.

Pathogenesis

Entry

The pathogen is easily transmitted. It is often carried in the nasopharyngeal region and can be transmitted by contaminated droplets or nonrespiratory epithelial cells. Open wounds are especially susceptible to infection.

Attachment

The bacterial F protein attaches to fibronectin receptors found on the host cells.

Avoiding host defenses

The pathogen avoids host defenses because the M protein of the cell wall is antiphagocytic.

Damage

Following insult, bacteria are introduced into the subcutaneous tissue. The enzymes hyaluronidase (which digests the extracellular matrix of cartilage) and collagenase (which digests connective tissue) enable the pathogen to digest fascia and rapidly spread to the adjacent tissue. Massive necrosis (tissue death) of the subcutaneous fat and fascia quickly follows, due to the pathogen's release of enzymes and toxins. Pyrogenic exotoxins cause mononuclear leukocytes to release tumor necrosis factor, interleukin-1, and interleukin-6, which in turn produce fever, shock, tissue injury, suppression of B-lymphocyte function, and cell death.

Clinical features

Early clinical findings may include an area with a small amount of redness and swelling, with rapid progression of tenderness out of proportion to the clinical appearance of the wound. Destruction of the vascular supply leads to death of the overlying skin. More advanced cases involve attacks on the muscle and bone by the bacteria. Patients rapidly deteriorate, with altered mental status, fever, septicemia, electrolyte abnormalities, and hemolytic anemia. In addition to the tissue decay, the rapid spread of the bacteria can cause total systemic shock, resulting in respiratory failure, heart failure, low blood pressure, and renal failure, which can lead to death.

Diagnosis

Clinical appearance

The appearance of the skin and presence of gangrenous changes (black or dead tissue) indicate necrotizing subcutaneous infection.

Laboratory

Specimen: A sample of pus or blood is obtained.

Tests: Streptococcus pyogenes can be identified by beta-hemolytic growth of gram-positive streptococci on blood agar. An ELISA can be used to identify group A streptococci.

Treatment

Early medical treatment is critical. Aggressive surgical debridement is required, with amputation in severe cases. Intense supportive care in the hospital is often necessary.

Streptococcus pyogenes is typically sensitive to β-lactam antibiotics. Penicillin is often used. Penicillin blocks formation of the peptide cross-bridges that link peptidoglycan together. As a result, the cell wall is not formed and the bacteria are killed by osmotic lysis.

Prevention

- The single biggest preventive measure is to simply keep the skin intact. By not puncturing the epidermis, the possibility of infection by the bacteria is greatly reduced. Small cuts and skin abrasions should be thoroughly cleaned, treated with antibiotic ointments, and covered.
- Individuals should wash their hands thoroughly, especially after coughing and sneezing and before preparing and eating food.

Hepatitis B Virus Infection

Hepatitis refers to any infection that leads to the inflammation and destruction of the liver. Although hepatitis is mostly caused by viruses, there have been cases in which the cause of disease was bacteria or other microorganisms. There are five different viruses that cause hepatitis; the focus here will be on hepatitis B virus (HBV). In the United States, 4,000 people die each year from HBV-related liver complications. Worldwide, HBV is the ninth leading cause of death by infectious disease.

Cause of the disease

HBV has a double-stranded circular DNA genome, a polyhedral capsid, and an envelope.

Transmission

Reservoir

Humans are the only reservoir.

Mode of transmission

Horizontal: Transmission is by the parenteral route. The pathogen requires blood-to-blood exchange.

Vertical: HBV can be passed between a mother and newborn child at birth.

Pathogenesis

The incubation period is 1 to 12 weeks.

Entry

In horizontal transmission, HBV is primarily spread by blood-to-blood exchange when intravenous-drug users share needles. Accidental needle sticks with contaminated blood in health care settings and tattooing, ear piercing, and acupuncture with contaminated needles have also been implicated. HBV is believed to be spread through homosexual and heterosexual contact, particularly in the presence of genital ulcers.

Attachment

Envelope proteins attach to receptors on liver cells.

Avoiding host defenses

The virus is an intracellular pathogen and initially avoids destruction by antibodies and cells of the immune system.

Damage

As the virus replicates, it destroys tissues in the liver, causing inflammation and physiological changes (hepatitis).

Exit

The virus exits via contaminated blood to infect a new host.

Clinical features

The majority of people do not have any symptoms at the onset of hepatitis B virus infection. Signs and symptoms include loss of appetite, nausea, diarrhea, fatigue, muscle or joint aches, and mild fever. HBV has been known to silently attack the liver, which leads to cirrhosis and possibly death from hepatic failure. Approximately 25 to 35% of those infected may have dark urine, jaundice, or light-colored stools. After 6 months of having HBV in the bloodstream, patients are considered to be carriers and are chronically infected.

Diagnosis

Specimen

A blood sample is used as a specimen.

Test

Common tests use monoclonal antibodies in ELISA and radioimmunoassay to detect HBV in the blood.

Treatment

The main treatment used for chronic hepatitis B virus carriers is high doses of alpha interferon. A few carriers, however, do not benefit from this treatment. A new drug, lamivudine, is being tested as a treatment for chronic HBV infection. While these drugs seem to help, neither is a cure.

Prevention

- The primary means of prevention of hepatitis B is the hepatitis B vaccine. The Centers for Disease Control and Prevention and the American Academy of Pediatrics recommend that all newborn infants and children (especially sexually active teenagers) be vaccinated against hepatitis B virus. Those who are already infected will not benefit from vaccination; however, infants born to infected mothers (or mothers who are carriers of HBV) can be protected.

Hepatitis C Virus Infection

Approximately 4 million Americans have been infected with hepatitis C virus (HCV), with about the same number being infected each year around the world.

Cause of the disease

HCV belongs to the family *Flaviviridae*. The virus is enveloped and has single-stranded RNA as its genetic information, protected by a polyhedral capsid.

Transmission

Reservoir
Human blood is the reservoir.

Mode of transmission
Horizontal: Horizontal transmission occurs by the parenteral route through sharing contaminated needles. Less common ways to transmit this virus include sexual contact and organ and blood donation.
Vertical: Mother-to-fetus transmission may occur.

Pathogenesis

Acute infection is cleared naturally through the bloodstream in 15 to 25% of infected people; however, most people develop chronic infection.

Entry
The pathogen most commonly entered through infected blood during blood transfusions given prior to 1992, before blood was screened to eliminate HCV-contaminated units. HCV is now transmitted by intravenous drug users sharing needles and by accidental needle sticks among health care workers.

Attachment
HCV attaches to the liver.

Avoiding host defenses
The virus is an intracellular pathogen and initially avoids destruction by antibodies and cells of the immune system.

Damage
As the virus replicates, it destroys tissues in the liver, causing inflammation and physiological changes (hepatitis). HCV causes inflammation and infection of the liver, which result in necrosis. The damage caused by HCV also includes cirrhosis of the liver and can induce primary liver cancer.

Clinical features

Most people with acute infections are asymptomatic; however, some people might experience jaundice, anorexia, abdominal pain, fatigue, and nausea. People with chronic infection normally do not show signs and symptoms until 10 to 20 years later, when complications involving the liver are reported.

Diagnosis

The primary way to diagnose HCV is through an ELISA, which is both accurate and sensitive.

Diagnosis of a chronic infection may include a liver biopsy to determine the presence and extent of fibrosis.

Treatment

There is no cure for HCV infection; however, antivirals can be used for treatment. Unfortunately, these drugs are not always effective, and therefore, they are used only for chronic infection. One of the drugs used is interferon, which represses HCV replication. Ribavirin is used with interferon in order to be more effective. The combination of these two drugs has a very high incidence of side effects, forcing many people to discontinue treatment, which usually lasts 6 months.

Prevention

- There is no vaccine for HCV infection, and there is no cure. Therefore, prevention efforts rely entirely on the behavior of people susceptible to HCV infection and health care workers.
- Safe injection practices in health care settings and screening of blood and organ donors help prevent infection.
- Those who should be tested include intravenous-drug users, people with known human immunodeficiency virus infection, and people who had a blood transfusion or organ transplant before 1992.

Measles

Worldwide, measles is the number six cause of death by infectious disease, with approximately 1 million deaths from 30 million infections annually. Most deaths occur in Africa and Southeast Asia in children under 5 years of age as a result of pneumonia or encephalitis caused by the measles infection.

In the United States, measles is primarily an imported disease. Infected individuals from other countries cause local outbreaks in people who are unvaccinated or inadequately vaccinated.

Cause of the disease

Measles virus is a member of the paramyxovirus family. It is an enveloped virus with a helical capsid containing single-stranded RNA with a negative-sense polarity.

Transmission

Reservoir

Symptomatic humans are the reservoir.

Mode of transmission

Airborne and droplet modes of transmission occur. Airborne viral particles are stable for 2 hours when suspended in the air but are quickly inactivated upon landing on surfaces.

Pathogenesis

Entry

The pathogen enters via inhalation of airborne particles or mucus droplets.

Attachment

Envelope proteins attach to the CD46 receptor on host cells in the respiratory epithelium.

Spread

The virus is carried by leukocytes to subepithelial and local tissues, multiplies in lymphoid tissues, and disseminates via the bloodstream throughout the body.

Avoiding host defenses

The virus replicates intracellularly, so it initially avoids circulating antibodies. The virus also destroys T cells, making it immunosuppressive.

Damage

The measles virus directly damages the host cell it infects. Most of the damage is done to the mucosal surface of the respiratory tract. Besides the direct damage, infection by the virus causes cells to fuse together into giant cells (syncytia). These cells can further restrict gas exchange and complicate measles pneumonia. As a result of the damage and immunosuppres-

sion, secondary bacterial infections are common. After initial infection, the virus travels to lymphoid tissue, causing a secondary viremia which spreads the pathogen to tissues under the skin. The resulting inflammatory response initiates rash formation.

Exit

The pathogen exits via the respiratory route and continues to do so for 3 or 4 days after the rash is gone.

Clinical features

The incubation period is typically 10 to 14 days, followed by an acute respiratory illness, including runny nose, fever, conjunctivitis, sensitivity to light, and cough. The fever rises steadily until the appearance of the rash 2 to 4 days later. A maculopapular rash (small red, slightly raised spots) begins on the head and spreads down to the trunk and outward toward the extremities. Koplik's spots (pinpoint blue-white spots on a red background) appear on the inside of the cheeks (buccal mucosa) of the mouth 1 or 2 days before the rash appears. Serious complications, such as pneumonia and encephalitis, occur in about 4% of cases.

Diagnosis

Clinical features are used to diagnose the disease. Koplik's spots, a maculopapular rash spreading from the head down, fever, and conjunctivitis indicate measles.

Treatment

There are no antiviral medications for inhibiting the measles virus. Treatment is symptomatic and commonly includes bed rest, intake of fluids and electrolytes to replace those lost from the fever, and over-the-counter medications, such as acetaminophen or ibuprofen, for fever and headache.

Prevention

- A highly effective live attenuated (immunogenic but not pathogenic) measles vaccine is given most commonly to children as the MMR vaccine, which protects against measles, mumps, and rubella.

- People who are infected should be isolated due to the highly contagious nature of the disease.

Pseudomonas aeruginosa Skin Infections

Pseudomonas aeruginosa is a common opportunistic pathogen (a disease-causing microbe that infects those with a compromised immune system) and a nosocomial (health care-acquired) pathogen. It is very common in patients with diabetes and burns. It is also the second most common cause of nosocomial pneumonia. Relatively recently, *Pseudomonas* folliculitis has emerged as a community-acquired skin infection The infection is caused by bacterial colonization of hair follicles after exposure to contaminated water from whirlpools, hot tubs, swimming pools, water slides, bathtubs, etc.

Cause of the disease

P. aeruginosa, a bacterial pathogen, is a gram-negative, rod-shaped bacterium that has a monopolar flagellum. It produces a blue-green pigment, pyocyanin.

The outer membrane of the cell has small porins, which can restrict the diffusion of many disinfectants and antibiotics into the cell. It can also carry a plasmid that codes for a transport protein that pumps many antibiotics out of the cell.

Transmission

Reservoir

P. aeruginosa is normally a common inhabitant of soil and water and is sometimes present on humans, but it typically does not cause disease in those with healthy immune defenses.

Mode of transmission

The pathogen can be spread in droplet mode by the respiratory route or by direct contact with an infected individual or an environmental surface contaminated with the pathogen. It is also a common contaminant of hospitals due to its resistance to disinfection. It is spread by fomites, such as respiratory equipment, food, sinks, taps, plants and flowers, and mops.

Pathogenesis

Entry

The pathogen is spread by several different routes and from a variety of environmental sites.

Attachment

The fimbriae of *Pseudomonas* adhere to the epithelial cells of the respiratory tract, burn wounds, or postoperative wounds and spread to other epithelial cells.

Avoiding host defenses

The pathogen has an antiphagocytic capsule.

Damage

Pseudomonas produces two extracellular proteases (elastase and alkaline protease), which together cause the inactivation of some components of the immune response. Two hemolysins, which destroy erythrocytes, are produced, as well as a cytotoxin, which kills a variety of cells. In addition, two extracellular toxins—one impairs phagocyte function, and one mimics the cytotoxic effects of diphtheria toxin—cause damage.

Exit

The pathogen exits through respiratory secretions, plus fomites or direct contact.

Clinical features

P. aeruginosa can cause folliculitis and often affects those with a suppressed immune system (burn victims, postoperative patients, hospital residents, acquired immune deficiency syndrome [AIDS] patients, and those with cystic fibrosis). Folliculitis is characterized by a red, itchy, pustular rash. The pus may have a blue-green coloration and a fruity smell.

Diagnosis

Specimen

A sample of pus serves as a specimen.

Tests

The pathogen is commonly isolated on blood agar plates and is further characterized by Gram staining, an inability to ferment lactose, a fruity odor, and the ability to grow at 42°C.

Treatment

P. aeruginosa is resistant to many antibiotics. Infections are often treated with a combination of antibiotics selected from a group of antipseudomonal penicillins and cephalosporins, imipenem, meropenum, and ciprofloxacin.

Prevention

- Health care-acquired infections can be prevented by proper hospital isolation procedures, aseptic techniques, and careful cleaning and monitoring of respirators, catheters, and other instruments.

- Topical therapy of burn wounds and postoperative patients with antibacterial agents can dramatically reduce incidence.

- Health care workers must follow strict infection control procedures.

- Waterborne outbreaks can be prevented with adequate chlorination of pools and hot tubs.

Ringworm

Ringworm is common and has a worldwide distribution. It occurs more often in hot, humid climates. Although ringworm occurs in all age groups, children and their care givers are more likely to be affected than other people.

Cause of the disease

Trichophyton, *Microsporum*, and *Epidermophyton* are genera of eukaryotic filamentous molds that cause body surface infections and ringworm.

Transmission

Reservoir

This mold is commonly found in humans and animals.

Mode of transmission

The pathogen is transmitted by direct contact with lesions of infected people or pets. Infection can also occur indirectly from infected people who contaminate shower stalls or floors.

Pathogenesis

Entry

The spore of the mold germinates on the epidermis of the skin.

Attachment

The hyphae (long filaments of the fungus) penetrate the stratum corneum of the epidermal layer of the skin.

Avoiding host defenses

The hyphae remain in the epidermal layer of the skin and avoid circulating antibodies and cells of the immune system.

Damage

The branched hyphae spread radially from the inoculation site through the stratum corneum and, if possible, will penetrate the hair shaft and grow down to an area where viable cells are present, resulting in inflammation and irritation.

Exit

The mold forms spores, which are sloughed off the skin.

Clinical features

The clinical features include dry or moist scaling, crusting, and an eczematous reaction on the surface of the skin. On hairless skin, a circular inflamed area becomes prominent about 3 weeks after infection. The red patches found on the surface of the skin are usually round and have raised, wavy edges. Either bald patches or patches of short broken hair with red scaly skin underneath form on the scalp.

Diagnosis

Specimen

A scraping of the infected tissue is taken.

Test

Microscopy of a hair or a scraping from a skin lesion which has been soaked in 10% potassium hydroxide is used as a test. The strong base dissolves the keratin from the skin cells, making it possible to see the filamentous fungus.

Treatment

Topical antifungal creams (azole derivatives) are used regularly for 2 to 4 weeks. Antifungals, such as clotrimazole, miconazole, or ketoconazole, are fungistatic. They block the synthesis of a key steroid found only in fungi, not in human cells, that is necessary for proper functioning of the fungal cell membrane.

Prevention

- Avoid pets that have a rash of unknown etiology.
- Select shoes that fit properly and try to keep your feet dry.
- Beware of possible transmission from shower floors.
- Practice good hand-washing techniques.
- Make sure that skin is thoroughly dried after washing.
- Avoid sharing personal items (combs, towels, and clothing).
- Vacuum carpeted areas and furniture that may have come in contact with the fungus.

Staphylococcus aureus Skin Infections

Staphylococcus aureus is a very common pathogen. About 25% of individuals are colonized persistently with *Staphylococcus aureus*. Health care workers, people with diabetes, and patients on dialysis all have higher rates of colonization. The nose is the predominant site of colonization. *Staphylococcus aureus* is a very versatile pathogen and can cause skin infections, such as folliculitis, furuncles, impetigo, wound infections, and scalded-skin syndrome. In addition, it can cause septic bursitis, septic arthritis, toxic shock syndrome, endocarditis (infection of the inside of the heart), osteomyelitis (infection of the bone), pneumonia, food poisoning, infections related to prosthetic devices, and urinary tract infections, and it is the leading cause of hospital-acquired infections.

Besides being a versatile pathogen, *Staphylococcus aureus* has shown an extraordinary ability to acquire resistance to antibiotics. Currently, fewer than 5% of clinical isolates remain sensitive to penicillin, and over half of methicillin-resistant isolates are sensitive only to vancomycin.

Cause of the disease

Staphylococcus aureus, a bacterial pathogen, is a gram-positive staphylococcus that is coagulase positive (it causes blood plasma to clot) and catalase positive (it breaks down H_2O_2 using the enzyme catalase). It is nonfastidious (able to grow on simple laboratory media), is a facultative anaerobe (capable of both anaerobic and aerobic growth), and can tolerate high-osmolarity environments.

Transmission

Reservoir

Humans and other animals are the reservoirs; it can also contaminate foods. *Staphylococcus aureus* is typically found in the perineum and skin and within the nose.

Mode of transmission

The pathogen can be passed from person to person by respiratory droplets, through direct contact, or by fomites. The organism survives drying and temperature changes, so it is a common pathogen in hospital settings (a nosocomial pathogen).

Pathogenesis

Entry

Staphylococcus aureus can cause boils by infecting hair follicles or enter the body through breaks in the skin. It also complicates infections by other pathogens, for example, causing secondary pneumonia in someone with a primary influenza virus infection.

Attachment

Staphylococcus aureus can attach to a variety of mammalian tissues by binding to plasma proteins and components of the extracellular matrix of a variety of cells (fibronectin and collagen).

Avoiding host defenses

Staphylococcus aureus produces a protein (protein A) that binds antibodies in such a way that the pathogen is not easily targeted for destruction by phagocytes. Some strains also have antiphagocytic capsules.

Damage

Staphylococcus aureus contains more mechanisms for causing tissue damage than any other pathogen. Damaging enzymes include coagulase, which causes blood clotting; lipases that hydrolyze cellular lipids; hyaluronidase, which breaks down the extracellular matrix of bone and cartilage; staphylokinase, which dissolves blood clots; and a nuclease that can break down DNA and RNA. Toxins include hemolysins that cause erythrocyte lysis; leukocidins that destroy leukocytes; delta-toxin, which acts like a detergent to solubilize cell membranes; six types of enterotoxins that cause food poisoning; epidermolytic toxin, which causes scalded-skin syndrome; and toxic shock syndrome toxin, which causes a life-threatening drop in blood pressure. The damage produced by enzymes and toxins is complicated by inflammation, causing edema (swelling) and a local fever.

Clinical features

Staphylococcus aureus is a very common and versatile pathogen. Some common diseases it causes are boils, impetigo, folliculitis, cellulitis (infection of the tissue under the skin), pneumonia, endocarditis, osteomyelitis, toxic shock syndrome, and food poisoning.

Diagnosis

A specimen from the infected site is obtained and grown on blood agar (it forms golden colonies) or mannitol salt agar (*Staphylococcus aureus* survives the high concentration of salt and ferments mannitol to acid products, causing the medium to turn yellow).

Treatment

If possible, treatment is determined after the clinical laboratory has characterized the pathogen's antibiotic sensitivity profile. *Staphylococcus aureus* is very adaptable, and different strains have developed resistance to nearly every drug used to treat infections. Once-useful drugs no longer can be used against most strains of *Staphylococcus aureus*; 90% of hospital isolates of *Staphylococcus aureus* are resistant to most of the β-lactams. In some cities, over 50% of isolates are resistant to the β-lactams that resist degradation by β-lactamase, the enzyme that is produced by most β-lactam-resistant cells. These variants are called MRSA because they are methicillin resistant due to a mutation that alters the enzyme (penicillin-binding protein) that is normally inhibited by the β-lactams. Therefore, MRSA strains are resistant to all but a few of the β-lactams.

In addition, *Staphylococcus aureus* has developed resistance to vancomycin, which is often viewed as the drug to use when most other drugs fail. Both intermediate- and high-level resistant strains of *Staphylococcus aureus* have been identified and are spreading.

Prevention

- Proper hygiene is most important in preventing the spread of *Staphylococcus aureus*. Frequent and thorough hand washing prevents the pathogen from being carried or spread on the hands.

- In a hospital setting, health care workers should change gloves prior to contact with a new patient, and contaminated surfaces in the hospital (stethoscopes, blood glucose monitors, weighing scales, and electronic thermometers) should be disinfected with 70% isopropyl alcohol and chlorine compounds.

Outbreaks of Multisystem Zoonoses
and Vector-Borne Diseases

> *You think Nature is some Disney movie? Nature is a killer.*
> *Nature is a bitch. It's feeding time out there 24 hours a day,*
> *every step you take is a gamble with death. If it isn't getting hit*
> *by lightning today, it's an earthquake tomorrow or some deer*
> *tick carrying Lyme disease. Either way, you're ending up on the*
> *wrong end of the food chain.*
>
> JEFF MELVOIN, *Northern Exposure* (1994)

Animals are important in the field of microbiology as reservoirs for pathogens that can also cross species lines and infect humans (zoonoses) and as vectors that transmit microbial pathogens into their human hosts (vector-borne diseases). Prevention of zoonoses requires separating the human population from the animal disease reservoir. As populations continue to grow and human habitation pushes into more and more natural environments, exposure to rodents and other wild animals increases. In urban areas with limited public services, accumulation of waste provides rodents with food and habitats, leading to zoonotic disease outbreaks.

Vector-borne diseases are prevented by controlling the population of insects or other arthropod vectors that transmit the disease. This requires a combination of community-wide and personal efforts. For example, publicly supported spraying of mosquitoes over large areas reduces the risk of an outbreak. In addition, individuals can avoid being outside during times of the day when the mosquitoes feed, use mosquito netting at night, and wear insect repellent containing DEET (*N*,*N*-diethyl-*m*-toluamide).

Worldwide, the lack of resources devoted to public health in many underdeveloped countries has resulted in several vector-borne diseases being among the top 10 killers. Malaria is the fifth leading cause of death by infectious disease, causing approximately 2 million to 3 million deaths per year. Dengue hemorrhagic fever (DHF), a complication of a double infection by any of several serotypes of dengue virus, is the 10th leading cause of death by infectious disease.

Although the number of deaths due to zoonoses is low relative to the number of deaths due to other infectious diseases, these zoonoses are important for several reasons. First, a number of zoonoses damage multiple organ systems, resulting in very high mortalities. Consequently, rapid diagnosis and aggressive intervention therapies are necessary to prevent loss of life. Also, several multisystem zoonoses are caused by pathogens that are among the nation's top concerns as bioterrorism agents. Ebola virus, *Yersinia pestis*, *Bacillus anthracis*, *Francisella tularensis*, and *Clostridium botulinum* neurotoxin are all category A biological agents—those that are considered the most dangerous potential bioweapons. Outbreaks of these pathogens may indicate the intentional release of a bioterrorism agent and must be thoroughly investigated.

Table VI.1 Selected outbreak-causing multisystem zoonotic and vector-borne pathogens

Organism	Key physical properties	Disease characteristics
Bacteria		
Bacillus anthracis	Gram-positive bacillus; aerobic; produces an antiphagocytic capsule and tissue-damaging cytotoxins	Naturally occurring anthrax typically affects the skin, causing cutaneous lesions.
Borrelia burgdorferi	Gram-negative spirochete	Lyme disease causes a rash and arthritis; late stages can cause nervous system and cardiac manifestations.
Brucella spp.	Fastidious gram-negative bacillus	Brucellosis can cause fever, lymphadenopathy, hepatosplenomegaly, and other physiological problems.
Francisella tularensis	Fastidious gram-negative bacillus	Tularemia causes skin ulcers, lymphadenopathy, fever, bacteremia, and pneumonia.
Rickettsia rickettsii	Obligate intracellular organism; very small	Rocky Mountain spotted fever causes fever, rash, and capillary damage.
Rickettsia prowazekii	Obligate intracellular organism; very small	Epidemic typhus causes fever and disseminated intravascular coagulation.
Yersinia pestis	Gram-negative bacillus	Plague causes localized lymphadenopathy (bubonic), highly lethal bacteremia, and pneumonia.
Viruses		
Dengue viruses	Enveloped polyhedral capsid with single-stranded RNA	Dengue fever and DHF cause intense joint pain, fever, headache, rash, muscle pain, and sometimes hemorrhagic fever/shock.
Filoviruses (Ebola virus, Marburg virus)	Enveloped helical capsid with single-stranded RNA	Disease causes hemorrhagic fever with high mortality; the reservoir is not known.
Hantaviruses	Enveloped helical capsid with single-stranded RNA	Infection causes pneumonia and hemorrhagic fever with renal dysfunction.
Yellow fever virus	Enveloped polyhedral capsid with single-stranded RNA	Yellow fever causes severe hepatitis and GI tract hemorrhages with a high mortality rate.

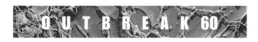

An Outbreak of Typhus

BURUNDI, 1997

An extensive ongoing outbreak of typhus occurred in refugee camps in Rwanda, Burundi, and Zaire. For people in the camps, daily living was an immense hardship. Following the outbreak of civil war in 1993, over 760,000 refugees lived in camps under appalling conditions. Sanitation and clean water were hard to find, and disease was rampant. Besides typhus, outbreaks of typhoid fever, dysentery, and malaria also affected the refugee communities. The United Nations World Food Program distributed emergency rations to curb malnutrition. In some refugee camps, the people were required to work like a chain gang, collectively, on a single tract of land at a time. Those that left the camps were assumed to be rebel forces and could be shot by government soldiers. The civil war between the two main tribes for control of the government degraded into a tit-for-tat massacre of civilians.

Against this background, a typhus epidemic emerged among the displaced population of Burundi. The outbreak may have begun among prisoners in a jail in N'Gozi in 1995. Clinical aspects of the disease included headache, chills, fever, prostration, confusion, photophobia, vomiting, and rash (generally starting on the trunk). There was a fatality rate of 15% among jail inmates. At the time, the disease was not recognized and was referred to as sutama. Reports of sutama among the civilian population date back to late 1995, and in association with body louse infestation, the disease subsequently swept across the higher and colder regions of the country.

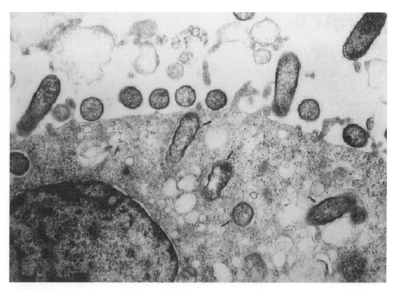

Figure 60.1 A transmission electron micrograph of the intracellular pathogen.

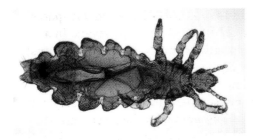

Figure 60.2 A body louse.

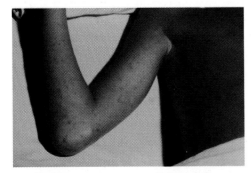

Figure 60.3 A rash caused by the pathogen.

During a field study in February 1997, 102 refugees with sutama underwent clinical examinations and interviews. Serum samples were collected, and infesting body lice were removed. Analysis of blood sera by immunofluorescence microscopy found antibodies present against the causative agent, a small obligately intracellular pathogen. Most of the 102 patients with sutama during initial assessment presented with typical manifestations of the disease. Up to September 1997, 45,558 cases were clinically diagnosed, most of which occurred in regions at an altitude of over 1,500 meters.

QUESTIONS

1. What pathogen caused the typhus outbreak?

2. How is the pathogen typically transmitted?

3. How does the pathogen cause the bleeding under the skin that leads to the rash?

4. What recommendations would you have made to treat this pathogen? Explain why.

5. Why would the disease be most common in higher altitudes of eastern Africa?

6. Why did the outbreak first appear among prisoners?

OUTBREAK 61

An Outbreak of Cyclic Fevers

INDIA, 2002

In India, a prolonged spell of heavy rain in 2002 created vast pools of stagnant water that preceded an outbreak of cyclic fevers. In a 6-week period, hundreds of thousands of people in India's northeastern Assam state became ill. The disease was characterized by fever that began with the patient feeling intensely chilled, followed by a high, dry fever and then drenching sweats. Some fevers cycled every 2 days and others every 3 days. Associated with the fever were vomiting, intense headaches, anemia, and an enlarged spleen and liver. In Assam state, 73 people died of the disease.

Examination of blood smears identified the protozoal pathogen. "At least 400,000 people tested positive," B. K. Baishya, Assam's disease control officer, told Reuters in Guwahati, the state's main city. Baishya said they had formed more than 150 rapid response teams made up of doctors, nurses, and pathologists to take care of the people affected.

Assam averages about 100 deaths from the disease every year. In 1995, however, more than 1,200 people died.

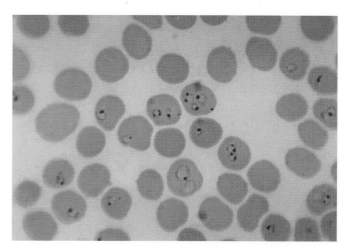

Figure 61.1 A blood smear showing the intracellular pathogen.

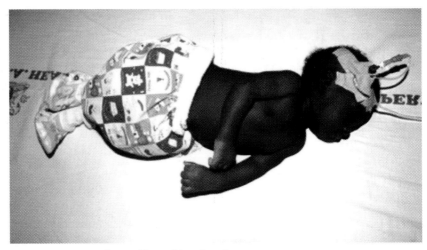

Figure 61.2 An infant affected by the disease.

QUESTIONS

1. Name the disease, and identify and describe the pathogenic agent(s) that caused the outbreak.

2. How would you have treated those affected by the disease?

3. Why did some affected individuals suffer from 2-day cycling fevers while others had 3-day cycling fevers?

4. How would you have stopped this outbreak and prevented future outbreaks from occurring?

5. What areas of the world are most affected by this pathogen?

An Outbreak of Encephalitis

NEW YORK, 1999

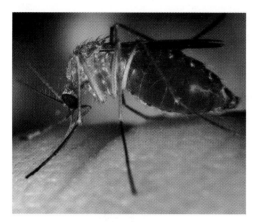

Figure 62.1 *Culex* mosquito vector.

An outbreak of mosquito-borne encephalitis was first recognized in New York City in late August 1999 and then was identified in neighboring counties in New York State. Although initially attributed to St. Louis encephalitis virus, the cause of the outbreak was confirmed as a West Nile-like virus based on the identification of the virus in human, avian, and mosquito samples. West Nile virus (WNV) is transmitted principally by *Culex* mosquitoes but can also be transmitted by species of the genera *Aedes*, *Anopheles*, and others.

On 23 August, an infectious-disease physician from a hospital in northern Queens contacted the New York City Department of Health to report two patients with encephalitis. On investigation, the New York City Department of Health initially identified a cluster of six patients with encephalitis, five of whom had had profound muscle weakness requiring respiratory support. Eight of the earliest case patients were residents of a 2- by 2-mile area in northern Queens.

Before and concurrent with this outbreak, local health officials observed increased fatalities among New York City birds, especially crows. Between 7 and 9 September, officials of the Bronx Zoo noted the deaths of a cormorant, two captive-bred Chilean flamingoes, and an Asian pheasant. Necropsies performed on the birds at the zoo revealed varying degrees of meningoencephalitis (swelling of the tissues lining the brain and the brain itself) and severe myocarditis (damage of the heart muscle). Tissue specimens from the birds and a crow with pathologic evidence of encephalitis from New York State were sent to the Centers for Disease Control and Prevention (CDC). Testing of the isolates by polymerase chain reaction (PCR) and deoxyribonucleic acid (DNA) sequencing at the CDC on 23 September indicated that the genomic sequences were identical.

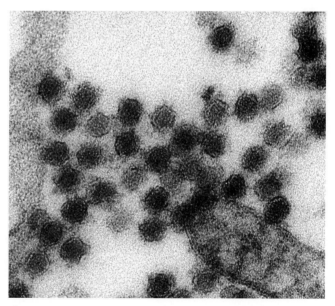

Figure 62.2 A transmission electron micrograph of the viral pathogen.

As of 28 September, a total of 37 human cases and four deaths were reported from New York City (25 cases) and the surrounding counties of Westchester and Nassau. The four deaths occurred among people aged 68 years or more. One case patient with onset in late August reported a history of travel to Africa completed in June 1999; none of the remaining case patients had traveled during the incubation period to areas where WNV is known to be endemic. Two of the Westchester County case patients had no reported travel history to New York City or other areas in which WNV had previously been detected.

WNV was first isolated in the West Nile Province of Uganda in 1937. The first recorded epidemics occurred in Israel from 1950 to 1954 and in 1957. Epidemics were reported in Europe in the Rhone Delta of France in 1962 and in Romania in 1996. The largest recorded epidemic occurred in South Africa in 1974.

QUESTIONS

1. Can WNV encephalitis be transmitted person to person?

2. List three important activities that would need to be accomplished to minimize the impact of WNV on the human population.

3. Would it be feasible or cost-effective to attempt to prevent the spread of the virus through the avian reservoir? Explain your answer.

4. Is there an antiviral agent for treating those seriously affected by a WNV infection?

5. How far has WNV now spread in the United States?

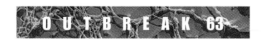
Yellow Fever in a Traveler Returning from Venezuela

CALIFORNIA, 1999

On 28 September 1999, a previously healthy 48-year-old man from California sought care at a local emergency department and was hospitalized with a 2-day history of fever (38.9°C), chills, headache, photophobia, diffuse myalgias (muscle pain), joint pain, nausea, vomiting, constipation, upper abdominal discomfort, and general weakness.

On admission to the hospital, physical examination revealed that the white areas of the eyes were yellow and the upper abdomen was tender. No enlarged liver or spleen or swollen lymph nodes were noted. Laboratory results indicated markedly elevated serum bilirubin and liver enzymes (indicating damage to the liver), leukopenia (decrease in the leukocyte count, indicating damage from infection), thrombocytopenia (decrease in platelets), and evidence of acute renal failure. A preliminary diagnosis of hemorrhagic fever syndrome was made. The patient was placed on doxycycline and ceftriaxone to combat bacterial infections that might be causing his illness.

Cultures of blood and urine were negative for bacterial pathogens. Blood smears for malaria were negative. Other tests were negative for dengue fever virus, *Leptospira,* New World arenaviruses, spotted fever group rickettsiae, and hantavirus.

Multiple red lesions consistent with recent mosquito bites were seen on the patient's lower legs and feet. Between 16 and 25 September, the patient had traveled with six companions to rainforests in southern Venezuela (Amazonas State). He experienced multiple mosquito bites during his visit despite using DEET-based repellents. Before his trip, the patient had received tetanus toxoid (the inactivated tetanus toxin that provides immunity to tetanus), typhoid vaccine, hepatitis A vaccine, and malaria prophylaxis, but not yellow fever vaccine. Of the six travel companions, none had become ill during or following the trip. Five had received yellow fever vaccine before travel.

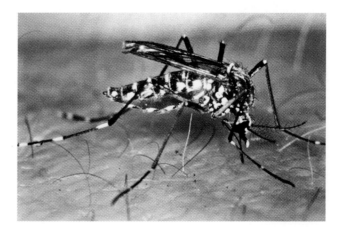

Figure 63.1 *Aedes* mosquito vector.

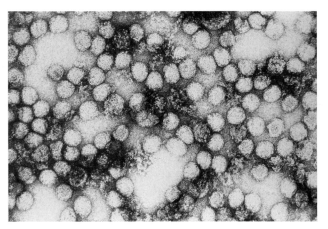

Figure 63.2 A transmission electron micrograph of the viral pathogen.

On 1 October, the patient developed general seizures and upper respiratory obstruction. He was placed on mechanical ventilation and transferred to the intensive care unit. His condition deteriorated rapidly, with formation of blood clots throughout his system and cardiac arrhythmias. He died on 4 October.

QUESTIONS

1. Why was the patient tested for the listed pathogens?

2. Based on the vaccination history and clinical signs and symptoms, diagnose the disease and describe the pathogenic agent.

3. Describe the risk of a future outbreak of this disease in California.

4. Describe a strategy for others in similar situations to reduce the risk of acquiring this disease.

A Hantavirus Pulmonary Syndrome Outbreak

VERMONT, 2000

On 17 February 2000, a 61-year-old previously healthy Vermont resident was hospitalized following three episodes of chills and fever (102°F, or 39°C), nausea, vomiting, and anorexia. On examination, the lungs were clear and a 2- by 2-centimeter (cm) nontender lymph node was identified at the angle of the left jaw. Chest radiographs were also clear. However, 1 day after admission, the patient's condition deteriorated, with onset of respiratory failure, profound hypoxemia (lack of oxygen), and hypotension (low blood pressure) requiring mechanical ventilation. Subsequent chest radiographs revealed fluid in the lungs consistent with acute respiratory distress syndrome. The patient also developed disseminated intravascular coagulation (blood clots forming throughout the body) and renal insufficiency.

During the 2 months preceding hospitalization, the patient, who resided in a house on four rural acres, had cleaned a mouse nest from a woodpile, observed mice in the basement, and trapped two mice under the kitchen counters.

Laboratory tests for bacterial pathogens, protozoal pathogens, influenza virus, adenovirus, and coronaviruses were negative. Using an enzyme-linked immunosorbent assay (ELISA), antibodies to Sin Nombre virus were detected in the patient's serum. Forty-three rodents were trapped around the home and also tested for traces of hantavirus infection. Two of five deer mice were positive for hantaviral antibodies; all other rodents were negative.

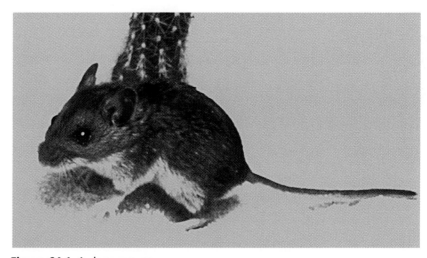

Figure 64.1 A deer mouse.

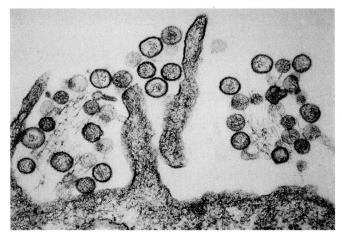

Figure 64.2 A transmission electron micrograph of Sin Nombre virus.

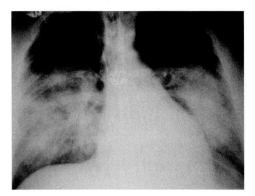

Figure 64.3 A chest X ray of a patient with hantavirus pulmonary syndrome.

QUESTIONS

1. Describe the pathogen that caused the disease.
2. How does Sin Nombre virus cause respiratory distress?
3. How is infection with this organism most commonly acquired?
4. How would you prevent an outbreak of this disease from occurring?

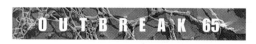

Cases of Rash and Fever, One Fatal, in a Family Cluster

KENTUCKY, 2003

In August 2003, two family members were treated after an outbreak of rash and fever. A male aged 2 years was taken to a pediatrician after 1 day of fever (101.0°F [38.3°C]) with a papular rash (small red bumps) on his legs, arms, trunk, and back. An unspecified viral syndrome was diagnosed, and the child was treated with nonsteroidal anti-inflammatory drugs. Over the next 2 days, the child had spiking fevers and variable rash. The child was examined in an emergency department at a local hospital and discharged with a diagnosis of viral infection. Four days after initial treatment, the child was again evaluated by a pediatrician because of lethargy and refusal to walk.

Laboratory tests showed thrombocytopenia (low platelet count), an elevated white blood cell count, and anemia (low hemoglobin levels). The next day, the child was admitted and treated with intravenous (i.v.) antibiotics. Two days later, the child was transferred to a tertiary care hospital. Physical examination at admission revealed a fine petechial rash (indicating capillary damage) on the groin, trunk, ankles, and palms. The patient was treated intravenously with vancomycin, cefotaxime, and doxycycline. His condition continued to deteriorate; 8 days after initial treatment, he died from multiple-system organ failure.

The child's mother, aged 40 years, was hospitalized 2 days before her son's death with 2 days of diplopia (double vision), dizziness, headache, and fever. Oral doxycycline and i.v. ceftriaxone were administered; she was discharged after 5 days.

Both the mother and child tested positive by indirect ELISA for antibodies to an intracellular tick-borne pathogen. The disease has a case fatality rate as high as 30% if untreated. Even with treatment, hospitalization rates of 72% and case fatality rates of 4% have been reported.

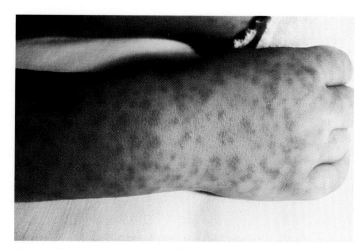

Figure 65.1 A rash caused by the pathogen.

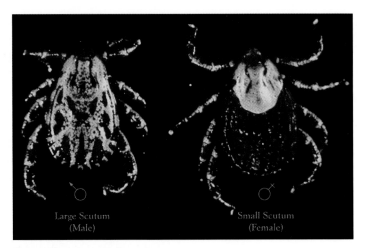

Large Scutum
(Male)

Small Scutum
(Female)

Figure 65.2 Dog ticks.

The family lived near a lake in the woods. The mother did not recall any recent tick bites, travel, or participation in outdoor activities by herself or her son prior to the onset of illness.

QUESTIONS

1. Based on the clinical presentation, diagnose the disease and describe the pathogenic agent.

2. How is this disease transmitted?

3. What property of the pathogen causes capillary damage and leads to such high mortality?

4. If the disease is recognized early, what is the treatment for those affected?

5. What recommendation would you have made to prevent an outbreak of this disease in other family members or others living in the same area?

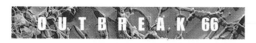

An Outbreak of Ebola Hemorrhagic Fever

UGANDA, 2000

On 8 October 2000, an outbreak of an unusual febrile illness with hemorrhagic complications and significant mortality was reported to the Ministry of Health in Uganda. Symptoms included diarrhea, anorexia, headache, nausea and vomiting, abdominal pain, and occasionally chest pain. Bleeding occurred in 20% of patients and primarily involved the gastrointestinal (GI) tract. During the initial surveillance of the outbreak, 62 cases were confirmed (36 [58%] died). Spontaneous abortions were reported among pregnant women. Patients who died usually exhibited a rapid progression of shock, increasing coagulopathy (blood clot formation causing damage to organs and tissues), and loss of consciousness. The incubation period of the disease was less than 21 days.

Laboratory tests included virus antigen detection, antibody ELISAs, and reverse transcriptase polymerase chain reaction. The pathogen was identified as Ebola virus, a virus with antisense single-stranded ribonucleic acid (RNA) and an enveloped helical capsid.

To prevent spread of the pathogen, isolation wards were established for suspected cases of the disease. However, 14 (64%) of 22 health care workers in Gulu were infected after the isolation wards were established.

Two distant outbreaks in the Mbarara and Masindi districts were initiated by movement of individuals who had been exposed to the disease to those districts.

Epidemiologic investigations identified the three most important means of transmission as (i) attending funerals of those that died of the disease, where ritual contact with the deceased occurred; (ii) being a family member of someone with the disease; and (iii) being a hospital caregiver for someone with the disease.

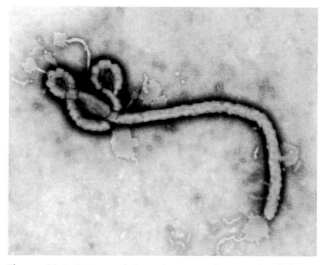

Figure 66.1 A transmission electron micrograph of the pathogen.

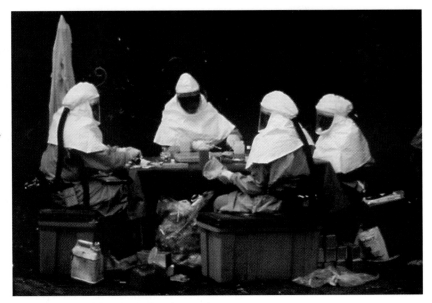

Figure 66.2 Field testing for the pathogen.

The combined area of the outbreak covered approximately 11,700 square miles with a population of about 1.8 million. Much of the area consisted of small villages in tropical jungles of Africa. Travel and communication between villages were not always possible and were generally difficult.

QUESTIONS

1. Identify the disease and describe the pathogenic agent.

2. What aspect of the pathogenesis of the virus causes the hemorrhagic manifestations of the disease?

3. Explain the rationale for the three main risk groups for acquiring the infection.

4. How would you have contained this outbreak?

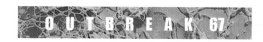

An Outbreak of Leptospirosis during EcoChallenge

MALAYSIA, 2000

A case of leptospirosis in a 35-year-old man was reported to the CDC. The illness was characterized by acute onset of high fever, chills, headache, and muscle aches. The patient had participated in the EcoChallenge Sabah 2000 Expedition Race, a multisport event held from 20 August to 3 September at various sites in Sabah in Malaysian Borneo.

The event involved jungle trekking, open-water swimming, river and ocean paddling, mountain biking, climbing across the rugged canyon terrain, scuba diving, and spelunking. Participating were 76 four-person teams from 26 countries, including 37 teams from the United States. Subsequently, 37 of 155 U.S. athletes reported having fever, and 12 (15%) were hospitalized. No deaths were reported.

Serum specimens were tested at the CDC by indirect ELISA. The test was positive for antibodies against *Leptospira*.

QUESTIONS

1. Describe the pathogenic agent.

2. How is the pathogen usually transmitted to the human population?

3. How would you have treated those who were ill and prevented illness in those exposed to the pathogen?

4. How would you have prevented the illness from spreading to the international community in contact with the EcoChallenge participants?

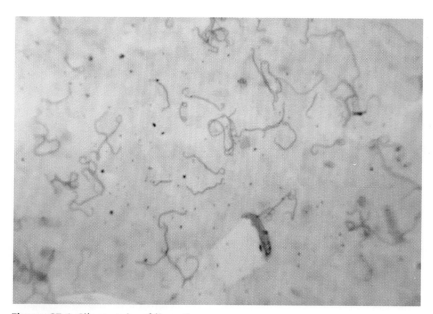

Figure 67.1 Silver stain of liver tissue.

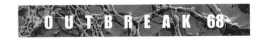

A Dengue Fever Outbreak

PUERTO RICO, 1998

Dengue fever is an acute viral disease characterized by fever, headache, myalgias (muscle aches), arthralgias (joint pain), rash, nausea, and vomiting. It is caused by any of the four dengue virus serotypes (DEN-1, DEN-2, DEN-3, and DEN-4). The principal mosquito vector is *Aedes aegypti*, which has a worldwide distribution in tropical and many subtropical areas. A small proportion of infected people may develop the severe form of disease, dengue hemorrhagic fever/dengue shock syndrome.

From 1 January through 29 August 1998, 4,677 laboratory-confirmed cases of dengue fever were reported in Puerto Rico (an additional 5,000 cases were suspected but not confirmed). At the peak of the epidemic, the number of cases reported was approximately six times that expected for the time of year, based on a 5-year average. The ages of the patients ranged from 0 to 98 years (median, 23 years). Age group-specific attack rates of reported disease were highest for persons aged 10 to 19 years and decreased with increasing age.

A total of 4,190 patients were hospitalized, and the case report forms of 2,888 of those infected (29.5%) noted some hemorrhagic manifestation. The highest rate of DHF occurred in people aged 55 to 59 years. Five people died.

Although a large survey in Puerto Rico in 1996 found high levels of awareness of dengue fever and the *Aedes aegypti* mosquito, most of the population were not taking action to control the vector. The principal barriers to action were lack of knowledge about how to locate and eliminate containers that could serve as larval habitats, the absence of external motivators to prompt the behavior, and the lack of positive feedback and other factors to encourage the public to carry out the necessary actions.

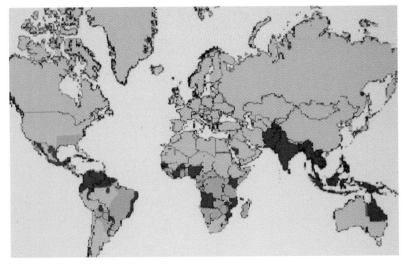

Figure 68.1 Range of *Aedes aegypti* (pink land areas) and areas where dengue fever is epidemic (red).

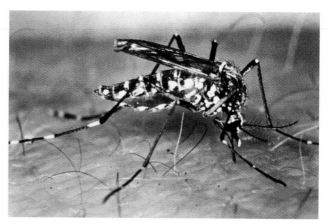

Figure 68.2 *Aedes* mosquito vector.

QUESTIONS

1. Why does dengue fever typically occur in seasonal patterns?

2. Where is *Aedes aegypti*'s habitat, and what time of day does it bite?

3. Is there a vaccine to prevent dengue fever?

4. Why does dengue hemorrhagic fever affect older persons while uncomplicated dengue fever primarily affects those who are younger?

5. How would you treat those with dengue fever?

6. How would you have decreased the cases of dengue fever from this outbreak?

An Outbreak of Lyme Disease

UNITED STATES, 1999

Lyme disease (LD) was first reported in Lyme, Connecticut, in 1972 and has since spread through most areas of the United States. Those affected by LD often have a target-shaped spreading rash that is ≥5 cm in diameter. For those without the rash, LD is diagnosed by an occurrence of at least one late manifestation of musculoskeletal, neurological, or cardiovascular disease with laboratory confirmation of infection.

In the years from 1990 through 1996, the numbers of reported LD cases were 7,943, 9,470, 9,908, 8,257, 13,043, 11,700, and 16,455, respectively. In 1999, 16,273 LD cases were reported (overall incidence, 6.0 per 100,000 population), a 3% decrease from the 16,801 cases reported in 1998 and a 21% increase from the 12,801 cases reported in 1997. Most cases were reported in northeastern, mid-Atlantic, and north central states. Nine states reported LD incidences higher than the national rate (i.e., Connecticut, 98.0; Rhode Island, 55.1; New York, 24.2; Pennsylvania, 23.2; Delaware, 22.2; New Jersey, 21.1; Maryland, 17.4; Massachusetts, 12.7; and Wisconsin, 9.3). These states accounted for 92.0% of the nationally reported cases. The highest county-specific incidence (950.7) occurred in Nantucket County, Massachusetts.

Cases of LD were relatively equally distributed among age groups and between men and women. Among 12,479 (76.7%) patients for whom the month of onset of the illness was reported, 7,161 (57.4%) had onset during June (28.5%) and July (28.9%); <5.8% reported onset during January, February, and December 1999.

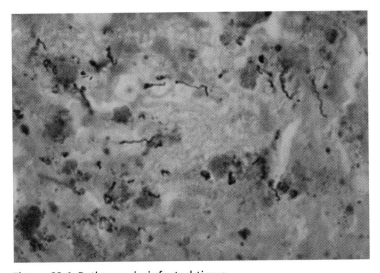

Figure 69.1 Pathogen in infected tissue.

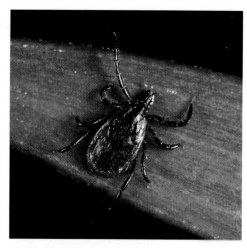

Figure 69.2 An *Ixodes* tick.

QUESTIONS

1. What pathogen causes LD, and how is the pathogen transmitted?

2. Why is the disease primarily distributed in the northeastern United States?

3. How can LD be prevented?

4. Explain why LD predominantly occurs in the summer.

5. How does the pathogen avoid the normal defenses of the immune system?

A Plague Outbreak

INDIA, 1994

The world's first plague pandemic was recorded in 543 in an area that is now Egypt. It spread to other continents and killed about 100 million people. The second pandemic, known as the Black Death, began in 1347 and killed at least 25 million people. In the third pandemic, at least 12.5 million people died, mostly in India, between 1889 and 1918. On 20 September 1994, a pneumonic plague epidemic broke out in Surat, India, and spread across the continent. Fear among the population was running so high that a man in New Delhi with plague symptoms committed suicide by jumping out of a hospital window.

Favorable clinical outcomes depend on prompt diagnosis and treatment. Streptomycin and gentamicin are the drugs of choice for treating plague; tetracyclines and chloramphenicol are highly effective alternatives. The penicillins and cephalosporins are not effective. Prompt and specific treatment reduces the case fatality rate from 60% or more to less than 15%. Tetracyclines, sulfonamides, and chloramphenicol may be used for prophylaxis (treatment of those exposed to others who have the disease).

In India, several complications developed that made controlling the epidemic difficult. First, plasmid-borne multidrug antibiotic resistance has developed in *Yersinia pestis*, the bacterium that causes plague. Scientists have discovered a strain of plague bacteria that shows high-level resistance to all the antibiotics usually used for plague prevention and therapy. David T. Dennis of the CDC's Division of Vector-Borne Infectious Diseases in Fort Collins, Colorado, has considered this to be a wake-up call for the international community and has stated that we need to be on alert for the possibility of the emergence of drug resistance in plague strains.

The resistant strain of *Yersinia pestis* was isolated in 1995 from a 16-year-old boy who survived the disease. The boy probably survived

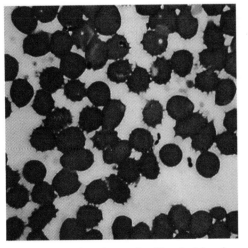

Figure 70.1 The plague bacillus in blood.

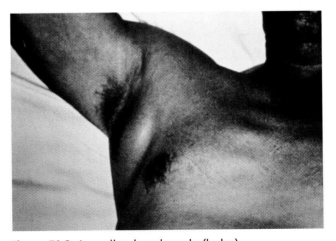

Figure 70.2 A swollen lymph node (bubo).

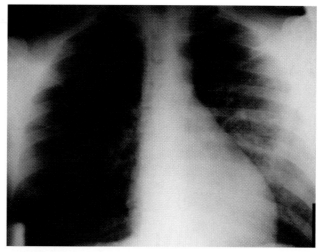

Figure 70.3 A chest X ray of a patient with plague pneumonia.

because he was treated with the antibacterial agent trimethoprim, which the strain was sensitive to. The strain is resistant to chloramphenicol, streptomycin, and tetracycline, drugs that have been the classical therapy for the disease. Another antibiotic mixture containing sulfonamides and tetracycline, which is usually given to people who have been exposed to the disease, also had no effect. Laboratory studies of this drug-resistant strain of *Y. pestis* indicated that it can transfer its resistance to other strains of plague bacteria.

The second complication that made abating the epidemic difficult was the Hindu religion. In Hinduism, the predominant religion in India, the rat is the steed of the vehicle of the elephant-headed god Ganesh, and few devout Hindus would deliberately kill a rat, believing it is sinful to do so.

Finally, the population of India is over 1 billion. Many people live in poverty. Homelessness, malnutrition, and lack of public health infrastructure (garbage disposal, sewage treatment, clean water supplies, and access to high-technology health care) are common in many areas. Given the government's limited resources, funds must be devoted to programs that will have the greatest effect on saving the most lives.

APPLICATION

Assuming you have been sent by the World Health Organization to advise the Indian government, how would you prioritize the expenditure of funds and resources?

1. What would be your first priority? Why?
2. What would be your second priority? Why?
3. What would be your third priority? Why?

Dengue Fever

Dengue fever is the most important mosquito-borne viral disease affecting humans. It is one of the top 10 killer infectious diseases worldwide. It is estimated that 2.5 billion people are at risk for acquiring dengue fever, and tens of millions of cases of dengue fever occur each year. The lethal version of the disease, DHF, affects hundreds of thousands per year, with a case fatality rate of about 5%.

Cause of the disease

The causative agent of dengue fever is a flavivirus, the dengue virus. The virus has single-stranded RNA inside an enveloped icosahedral capsid (a protein shell with 20 sides). There are four different serotypes of dengue virus: DEN-1, DEN-2, DEN-3, and DEN-4.

Transmission

Reservoir

The virus survives in either a human-mosquito or monkey-mosquito cycle. The disease is typically found in tropical and subtropical areas of the world.

Mode of transmission

Dengue fever is a vector-borne disease that is transmitted to humans by the bite of a female *Aedes aegypti* mosquito, a domestic, day-biting mosquito that prefers to feed on humans.

Pathogenesis

Entry

The pathogen is introduced directly into the blood by the bite of an infected mosquito.

Attachment

The virus attaches to mononuclear phagocytes.

Avoiding host defenses

The virus is an intracellular pathogen that initially avoids circulating antibodies and cells of the immune system. The virus destroys cells of the immune system.

Damage

Infection of monocytes results in an increase in the activation of complement and the release of kinins, which produces the systemic features of the disease. DHF is caused by a second infection of the dengue virus (especially DEN-2). The antibodies produced to fight off the first infection actually enhance the infection of monocytes during the second infection. The greater proportion of infected cells results in greater virus production. It is hypothesized that the infected monocytes release vasoactive mediators, resulting in the increased vascular permeability and hemorrhagic manifestations that characterize dengue hemorrhagic fever or dengue shock syndrome.

Clinical features

The incubation period is typically 5 to 8 days. Infection with dengue viruses produces a spectrum of clinical illness ranging from a nonspecific viral syndrome to severe and fatal hemorrhagic disease.

Symptoms of dengue fever include sudden onset of fever that lasts 2 to 7 days, severe headache, bone and joint pain, weakness, anorexia, nausea, vomiting, and a rash. Dengue hemorrhagic fever is characterized by dengue fever plus hemorrhagic manifestations: a tendency to bruise easily, bleeding nose or gums, and possibly internal bleeding, which may lead to failure of the circulatory system and shock, followed by death.

Diagnosis

Clinical

Dengue fever is often misdiagnosed as influenza, measles, typhoid fever, or malaria.

Laboratory

Specimen: A blood serum sample is used as a specimen.

Test: Anti-dengue immunoglobulin M (IgM) and IgG are detected by indirect ELISA. Specific serotypes can be identified by indirect fluorescent-antibody testing.

Treatment

There are no antiviral medications to inhibit the dengue virus.

Analgesics with acetaminophen are used to reduce pain and fever. Aspirin and nonsteroidal anti-inflammatory drugs, such as ibuprofen, should be avoided because of their anticoagulant properties. Other symptomatic therapies include bed rest and either oral or i.v. fluids and electrolytes.

Prevention

- There is no vaccine for dengue fever.
- The focus for prevention is to eliminate the places where the mosquito lays her eggs—primarily artificial

containers that hold water (i.e., plastic containers, 55-gallon drums, buckets, pet water bowls, flower vases, or used automobile tires).

- The risk of being bitten by mosquitoes indoors is reduced by utilization of air conditioning or windows and doors that are screened, application of mosquito repellents containing DEET, and wearing long-sleeved shirts and pants that are tucked into socks.

Ebola Hemorrhagic Fever

From the scraps of information he had been able to obtain about the situation in Sudan and Zaire, they were dealing with a plague virus that was tremendously lethal and that could be spreading from person to person in a manner not previously seen with such a lethal virus. The cardinal issue was now lucid, if starkly frightening. Is this virus going to turn out to be transmitted by sneezing and coughing in a manner similar to influenza? If you have an infection that is virtually fatal, as this turned out to be, and transmitted by that mechanism, now, suddenly you have a threat to the entire human species.

Karl Johnson, head of the Special Pathogens Branch of the CDC, on his way to investigate the first Ebola hemorrhagic fever outbreak in Zaire

Cause of the disease

Ebola virus is the causative agent of Ebola hemorrhagic fever. It is an enveloped virus with a helical capsid that is elongated and twisted on one end like a shepherd's crook. The virus contains single-stranded, negative-stranded RNA for genetic information.

Transmission

Reservoir

The exact origin, locations, and natural habitat of Ebola virus remain unknown. Researchers believe that the virus has a reservoir where it is maintained in an animal host that is native to the African continent. The virus has been acquired from ill chimpanzees in the jungles of the Congo and Gabon.

Mode of transmission

The pathogen is primarily transmitted by direct contact with infected fluids, such as blood, secretions, organs, or semen of infected persons. Health care workers have frequently been infected while attending patients.

Pathogenesis

The pathogenesis of Ebola hemorrhagic fever is not completely characterized. The disease is rare and occurs in remote areas of Africa. Due to the extreme danger of working with the virus, research is done only in a level IV biohazard facility.

Damage is caused by destruction of endothelial tissue. As a result, capillaries throughout the body are damaged, leading to massive tissue damage and fluid loss from all internal organs.

Clinical features

Incubation ranges from 2 to 21 days after infection. Ebola hemorrhagic fever is often characterized by the sudden onset of fever, weakness, muscle pain, headache, and sore throat, followed by vomiting, diarrhea, rash, limited kidney and liver functions, and both internal and external bleeding.

Diagnosis

Laboratory tests for Ebola hemorrhagic fever are done in high-level biohazard facilities, using ELISA to identify viruses or antibodies to the virus in the blood. PCR can also be used to detect Ebola virus genetic information.

Treatment

No specific treatment exists for Ebola hemorrhagic fever. Severe cases require intensive supportive care, as patients are frequently dehydrated from excessive internal bleeding and in need of careful monitoring of blood components to attempt to balance fluids, electrolytes, and blood components using intravenous therapy.

Prevention

- Containment: patients with suspected cases should be isolated from other patients, and strict barrier nursing techniques should be practiced. Hospital staff should have individual gowns, gloves, and masks. Gloves and masks must not be reused unless they are disinfected.

- Prompt burial: patients who die from the disease should be promptly buried or cremated.

- Contact tracing: as the primary mode of person-to-person transmission is contact with contaminated blood, secretions, or body fluids, any person who has had close physical contact with patients should be kept under strict surveillance, i.e., body temperature checks twice a day with immediate hospitalization and strict isolation recommended in cases of temperatures above 38.3°C (101°F).

- Casual contacts should be placed on alert and asked to report any fever.

- Surveillance of suspected cases should continue for 3 weeks after the date of their last contact. Hospital personnel who come into close contact with patients or contaminated materials without barrier nursing attire must be considered exposed and put under closely supervised surveillance.

Hantavirus Pulmonary Syndrome

Hantavirus pulmonary syndrome was first characterized during an outbreak in 1993 in the Four Corners area of the southwestern United States. Although most cases are found in the southwestern United States, the pathogen is more widely distributed by its rodent hosts.

Cause of the disease

The causative agent of hantavirus pulmonary syndrome is Sin Nombre virus, a hantavirus. The virus has an enveloped, icosohedral capsid (a protein shell with 20 sides) with single-stranded RNA for genetic information.

Transmission

Reservoir

The disease is a zoonosis. Four species of rodents are reservoirs for the virus: the deer mouse, the cotton rat, the rice rat, and the white-footed mouse.

Mode of transmission

The virus is airborne and is typically transmitted by inhaling aerosols from dried rodent urine or feces from rodents that were infected by the virus. The pathogen is not transmitted person to person.

Pathogenesis

Entry

The virus enters the lungs as an airborne pathogen.

Attachment

The pathogen probably attaches to alveolar macrophages and endothelial cells.

Avoiding host defenses

The virus is an intracellular pathogen, so it initially avoids circulating antibodies and cells of the immune system.

Damage

The damage caused by the virus results in a complex pathophysiology. One key to the damage is that the virus destroys endothelial cells, causing hemorrhaging and fluid loss. This causes a sudden life-threatening pneumonia.

Clinical features

Early signs and symptoms include fever, fatigue, and muscle aches and can include headaches, dizziness, chills, and abdominal problems. Later features occur as fluid accumulates in the lungs: coughing, difficulty breathing, and shortness of breath.

Diagnosis

Clinical

Hantavirus pulmonary syndrome is a difficult disease to recognize as early symptoms appear, since the symptoms resemble those of common illnesses that are treatable. The disease progresses rapidly after early symptoms develop, necessitating hospitalization and often ventilation. The fever, headaches, and myalgia are followed by a nonproductive cough with rapid onset of respiratory failure.

Laboratory

Specimen: A blood serum sample is used as a specimen.

Tests: Detection of viral proteins is evaluated by ELISA or the detection of viral RNA sequences in blood or tissue by reverse transcriptase polymerase chain reaction.

Treatment

Intense supportive care in a hospital is needed to manage fluid loss and lung damage. Broad-spectrum antibiotics have been used to prevent secondary bacterial infections that may further complicate the disease.

Prevention

- Prevention focuses on reducing suitable environments for rodents in and around homes.
- Food should be stored in tightly sealed, rodent-proof containers.
- All garbage should be discarded in rodent-proof containers and disposed of regularly.
- Habitats for rodents, such as brush or wood piles near homes, should be removed or moved.
- Traps can be set both inside and outside the home.
- Since sweeping or vacuuming can bring about aerosolization of dried rodent urine or feces, contaminated areas should first be wetted with disinfectant.

Leptospirosis

Leptospirosis is considered the most widespread zoonotic disease in the world. One hundred to 200 cases occur in the United States per year, about half in Hawaii. Leptospirosis is most common in young males during the summer and early fall.

Cause of the disease

Leptospira interrogans, a bacterial pathogen, is a gram-negative, long, thin spirochete that is highly motile. It can be free living or associated with animal hosts (humans and other animals).

Transmission

Reservoir

The pathogen survives well in freshwater, soil, and mud in tropical areas. Outbreaks are caused by exposure to water, food, or soil contaminated with the urine of infected animals.

Mode of transmission

Ingestion of the pathogen or direct contact with skin, especially broken skin, or mucosal surfaces of the eyes or nose introduces the pathogen into its host.

Pathogenesis

Entry

The pathogen enters by ingestion (i.e., drinking contaminated water); through abraded skin, lacerations, or intact mucous membranes in contact with the pathogen; and/or through intact skin after prolonged immersion in contaminated water.

Attachment

The helically shaped cell cylinder and two flagella enable the leptospires to burrow into tissue. Leptospires enter the bloodstream, disseminate throughout the body, and invade and multiply in numerous body tissues.

Overcoming host defenses

Leptospires can have a symbiotic relationship with hosts by staying in the renal tubules without producing disease or pathologic changes in the kidney.

Damage

Leptospires produce toxins.

Exit

The pathogen exits through urine.

Clinical features

There is about a 7-day incubation period (with a range between 2 and 20 days); the illness lasts up to about 3 weeks, but without treatment it can last months. Symptoms include high fever, severe headache, chills, muscle aches, vomiting, jaundice, red eyes, abdominal pain, diarrhea, and/or rash. If the disease is not treated, kidney damage, meningitis, liver failure, and respiratory distress can develop, and in rare cases, death can occur.

Diagnosis

Clinical

Leptospirosis is difficult to diagnose in the laboratory or clinic and is often overlooked because it shares the symptoms of many diseases (e.g., influenza) and can be easily mistaken for one of them, especially in the early stages.

Laboratory

Specimen: Blood samples are obtained.

Test: Microscope agglutination is the standard serologic test. Positive tests are confirmed by state health departments and the CDC.

Treatment

The drug commonly used to treat leptospirosis is doxycycline. Doxycycline inhibits the elongation of protein synthesis on 70S ribosomes. For young children, penicillin is commonly used. Penicillin prevents cross-linking of the peptidoglycan in the cell wall, causing osmotic lysis of the cell. Hospital care and intravenous medication are needed in serious cases.

Prevention

- There is no approved vaccine in the United States.
- Reducing the risk for acquiring the disease involves avoiding high-risk areas, i.e., areas with stagnant water, especially in tropical places, and not drinking the water in high-risk areas.
- Doxycycline has been used for prophylaxis to prevent getting the disease after exposure.
- Wearing shoes when outside in high-risk environments prevents entry of the pathogen through the feet when walking on contaminated soil.

Lyme Disease

Lyme disease was first described in Europe and was probably imported to the United States. The disease got its name from characterization of the first outbreak in the early 1970s in the Lyme, Connecticut, region. Lyme disease is now common in the United States from Maryland to Maine and in Wisconsin and Minnesota, with a smaller focus in northern California. The highest rates are in areas where there has been a large increase in deer and tick populations and where contact with humans has increased as people move into deer habitats. Approximately 90% of the approximately 10,000 annual cases are reported from the states between Maryland and Maine.

Cause of the disease

Lyme disease is caused by *Borrelia burgdorferi,* a bacterial pathogen. *Borrelia burgdorferi* is a gram-negative spirochete that moves using axial filaments. It has a unique genome consisting of a 950-kilobase linear chromosome, 9 linear plasmids, and 12 circular plasmids.

Achromosomal genes determine the antigenic identities of these organisms and presumably enable the bacterium to adapt to and survive in ticks and different mammalian hosts.

Transmission

Reservoir

The reservoirs for *Borrelia burgdorferi* are small mammals (primarily white-footed mice) and deer.

Mode of transmission

The pathogen enters by the parenteral route via the bite of a tick. Lyme disease is vector borne. The pathogen is carried and introduced by *Ixodes* ticks (deer ticks).

Pathogenesis

Entry

The tick normally must feed for 1 to 2 days in order for the pathogen to be transmitted.

Attachment

The pathogen attaches to fibronectin receptors and multiple other proteins, glycoproteins, and carbohydrates.

Avoiding host defenses

Infection by *Borrelia burgdorferi* produces a negative or delayed immune response to the pathogen. The pathogen also migrates to protected sites, such as joints and the central nervous system.

Damage

An inflammatory response occurs as the pathogen migrates in waves from the initial site of infection, causing a target-shaped rash. Systemic effects are caused by *Borrelia* initiating a series of events that stimulate release of tumor necrosis factor and interleukin-1. Both products stimulate endotoxic-shock symptoms.

Clinical features

After infection, there is typically a 7- to 14-day incubation period. Lyme disease is a multisystem, multistage, inflammatory illness. It begins with flu-like symptoms, which are often accompanied by an expanding target-shaped rash at the site of the tick bite. Arthritis also develops from joint inflammation. If untreated, the pathogen enters the central nervous system and can cause seizures, coma, and death.

Diagnosis

Clinical

If the characteristic rash does not develop, diagnosis by clinical signs alone is difficult, as the disease can be mistaken for influenza, arthritis, or multiple sclerosis.

Laboratory

Specimen: A blood sample is taken.

Tests: An ELISA or an indirect fluorescent-antibody test is used to detect antibodies against the pathogen. Diagnosis is confirmed by Western immunoblotting (monoclonal antibodies detect *Borrelia*-specific proteins after electrophoresis) to corroborate equivocal or positive results obtained with the first test.

Treatment

If infection is detected early, excellent results have been obtained with antibiotic treatment for 3 to 4 weeks. Doxycycline or amoxicillin is generally effective. Doxycycline blocks elongation of protein synthesis on 70S ribosomes. Amoxicillin is a β-lactam that blocks peptidoglycan cross-linking, causing osmotic lysis of the cell.

Prevention

- Avoid tick bites.
- Avoid tick-infested areas.
- Wear light-colored clothing outdoors to make ticks more easily visible.
- Wear long pants tucked into socks; a tucked-in, long-sleeved shirt; and a broad-brimmed hat.
- Use insect repellent containing DEET.
- Perform a tick check after spending time in a tick-infested area.
- Remove any biting ticks promptly.
- Control deer populations.
- Reduce tick populations near residential areas by removing leaf litter, brush, and woodpiles around houses and at the edges of yards and by clearing trees and brush to admit more sunlight, thus reducing deer, rodent, and tick habitats.
- Although it is effective and approved by the Food and Drug Administration, the vaccine against Lyme disease is no longer being distributed.

Malaria

Worldwide, malaria is the fifth most common cause of death from infectious disease (after pneumonia, tuberculosis, diarrhea, and acquired immune deficiency syndrome [AIDS]). An estimated 400 million clinical cases of malaria occur each year, with 2.6 million deaths; 70% of those who die of the disease are children. Malaria kills one child every 30 seconds.

Cause of the disease

Malaria is caused by *Plasmodium* spp., including *Plasmodium vivax*, *Plasmodium ovale*, *Plasmodium malariae*, and *Plasmodium falciparum*. *P. falciparum* is the most lethal species. *Plasmodium* is a eukaryotic protozoan with a complex life cycle that includes the formation of sporozoites.

Transmission

Reservoir

The parasite exists in a human-mosquito-human cycle.

Mode of transmission

Malaria is a vector-borne disease. The mode of transmission is the parenteral route by the bite of the *Anopheles* mosquito. The mosquito is a biological vector; the malarial parasite undergoes part of its developmental cycle within the mosquito host.

Pathogenesis

Entry

The pathogen enters by the parenteral route through the bite of an anopheline mosquito.

Attachment

Plasmodium attaches to and replicates in hepatocytes (liver cells) initially and is then released to infect erythrocytes.

Avoiding host defenses

The pathogen undergoes antigenic shifting as it progresses through its life cycle: trophozoites, schizonts, merozoites, sporozoites, and gametes.

Damage

The developmental cycle in erythrocytes ends with rupture and the release of merozoites to infect new erythrocytes. The rupture of erythrocytes causes severe anemia, capillary hemorrhage, and blood clots.

In *P. falciparum* infections, erythrocytes become sticky and block the capillaries in the brain, resulting in hemorrhages and necrosis.

Exit

The female anopheline mosquito removes blood that contains plasmodial gametes; the gametes fuse to form zygotes and then develop into sporozoite cysts in the mosquito.

Clinical features

Malaria is characterized by cyclic fevers that have 3- or 4-day cycles, depending on the infecting species. The cycle begins with a victim feeling cold and shivering, followed by a hot, dry fever and drenching sweats. This is accompanied by joint pain, intense headache, severe anemia, and repeated vomiting. Enlargement of the spleen and liver occurs with chronic infections. *Plasmodium falciparum* causes cerebral hemorrhaging, resulting in generalized convulsions, coma, and death.

Diagnosis

Microscopic analysis of blood samples allows the identification of different species of *Plasmodium* as they are undergoing development in erythrocytes.

Treatment

Chloroquine and phosphochloroquine are used to treat malaria. The toxic drugs accumulate preferentially in *Plasmodium*-parasitized erythrocytes. Since most strains are drug resistant, the older treatment drug, quinine, must often be used, even though it causes more side effects.

Prevention

- The key to prevention is to control the mosquito populations. Community efforts include public spraying, reducing breeding sites by draining the small sunlit pools of water that the *Anopheles* mosquito uses to reproduce, eliminating open water containers, and destroying old tires.

- Personal efforts include using an insecticide containing DEET, using mosquito netting, and avoiding exposure at times when mosquitoes feed.

- Prophylaxis with chloroquine is used to prevent malaria when traveling to areas where malaria is endemic.

Plague

Worldwide, there are 1,000 to 2,000 cases of plague each year. Almost all of the cases reported from 1995 to 2005 were rural and occurred among people living in either small towns and villages or agricultural areas.

Cause of the disease

Yersinia pestis, a bacterial pathogen, is a gram-negative, rod-shaped bacterium with an antiphagocytic capsule. It is a facultative intracellular pathogen.

Transmission

Reservoir

Plague is a multisystem zoonosis that has an animal reservoir, primarily the small-mammal population.

Mode of transmission

Plague is transmitted by the parenteral route from animal to animal and from animal to human by the bites of infective fleas. An uncommon mode of transmission is by inhaling infected droplets expelled by coughing from a person or animal with pneumonic plague.

Pathogenesis

Entry

The bites of infected fleas cause itching near the site of the break in the skin. Scratching the irritated area causes the feces carrying the pathogen from the fleas to be introduced into the blood.

Attachment

The ability of *Yersinia pestis* to attach to and enter macrophages is a key determinant of pathogenicity.

Avoiding host defenses

The pathogen synthesizes a capsule that is antiphagocytic.

Damage

The pathogen is carried to the lymph nodes that drain the area of the flea bite, where the bacteria multiply, causing inflammation and invasiveness. The pathogen produces coagulase (which produces clots) and fibrinolysin (which degrades blood clots), endotoxin that can cause shock and disseminated intravascular coagulation, and V and W antigens that enable the pathogen to cause an overwhelming septicemia.

Exit

The pathogen may be spread to another human via respiratory droplets if the pathogen spreads to the lungs and causes pneumonia.

Clinical features

There is an incubation period of 2 to 6 days after infection. Plague begins with a fever, headache, and general illness before the development of painful, swollen regional lymph nodes (buboes). Plague septicemia follows, with rapid invasion of the bloodstream, producing severe illness, prostration, and extreme exhaustion. The pathogen may also spread to the lungs, causing an overwhelming pneumonia with high fever, cough, bloody sputum, and chills.

Diagnosis

Specimen

Blood or pus from an infected bubo is used as a specimen.

Tests

Gram staining is used to identify irregularly stained gram-negative rods that appear as safety pin shaped. Direct fluorescent-antibody assays are used to confirm the diagnosis.

Treatment

Antibiotic therapy begins as soon as plague is suspected. Several aminoglycosides are effective at treating plague. Aminoglycosides, such as streptomycin, are bacteriocidal and block the formation of 30S initiation complexes during the initiation of protein synthesis. Where cost is important and the health care infrastructure is poorly developed, tetracyclines are also effective and can be delivered orally. Tetracyclines block aminoacyl-transfer RNA (tRNA) binding to 70S ribosomes during the elongation of protein synthesis.

Prevention

- As soon as a diagnosis of suspected plague is made, the patient should be isolated to prevent spread to others.
- Those who have had contact with the plague patient are traced and given prophylactic antibiotics.
- Insecticides can be used to control the flea population.
- Public health education can be used to instruct home owners to eliminate food and shelter for rodents.
- Vaccination is available to prevent infection in at-risk groups, including people working with the plague bacterium in the laboratory or in the field and people working in plague-affected areas.

Rocky Mountain Spotted Fever

Rocky Mountain spotted fever was first recognized in 1896 in the Snake River Valley of Idaho and was originally called "black measles" because of the characteristic rash. It was a dreaded and frequently fatal disease until the discovery of tetracycline and chloramphenicol in the late 1940s. Untreated, as many as 30% of people infected with *Rickettsia rickettsii* died. Contrary to what the name implies, the disease can be found throughout the United States.

Cause of the disease

Rickettsia rickettsii, a bacterial pathogen, is a small gram-negative coccobacillus. *Rickettsia rickettsii* is an obligate intracellular pathogen that cannot replicate outside of a host cell.

Transmission

Reservoir
Ticks of the genus *Ixodes*, such as the Rocky Mountain wood tick and the American dog tick, serve as the main reservoirs for the disease.

Mode of transmission
Rocky Mountain spotted fever is a vector-borne disease that is transmitted via the bite of a tick. As a result, the disease is seen mostly in the late spring and during the summer months, when people are camping and spending time in the woods. Person-to-person transmission does not occur.

Pathogenesis

Entry
An infection can occur when the vector releases organisms from its salivary glands approximately 4 to 6 hours after feeding or when the tick is crushed in an attempt to remove it from human skin.

Attachment
The pathogen attaches to the vascular endothelium.

Avoiding host defenses
The bacteria avoid the body's defenses by living intracellularly.

Damage
The pathogen causes damage to cells, resulting in increased vascular permeability, which leads to fluid loss from the capillaries. This causes swelling and hypotension that can lead to shock and death. Invasion of and damage to the vascular endothelium of capillaries under the skin provide the basis for the skin rash.

Clinical features

Symptoms appear 2 to 14 days after exposure. Rocky Mountain spotted fever involves a sudden onset of moderate to high fever, muscle aches, severe headache, appetite loss, a general feeling of being run down, respiratory problems, a rash, muscle pain, sensitivity to light, and chills. Abdominal pain may occur with nausea, vomiting, tenderness, and diarrhea. The rash appears on the extremities by the third day, starting at the wrists and ankles and eventually spreading to the rest of the body.

Diagnosis

Clinical
The progress of the rash is unique and serves as a basis for clinical diagnosis.

Laboratory
Specimen: A blood serum sample is taken.
Test: The indirect immunofluorescence assay is generally considered the reference standard in Rocky Mountain spotted fever serology and is the test currently used by the CDC and most state public health laboratories.

Treatment

Doxycycline and tetracycline are the antibiotics of choice. Chloramphenicol is used for children under 7 years of age. The drugs diffuse well into the host cells and inhibit protein synthesis by the intracellular pathogen.

Prevention

- Prevention focuses on avoiding the vectors that carry the pathogen.
- Woods and fields where ticks are found should be avoided when possible.
- Tick repellent should be used, and long-sleeved shirts and long pants that are tied around the waist, wrists, and ankles should be worn.
- When one is camping or working in the woods, checks for ticks should be done at least twice daily and again upon leaving the wooded area.
- If a tick is found, it should be removed by gently grasping it with a pair of tweezers as close to the skin as possible and carefully removing it. After handling a tick, the hands should be washed thoroughly with soap and water.

Typhus

Epidemic typhus occurs in Central and South America, Africa, and parts of Asia. Outbreaks are associated with conditions that favor the lice that transmit the bacterium.

The pathogen can cause widespread capillary damage, leading to gangrene and the loss of digits or limbs, multisystem organ failure, and death. If the disease is untreated, the mortality rate ranges between 20% in healthy individuals and 60% in elderly or debilitated people. With antibiotic therapy, mortality drops to 4%.

Cause of the disease

Rickettsia prowazekii, a bacterial pathogen, is a short, pleomorphic (having many different shapes), gram-negative bacterium that is an obligate intracellular pathogen.

Transmission

Reservoir
Infected humans are the reservoir.

Mode of transmission
Vector-borne transmission occurs via the human body louse *Pediculus humanus*. A person with typhus cannot directly infect another person.

Pathogenesis

Entry
Epidemic typhus is most prevalent during war, famines, and other situations that promote unsanitary conditions in which body lice flourish. The lice jump from human to human to feed on their blood. Two to 3 days after their meal, the lice begin to defecate on the host's skin. The bites itch, and when humans scratch, the infected feces fall into the wound, where the bacteria begin to multiply.

Attachment
The bacteria travel through the body until they reach the circulatory system, where they attach to endothelial cells (cells that line small blood vessels and capillaries).

Avoiding host defenses
The bacteria avoid the body's defenses by living intracellularly.

Damage
The bacteria cause endothelial cells to enlarge and burst, causing widespread capillary damage and releasing *R. prowazekii* into the blood to infect other cells.

Exit
The pathogen exits when non-pathogen-carrying lice make a meal from the blood of an infected human.

Clinical features
Patients become ill after an incubation period of 8 to 12 days. Infected people experience photosensitivity, severe headache, high fever, chills, falling blood pressure, stupor, delirium, and cough. Severe muscle pain and severe exhaustion, alternating with agitation, are also observed. A rash appears on the fifth or sixth day, beginning on the chest and spreading to the rest of the trunk and extremities, but not the palms, the soles of the feet, or the face. The early rash is faint and rose colored and fades with pressure. Later, the lesions become dull and red and do not fade.

Diagnosis
Typhus can be confirmed by performing a biopsy of the skin rash. The rash can lead to diagnosis by use of a direct fluorescent-antibody assay showing the presence of rickettsiae in the tissue.

Treatment
Typhus is generally treated with a single dose of doxycycline. Tetracyclines are bacteriostatic inhibitors of protein synthesis that block the binding of aminoacyl-tRNAs to the ribosome, preventing the addition of amino acids to the growing peptide chain.

Prevention
- Pesticides can be used to treat individuals or large groups infested with body lice.
- Louse-infested clothing can be treated to remove potential pathogens by washing and then drying the clothes at a minimum 70°C for 1 hour.

West Nile Encephalitis
West Nile virus was discovered in 1937 in the West Nile district of Uganda. West Nile encephalitis is common in the Middle East, Asia, and Africa. For example, approximately 50% of children in Egypt test positive for having been infected by the virus. West Nile encephalitis is the most common cause of viral aseptic meningitis or encephalitis in patients presenting to emergency departments in Cairo.

West Nile virus emerged in the United States for the first time in the New York City area in August 1999 and has now spread throughout the United States. Although most infections are asymptomatic, West Nile virus can cause life-threatening encephalitis, especially in the elderly.

Cause of the disease

West Nile encephalitis is caused by West Nile virus, a flavivirus. This virus has a positive-sense, single-stranded RNA surrounded by an icosahedral capsid (a protein shell with 20 sides) with an envelope.

Transmission

Reservoir

The pathogen is primarily found in birds.

Mode of transmission

West Nile encephalitis is a vector-borne disease. The *Culex* mosquito is the common vector. It becomes infected when it feeds on infected birds. Infected mosquitoes can then transmit West Nile virus to humans and animals while biting to take blood. In rare instances, the virus has been spread by blood transfusion.

Pathogenesis

Entry

The virus enters by the parenteral route via the mosquito vector.

Avoiding host defenses

The virus is an intracellular pathogen, so it initially avoids circulating antibodies and cells of the immune system.

Damage

The pathogen multiplies in the person's blood system and crosses the blood-brain barrier, after which it can cause inflammation of brain tissue.

Exit

The virus exits by the bite of a mosquito.

Clinical features

Most infections are asymptomatic. About 20% develop into West Nile fever after an incubation period of 3 to 14 days. Less than 1% develop into meningoencephalitis (swelling of the brain and the protective tissues surrounding the brain and spinal cord). Advanced age is the primary risk factor for severe neurological disease and death. The disease presents as a mild dengue-like illness with sudden onset, including fever, lymphadenopathy (swollen lymph nodes), headache, abdominal pain, vomiting, rash, conjunctivitis, eye pain, and anorexia. The disease typically lasts 3 to 6 days.

Diagnosis

Specimen

Blood or cerebrospinal fluid is used as a specimen.

Test

An indirect ELISA is used to measure serum IgM antibodies made early in the response to a West Nile virus infection.

Treatment

There are currently no effective antiviral agents to inhibit the growth of West Nile virus. Treatment focuses on supportive care. About 25% of patients require intensive care, including mechanical ventilation.

Prevention

- The key to prevention is to control mosquito populations. Community efforts include public spraying and reducing breeding sites and habitats.
- Personal efforts include using an insecticide containing DEET, using mosquito netting, and staying inside when mosquitoes feed.

Yellow Fever

Yellow fever transmission predominantly occurs in areas of sub-Saharan Africa and South America near the equator. These epidemics commonly involve 30 to 1,000 cases and have fatality rates of 20 to 50%. The highest incidence of yellow fever is in areas of West Africa, with an estimated 200,000 cases annually. In today's culture, almost all cases of yellow fever are found in those who work outdoors in agriculture and forestry. As a result, they are exposed to mosquitoes that have acquired the virus from monkeys with the disease.

Cause of the disease

The causative agent of yellow fever is the yellow fever virus. The pathogen has positive-stranded, single-stranded RNA as genetic information; a polyhedral capsid; and an envelope.

Transmission

Reservoir

The primary reservoir is monkeys.

Mode of transmission

Yellow fever is a vector-borne disease that is transmitted primarily in a monkey-mosquito cycle. It can enter the human population, and if enough people are infected, a human-mosquito cycle can begin. *Aedes aegypti* is the primary vector in urban epidemics.

Pathogenesis

Entry

The pathogen enters via the parenteral route from the bite of an *Aedes* mosquito.

Attachment

The virus attaches to leukocytes, platelets, and endothelium.

Avoiding host defenses

The virus is an intracellular pathogen, so it initially avoids circulating antibodies and cells of the immune system. It also infects and destroys leukocytes, causing immunosuppression.

Damage

The pathogen causes direct damage through cell lysis. Damage of liver cells causes jaundice. Destruction of platelets causes hemorrhagic manifestations, especially in the GI tract. Destruction of the endothelium causes fluid loss and shock. The pathogen may also cross the blood-brain barrier to cause encephalitis symptoms.

Indirect damage is caused by the release of cytokines to trigger fever and flulike symptoms.

Clinical features

The disease has an incubation period of 3 to 6 days. This is followed by a sudden onset of fever; an intense frontal headache; and muscle aches, flushing of the skin, anorexia, conjunctivitis, and prostration. Yellow fever results in severe jaundice due to liver damage and massive gastrointestinal hemorrhage. Fluid loss can cause hypotension, dehydration, kidney failure, and shock. The disease has a mortality rate of about 30%.

Diagnosis

Clinical

Early stages of yellow fever are easily confused with malaria, hemorrhagic fevers, and typhoid.

Laboratory

Specimen: A blood serum sample is taken.

Test: Serologic assays are used to screen for yellow fever virus antibodies in the blood.

Treatment

There are no effective antiviral agents to inhibit replication of the virus. Treatment focuses on providing supportive care, including rehydration with fluids and electrolytes, providing antibiotics to prevent secondary bacterial infections, and intensive supportive care in a hospital.

Prevention

- There is an effective vaccine that is recommended for all people 9 months of age or older traveling to areas of Africa, South America, or India where yellow fever is endemic. Immunity lasts for about 10 years.

- The key to widespread prevention is to control the mosquito populations. Community efforts include public spraying and reducing breeding sites and habitats. Personal efforts include using an insecticide containing DEET, using mosquito netting, and avoiding exposure during times when mosquitoes feed.

Outbreaks of Diseases of the Central Nervous System

I died last night of my physician.
MATTHEW PRIOR, *The Remedy Worse than the Disease* (1714)

The central nervous system (CNS) is well protected by very restrictive permeability barriers. CNS pathogens that have escaped the formidable defenses of the skin and blood still have to cross the blood-brain barrier. The capillaries in the brain lack pores and are surrounded by astrocytes, resulting in a double cell layer that restricts the movement of hazardous chemicals and pathogens into the nervous tissue. Although the capillaries next to the choroid plexus have pores, the cells of the choroid plexus are tightly linked to prevent easy entry into the cerebrospinal fluid. As a result, most CNS pathogens are rare complications of infections at other sites. Few pathogens pass through the CNS during their normal pathogenesis.

Microbes that infect the CNS have several strategies to bypass host defenses. *Streptococcus pneumoniae* causes pneumonia. *Neisseria meningitidis* can live in nasal mucosa. Both bacteria can cause pharyngitis. If the damage caused by such an infection allows entry of the bacteria into the blood, they may also cause meningitis. *Streptococcus pneumoniae* and *Neisseria meningitidis* produce antiphagocytic capsules and a protease that degrades immunoglobulin A antibodies. As a result, they are more likely to avoid mucosal immune defenses and survive attack by leukocytes in the blood. Other pathogens, such as poliovirus and rabies virus, enter peripheral neurons and migrate to the CNS. As intracellular pathogens, they are protected from circulating antibodies.

The consequences of a microbial infection of the CNS are serious. Untreated, meningitis caused by *Neisseria meningitidis* is fatal. Even with antibiotic therapy, *Neisseria meningitidis* has about a 10% mortality rate. Rabies virus is lethal without postexposure vaccination.

Even when infections of the CNS are not lethal, they can still have major health consequences, such as paralysis, seizures, mental retardation, blindness, and/or deafness.

In a college setting, the most common CNS pathogen is meningitis-causing microbes that are spread as respiratory pathogens. This section emphasizes the importance of rapid treatment and prevention strategies to decrease the spread of infections that can be lethal.

Table VII.1 Selected outbreak-causing pathogens of the nervous system

Organism	Key physical properties	CNS characteristics
Bacteria		
Clostridium botulinum	Anaerobic, gram-positive, endospore-forming bacillus that produces a potent neurotoxin, which causes muscle paralysis	Botulism, flaccid paralysis
Clostridium tetani	Anaerobic, gram-positive, endospore-forming bacillus that produces a neurotoxin that causes continuous muscle contraction	Tetanus
Haemophilus influenzae type b	Fastidious, gram-negative bacillus that produces an antiphagocytic capsule	Meningitis in unvaccinated infants and young children
Neisseria meningitidis	Gram-negative diplococcus; oxidase positive	Meningococcal meningitis
Streptococcus pneumoniae	Gram-positive streptococcus; alpha-hemolytic on blood agar; catalase negative	Meningitis
Fungi		
Cryptococcus neoformans	Yeast with a large capsule	Meningitis
Protozoa		
Plasmodium falciparum	Sporozoa that infect red blood cells	Cerebral malaria, cyclic fevers, encephalitis
Toxoplasma gondii	Large cysts in tissue	Toxoplasmosis; encephalitis and abscesses
Viruses		
Enteroviruses	Nonenveloped polyhedral capsids with single-stranded RNA	Most are asymptomatic, but can cause fever and rash or viral meningitis (aseptic meningitis)
Polioviruses	Nonenveloped polyhedral capsids with single-stranded RNA	Polio causes motor neuron damage and paralysis
Rabies virus	Enveloped helical capsid with single-stranded RNA	Rabies causes periods of agitation and calm, paralysis of the swallowing reflex, and lethal encephalitis

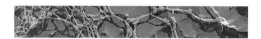

An Outbreak of Acute Flaccid Paralysis

CAPE VERDE, 2000

Between 16 August and 17 October 2000, 33 cases of acute flaccid paralysis, including 7 (21%) deaths, were reported in Cape Verde, an archipelago of 10 islands west of Senegal and Mauritania. The first patient was a child aged 2 years from the capital city of Praia; the onset of paralysis occurred on 16 August. Twenty-two cases were reported from the island of São Tiago, seven from Sal, three from São Vicente, and one from Maio. The ages of the acute flaccid paralysis patients ranged from 3 months to 38 years.

The estimated population of Cape Verde in 2000 was 437,500 (World Health Organization, unpublished data, 2000). The reported routine vaccination coverage had been <80% every year since 1995.

In addition to paralysis, those who were affected had experienced stiffness in the neck, flu-like symptoms, and diarrhea. The viral pathogen, identified by enzyme-linked immunosorbent assay, was a positive-sense, single-stranded ribonucleic acid (RNA) virus with a polyhedral capsid belonging to the picornavirus family (Fig. 71.1).

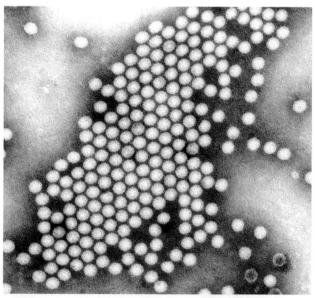

Figure 71.1 A transmission electron micrograph of the virus that caused the paralysis.

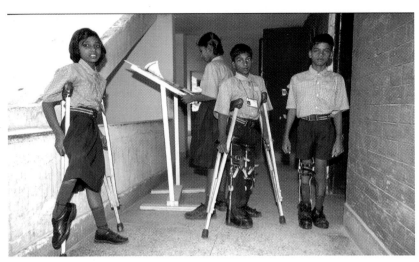

Figure 71.2 Paralysis in children affected by the pathogen.

QUESTIONS

1. What disease was involved in this outbreak?

2. Identify the pathogen and describe how it is typically transmitted.

3. How does the virus cause paralysis?

4. Would you have expected more than 33 people to have been infected by this virus during the outbreak?

5. In order to minimize the number of deaths and cases of the disease, how would you have managed the outbreak?

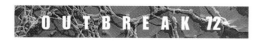

An Outbreak of Paralysis from Eating Fermented Beaver Tails

ALASKA, 2001

On 18 January 2001, the Alaska Division of Public Health was informed by a local physician of a village in southwest Alaska where 14 people became ill after eating fermented beaver tails and paws on 17 January. Approximately 20 hours after the meal, 3 of the 14 had symptoms, including dry mouth, blurry vision, and general weakness. Two patients developed respiratory failure and required mechanical ventilation. One of the two patients suffered cardiac arrest and underwent successful cardiopulmonary resuscitation. They subsequently were evacuated to an intensive-care unit (ICU) in Anchorage. Two patients recovered without further complications. The third required tracheotomy tube placement and mechanical ventilation for 1 month. Of the other 11 exposed persons, 4 reported minor symptoms, including dry mouth and nausea.

Beavers are hunted in southwest Alaska, and certain parts are often fermented and eaten later. In traditional fermentation, food is kept in a grass-lined hole in the ground or a wooden barrel sunken into the ground or is placed in a shady area above ground for several weeks to months. Since the 1970s, however, plastic or glass containers have been used and fermentation has been done above ground or indoors. In this outbreak, the tail and paws had been wrapped in a paper rice sack and stored for up to 3 months in the entry of a patient's house. Some of the beaver tails and paws had been added to the sack as recently as 1 week before they were eaten. Clinical specimens from the 14 exposed people were tested at the Centers for Disease Control and Prevention (CDC) laboratory. Serum specimens from two of the ICU patients and in stool from the third were positive for a neurotoxin. The toxin was also detected in three beaver paws from the implicated meal.

Bacteria were cultured from the fermentation containers. The cultures grew only under anaerobic conditions. Laboratory tests indicated a gram-positive, endospore-forming bacillus as the causative agent.

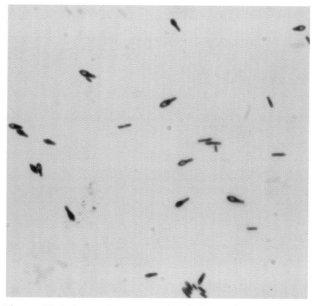

Figure 72.1 An endospore stain of the pathogen.

QUESTIONS

1. What pathogen caused the outbreak?

2. Describe the typical course of the disease.

3. What features of nontraditional fermentation practices allow the growth of this toxin-producing bacterium?

4. How would you have treated those seriously affected by the disease?

5. How could you prevent future outbreaks within the Alaskan Native population?

6. Describe the pathogenesis of the disease.

Rabies Infections from Organ Donor Tissues

MULTISTATE, 2004

An Arkansas man who visited two hospitals in Texas with severe mental status changes and a low-grade fever became an organ donor after his death. Neurological imaging indicated findings consistent with a subarachnoid hemorrhage (bleeding in the space between the brain and the skull) leading to death. Donor eligibility screening and testing did not reveal any contraindications to transplantation, and the kidneys and liver were recovered and transplanted into three recipients at a transplant center in Texas.

The liver recipient was a man with end-stage liver disease. The first kidney recipient was a woman with end-stage renal disease caused by hypertension and diabetes. The second kidney recipient was a man with lethal renal disease. The patients did well immediately after transplantation and were discharged after an initial recovery period in the hospital. Three to four weeks after transplantation, the patients were readmitted with neurological problems. The patients' neurological status deteriorated rapidly, with deteriorating mental status, seizures, and respiratory failure. The patients eventually required critical-care support. Magnetic resonance imaging showed severe cerebral edema (swelling). One to two weeks after admission, the patients died of encephalitis.

In all three patients, histopathologic examination of CNS tissues at the CDC revealed encephalitis with viral inclusions suggestive of Negri bodies; the diagnosis of rabies in all three recipients was confirmed by immunohistochemical testing and by the detection of rabies virus antigen in fixed brain tissue by direct fluorescent-antibody tests. Rabies virus antibodies were demonstrated in blood from two of the three recipients and the donor.

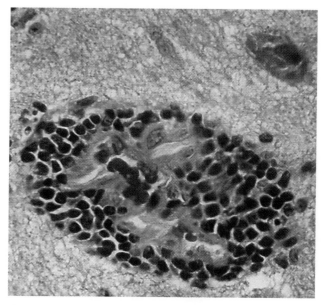

Figure 73.1 A Negri body in CNS tissue.

QUESTIONS

1. How did these individuals probably acquire the rabies virus infections?

2. How are the majority of rabies cases transmitted in the United States?

3. Explain why postexposure vaccination can prevent rabies in someone who has been infected.

4. Why is it necessary to begin the vaccination process quickly?

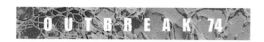

A Tetanus Outbreak

PUERTO RICO, 2002

Case 1

On 19 December 2001, a man aged 86 years with a history of hypertension and coronary artery disease sustained a splinter in his right hand while gardening. On 22 December, the patient saw a physician for wound care. On 26 December, the patient received treatment for pharyngitis (sore throat) from a local physician. On 29 December, he presented to an emergency department (ED) with difficulty talking, swallowing, and breathing and with chest pain and disorientation of 2 days' duration. He was admitted to a general-medicine ward with a preliminary diagnosis of stroke. On 2 January 2002, the patient had neck rigidity and respiratory failure requiring tracheotomy and mechanical ventilation and was transferred to the ICU, where tetanus was diagnosed. His hospital course was complicated by two myocardial infarctions, congestive heart failure, a stroke, and pneumonia. He died on 2 February.

Case 2

On 18 April 2002, a man aged 68 years with a history of diabetes mellitus, coronary artery disease, and heart valve replacement sustained a puncture wound in his right foot from stepping on a rusted nail. His spouse cleaned the wound with a surface antiseptic containing benzalkonium chloride. The following day, the patient sought care from a primary-care physician, who administered intravenous cefazolin and prescribed oral ciprofloxacin and oxycodone. On 22 April, the patient presented to an ED complaining of difficulty swallowing, mild shortness of breath, abdominal pain, throat pain, and stiff jaw muscles (mandibular rigidity). On physical examination, he had muscular rigidity and difficulty speaking. He was admitted to the ICU with diagnoses of suspected tetanus and right foot cellulitis (infection of the tissue under the skin). He was treated with metronidazole,

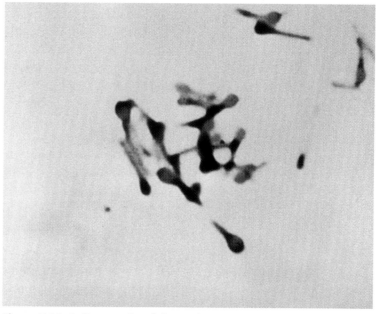

Figure 74.1 A Gram stain of the pathogen.

223

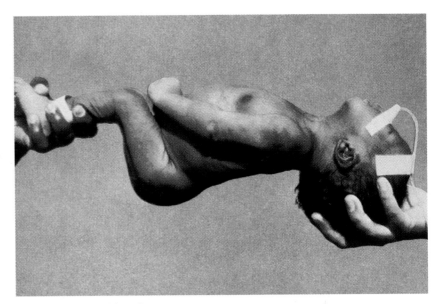

Figure 74.2 A child with tetanus.

ciprofloxacin, and midazolam by continuous intravenous infusion. On 23 April, the patient had seizures and respiratory failure requiring mechanical ventilation. He died on 27 April.

Case 3

On 10 April 2002, a man aged 76 years with a history of hypertension sustained a splinter wound in his right hand. On 18 April, the patient experienced weakness and difficulty speaking. At that time, he was treated for otitis media. On 20 April, the patient presented to an ED with difficulty walking, talking, and swallowing. He did not report any wound history to the attending physician. He was treated with an intramuscular corticosteroid injection and an antihistamine. On 21 April, the patient sought care at another ED. He was admitted to the ICU with diagnosed tetanus and put on mechanical ventilation preemptively. On 22 April, he received 3,000 units of tetanus immunoglobulin and was started on metronidazole. His course was complicated by methicillin-sensitive *Staphylococcus aureus* pneumonia and pseudomembranous colitis. He was released from the hospital on 17 June.

QUESTIONS

1. What pathogen causes tetanus?

2. Is there any danger of the disease spreading to family members or health care workers?

3. What characteristic of the pathogen makes puncture wounds like the ones described above particularly susceptible to the tetanus-causing pathogen?

4. How is the disease prevented?

5. What recommendations would you have made to the Puerto Rican health care community to decrease the number of tetanus cases?

An Outbreak of Aseptic Meningitis among Recreational Vehicle Campers

CONNECTICUT, 2003

Aseptic meningitis is an inflammation of the tissues covering the brain and spinal cord and is caused by a virus. In August 2003, an investigation by the Connecticut Department of Public Health identified 12 viral meningitis cases among recreational vehicle campers staying at a campground in northeastern Connecticut.

A meningitis patient in this outbreak was defined as a seasonal camper with headache and either neck stiffness or photophobia, with illness onset between 16 July and 17 August 2003. Other acute, self-limited illnesses consistent with enteroviral infections were also identified during the outbreak period. A case of enterovirus-like illness was defined clinically as an acute illness in a seasonal camper with illness onset between 16 July and 17 August with any one of the following symptoms: headache, neck stiffness, photophobia, sore throat, chills, or an acute generalized skin rash. Among 201 seasonal campers, 12 cases of meningitis and 24 other cases of enterovirus-like illness were identified. Four meningitis patients were hospitalized.

The following factors were associated with illness.

1. The dates of onset of illness for meningitis and other enterovirus-like illness cases were similar and clustered in four peaks 6 to 8 days apart. (For example, two enterovirus-like illnesses occurred in campers from a single campsite. The first illness preceded the second illness peak by 8 days). Four children hospitalized with laboratory-confirmed aseptic meningitis came from four different campsites. The mothers of three of these children had an enterovirus-like illness with onset 6 to 8 days before the onset of their child's illness.

2. Attack rates were higher at campsites with more campers per site: 1 or 2 campers per site, 6% (2 of 36); 3 or 4 campers, 16% (12 of 74); 5 or 6 campers, 17% (8 of 47); 7 or 8 campers, 21% (6 of 28); 9 or 10 campers, 50% (8 of 16).

3. Increasing frequency of submerging one's head in the campground pool during the outbreak period was associated with increased risk for primary illness of either type. Campers reported that the pool often was crowded at midday, particularly during weekends. Chlorine levels were checked twice a day (i.e., at approximately 7 a.m. and 8 p.m.) with a handheld test kit. According to written records, chlorine levels were low (0.5 to 1.0 milligram [mg]/liter versus the required level of >1.5 mg/liter) almost every evening throughout late July and August.

QUESTIONS

1. What types of viruses most frequently cause viral meningitis?

2. What was the attack rate for aseptic meningitis? For any enterovirus illness?

3. Why were the attack rates higher in campsites with more campers?

4. How would you explain the link between pool use and illness?

5. Why were the outbreaks clustered 6 to 8 days apart?

6. How would you have stopped this outbreak and prevented future outbreaks?

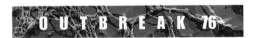

A Mad Cow Disease Outbreak in Humans and Cattle

UNITED STATES, CANADA, EUROPE, AND JAPAN, 2005

The U.S. response to a second case of mad cow disease in Canada was closely monitored in Japan, a major importer of U.S. beef. The Canadian government said that the dairy cow from the western province of Alberta which was found to have the disease was born in 1996 and was probably infected before strict prevention measures were put in place in 1997. Canada assured its trading partners that its beef was safe and that the country had a strong regulatory regime in place to stop the spread of bovine spongiform encephalopathy (BSE), also known as mad cow disease. The United States had banned the import of live Canadian cattle after the discovery of a case of mad cow disease, also in Alberta, in 2003.

Japan confirmed its first human case of variant Creutzfeldt-Jakob disease (vCJD), the human version of mad cow disease, after the death of a man in his fifties who had shown symptoms of the fatal brain-wasting illness. He might have contracted the disease while living in Great Britain for a period of at least 1 month in 1989. During that period, Britain began taking measures to check the world's worst outbreak of vCJD. Japan was already facing a national beef scare related to a limited outbreak of the disease in its domestic cattle herds, in which 15 cases were detected. From 1995 to 2004, 148 people have died of vCJD, almost all in Britain. As a result, Europe imposed a total ban on feeding of meat and bone meal to livestock in January 2001.

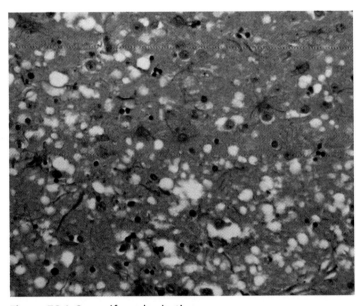

Figure 76.1 Spongiform brain tissue.

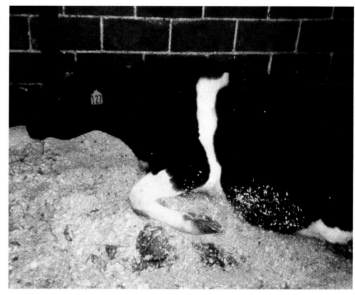

Figure 76.2 Lack of muscle control in an infected cow.

Once the largest importer of U.S. beef, Japan banned beef products from the United States after a cow in Washington State was determined to have the disease in December 2003. Although the ban was lifted at the end of 2005, Japanese consumers are hesitant to eat U.S. beef products because of fear of disease. Before the ban, Japan imported about $1.7 billion in beef products per year. The U.S. cattle industry is about a $30 billion industry.

In response to the news of the human and bovine cases of the disease, United Nations Food and Agriculture Organization expert Andrew Speedy stated that the recent cases "are isolated incidents."

QUESTIONS

1. What type of pathogen causes vCJD and mad cow disease?

2. How is vCJD contracted?

3. What are the clinical signs and symptoms of the disease in cattle? In humans?

4. How did the outbreak in Canada affect the Japanese import of cattle from the United States?

5. Do you agree that the Canadian cases were isolated incidents and that they did not endanger the U.S. beef supply?

6. If so, how would you argue the position with Japan, which has some of the highest food standards of any country in the world?

Meningitis Outbreaks Traced to Raves and Clubs

MICHIGAN AND ARGENTINA, 2000

Scientists traced several outbreaks of meningitis to local bars and dance clubs in the United States and Argentina. In all cases, the pathogen was a gram-negative, diplococcus-shaped bacteria. Common clinical features included symptoms of high fever, headache, a stiff neck, nausea, vomiting, confusion, sleepiness, and sometimes a rash.

In the United States, state health officials in Michigan reported that hundreds of students might have been exposed to meningitis at a "rave" party. Officials were concerned that the disease could have been passed among the partygoers when many of them shared a pacifier that had been dipped in the drug ecstasy. A side effect of ecstasy use is clenching and grinding of the teeth. As a result, candy pacifiers are used and were shared among those at the party. One young woman was diagnosed with meningitis after attending a rave party and had close contact with many of those at the party. One complication in determining who might have been exposed was that many of the students in attendance had not told their parents about the party. Therefore, the parents of those who became ill at home might not have recognized the need for quick treatment.

In Argentina, an outbreak of meningitis was traced to a popular disco. Researchers there examined eight patients hospitalized with symptoms of meningitis in a city in northeastern Argentina. All of the patients had resided in the city for more than 10 days before developing symptoms. Each patient was compared with four controls, individuals who had not developed meningitis but who were similar to the patients in gender and age.

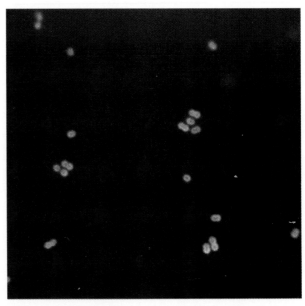

Figure 77.1 Direct fluorescent-antibody assay for *Neisseria meningitidis.*

The researchers collected data on each study subject, including risk factors for infection, such as the number of people living in the household, the size of the house, vaccination status, contact with others with respiratory symptoms, and exposure to public places. Those who had meningitis had attended one particular disco where it was popular to share maté, a drink that is served to groups with the use of a communal straw.

QUESTIONS

1. What pathogen caused the outbreaks of meningitis at the dance venues?

2. What are the key features of the disease that indicate it is meningitis and not simply a case of the "flu"?

3. How was the disease transmitted in these settings?

4. Why is it important to quickly identify close contacts of those who come down with meningitis?

5. What resources would you have mobilized to help identify those students who had attended the rave party in Michigan?

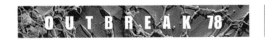 GLOBAL PERSPECTIVE

Meningitis among Travelers Returning from Saudi Arabia

UNITED STATES, 2000

Eleven thousand pilgrims were reported to have traveled from the United States to Saudi Arabia for the hajj (pilgrimage to Mecca), which concluded on 17 March 2000. On 9 April 2000, the CDC was notified by national public health agencies in several European countries of cases of meningitis among pilgrims returning from the hajj in Mecca and their close contacts (199 cases were reported within Saudi Arabia).

As of 20 April 2000, the New York City Department of Health had reported three cases of meningitis in the United States. A rash was apparent in one meningitis case. One patient was a returning pilgrim who had been vaccinated with the meningococcal quadrivalent polysaccharide vaccine that normally provides immunity to serogroup A of *Neisseria meningitidis*. A second case was a household contact of a returning pilgrim who did not show symptoms of the disease. The third patient did not participate in the hajj and had no household members or other close contacts who had traveled to Mecca; however, 5 days before the onset of illness, the patient might have interacted with returning pilgrims or their families. The three patients had no identified shared friends or associations. Samples were taken, and laboratory tests were performed to identify the pathogen, *Neisseria meningitidis*.

Prompted by a serogroup A meningococcal-disease outbreak associated with the 1987 hajj, Saudi Arabia began to require meningococcal vaccine for all entering pilgrims; however, the vaccine formulation varies by country. Most U.S. pilgrims probably received the quadrivalent polysaccharide vaccine covering serogroups A, C, Y, and W-135,

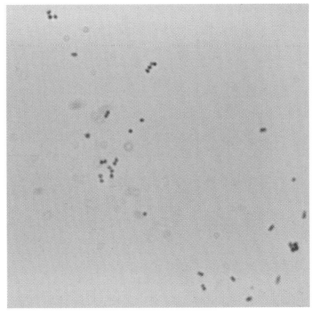

Figure 78.1 A Gram stain of the pathogen.

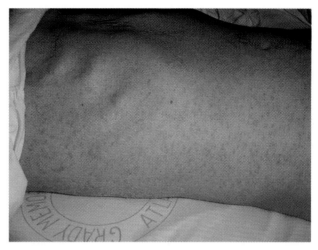

Figure 78.2 A rash associated with meningitis.

because it is the only meningococcal vaccine distributed in the United States. Meningococcal serogroup A and C polysaccharide vaccines have clinical efficacies of 85 to 100%. Vaccination with W-135 polysaccharide induces a bactericidal antibody, although clinical protection has not been documented. In addition, the polysaccharide vaccine does not prevent or eliminate carriage of the pathogen in the nasopharynx.

QUESTIONS

1. Which serotype would you expect the pathogen to be (given the information about the effectiveness of the vaccine)?

2. Describe the signs and symptoms of meningococcal meningitis.

3. What is the end result of the disease if a patient is not treated?

4. How would you have treated the three cases described?

5. What actions would you have taken to try to prevent a meningitis outbreak in New York?

6. What recommendations would you make to travelers to Saudi Arabia during the next hajj?

APPLICATION

Assume that you have been put in charge of grant distribution at the CDC branch that is to prevent future meningococcal-meningitis epidemics in the United States. Your primary goal is to minimize the number of deaths due to the pathogen. The director has given you only $1,000,000 to distribute. Discuss how you would distribute the funds at your disposal and justify your funding decisions to the CDC director. (You can fund one program or several programs or give a little to all the programs as you see fit. You may also request a proposal from another source if you believe it is necessary to meet your objective.) Requests have come in from the following sources.

1. The NIH emerging pathogens group has requested funds for a new vaccine development study.

2. The Public Health Service has requested additional staff to run contact tracing for those who might have been exposed to the pathogen.

3. A local hospital has requested additional funds to pay for a study to determine how best to treat the disease.

4. The local Saudi community has requested funds for education efforts on how to prevent the transmission of the pathogen and how to recognize early signs and symptoms of the disease.

5. The state university has requested to study the genetic fingerprints of the pathogens and compare them to others in the United States and those found in Saudi Arabia.

6. A large biotechnology firm has requested to develop a rapid screening kit that would enable 10-minute identification of the pathogen in a clinical setting.

7. The county health care clinic has requested funds to take a throat sample from anyone who requests it for the purpose of identifying whether they are carrying the pathogen.

Botulism

There are almost 1,000 cases of food-borne botulism worldwide each year, with approximately 10 outbreaks per year in the United States. There are about 60 cases of infant botulism worldwide each year.

Cause of the disease

Clostridium botulinum, a bacterial pathogen, is a gram-positive, rod-shaped bacterium commonly found in soil and sediments. It forms endospores that allow the obligate anaerobe to survive in an O_2 environment. The endospores are also heat resistant, allowing the pathogen to survive in foods that are not correctly processed. *Clostridium botulinum* produces a potent neurotoxin.

Transmission

Reservoir
Clostridium botulinum is commonly found in the soil and in anaerobic sediments of aquatic environments.

Mode of transmission
Botulism is caused by ingestion of food contaminated with the toxin (adult, or food-borne, botulism), by an infant without a completely developed intestinal flora ingesting contaminated food (infant botulism), or by having a wound with poor circulation infected with botulism endospores (wound botulism).

Pathogenesis

Entry
The pathogen or toxin enters through ingestion. Wound botulism occurs when the pathogen infects a puncture wound.

Attachment
The toxin attaches to the neuromuscular junctions. The bacteria, if ingested, may attach to the large intestine.

Avoiding host defenses
The toxin is acid stable and survives passage through the stomach. It also avoids defenses because it is able to cause disease at a concentration that is too low to be immunogenic. The bacteria normally cannot outcompete the flora of the large intestine for an anaerobic microenvironment. However, infants are susceptible to *Clostridium botulinum* infection, since the normal flora is incompletely developed.

Damage
The bacteria produce botulism toxin, which blocks neurotransmitter release at the neuromuscular junction, causing paralysis.

Exit
The disease is noncommunicable—it is not spread person to person.

Clinical features

Symptoms usually occur within 18 to 36 hours after infection. Symptoms include general weakness, dizziness, double vision, trouble speaking or swallowing, difficulty breathing, weakness of other muscles, abdominal distension, and constipation. The disease may progress to respiratory failure, complete paralysis, and death.

Diagnosis

Botulism is diagnosed by demonstrating the presence of the toxin in the serum or feces of the patient or in the food which the patient consumed. The toxin is detected by using a mouse bioassay.

Treatment

Botulism antitoxin injections can be helpful in preventing the condition from getting worse if given soon after symptoms begin. The antitoxin is derived from horse serum and is available through the CDC. Intensive supportive treatment is required, and a respirator may be necessary. Intravenous fluids and foods may be necessary during hospitalization because of difficulty in swallowing.

Prevention

- Infant botulism is often associated with children under 1 year old eating unpasteurized honey. Therefore, avoiding feeding raw honey to infants can reduce the risk of botulism.

- Most outbreaks of food-borne botulism result from spores infiltrating improperly prepared home-canned vegetables, sausages, and meat and seafood products. The endospores can be killed only through a sterilization process. Pressure cooking home-canned foods for an appropriate time at appropriate temperature and pressure effectively kills the endospores. Improper canning provides an ideal anaerobic environment loaded with nutrients for the spores to germinate and the bacteria to produce toxin. If a can is bulging or the contents have a peculiar color or odor, or cotton-like mold growth, the food should not be tasted.

- Jams and jellies have a high sugar concentration and thus plasmolyze (remove water through osmosis) *Clostridium botulinum*.
- Properly pickled foods have an acidic pH, which inhibits endospore germination.
- Wound botulism is prevented by prompt disinfection, treatment, and care of puncture wounds and deep lacerations.
- Heating food for 30 minutes at 80°C destroys the toxin.

Creutzfeldt-Jakob Disease

An epidemic of mad cow disease (BSE) led to the destruction of more then 160,000 cattle in Britain. This new disease is thought to be caused by the addition of meat and bone meal dietary supplements that were contaminated with scrapie-infected sheep products (scrapie is a prion-caused disease in sheep) and those of other cattle with BSE. The prion can be transmitted to humans through the consumption of contaminated meat. In humans, the prion causes vCJD.

Cause of the disease

vCJD is caused by a prion, an infectious agent made of protein only. It does not contain any genetic information.

Transmission

Reservoir

The reservoir is infected nervous tissue of cattle, sheep, and other farm and wild animals.

Mode of transmission

The prion is transmitted by the ingestion of infected tissue.

Pathogenesis

Entry

Most cases of vCJD are transmitted by eating beef from cattle infected with the prion that causes mad cow disease. How prions reach the brain has not been precisely determined. It may involve two pathways: one mediated by the presence of B lymphocytes and one involving the vagus cranial nerve.

Attachment

The spleen and lymph nodes have been demonstrated to be the first sites of replication of the prion,

indicating that the prion must attach to cells of the immune system.

Avoiding host defenses

The prion invades cells of the CNS, an environment protected from circulating antibodies and cells of the immune system.

Damage

In humans, a normal protein called PrP (a glycosylphosphatidylinositol-anchored cell surface glycoprotein) is found in high concentrations in CNS tissues. Its exact function is not known, but it may have a role in copper transport or metabolism. The protein is highly conserved among mammals and is found in all vertebrates. The secondary structure of this protein is about 40% alpha helix and about 3% beta sheet. The prion that causes vCJD and BSE induces a structural change in the protein to about 45% beta sheet and 30% alpha helix. This structural change makes the protein highly resistant to degradation by proteases, and the altered proteins can bind to other proteins and alter their structures. This leads to neuron damage in the CNS.

Clinical features

vCJD is characterized by a rapidly progressive dementia, behavioral abnormalities, increased brain dysfunction, visual abnormalities, and spasmodic muscle contraction. vCJD is a progressive disease that leads to death; it has a mean duration of 16 months.

Diagnosis

Clinical

Diagnosis is by characteristic neuropathology.

Laboratory

Diagnosis is by isolation of protease-resistant PrP by Western blotting from CNS tissue.

Treatment

There is no treatment for vCJD.

Prevention

- Most countries now have strict guidelines for the management of infected cows and strict restrictions regarding what cattle are fed to avoid the potential for transmission of vCJD to humans.
- Equipment must be sterilized to inactivate prions that may cause the disease.

Aseptic Meningitis

Meningitis is characterized by inflammation of the tissues that cover the brain and spinal cord (the meninges). The most common type of meningitis is "aseptic" meningitis, caused by several types of viruses. In the United States, there are between 25,000 and 50,000 hospitalizations due to viral meningitis each year.

Cause of the disease

The causative agents of about 90% of cases of viral meningitis are enteroviruses. Enteroviruses are small nonenveloped viruses with a polyhedral capsid containing single-stranded, positive-sense RNA as genetic information.

Transmission

Reservoir

The common reservoir is the gastrointestinal tracts of infected individuals.

Mode of transmission

The typical mode of transmission is direct contact with respiratory secretions (e.g., saliva, sputum, or nasal mucus) of an infected person. The virus may also be transmitted by fomites, nonliving intermediates that carry the virus. Fomite transmission may occur by touching something an infected person has handled and then rubbing the nose or mouth.

Pathogenesis

Entry

The pathogen is introduced into the upper respiratory tract by ingestion or inhalation of contaminated secretions of saliva or mucus.

Attachment

The pathogen attaches to and replicates in the nasopharynx. It is released into the saliva and swallowed.

Avoiding host defenses

The pathogen is acid stable, enabling it to survive the acidity of the stomach and pass into the cells lining the intestines, where it continues replication. The virus is also an intracellular pathogen and initially avoids circulating antibodies and cells of the immune system.

Damage

As a result of damage caused in the intestines, the virus is able to enter the bloodstream. In a small number of cases, the virus crosses the blood-brain barrier and infects the CNS. Infection of CNS tissues causes an inflammatory response. Swelling in the cranium and spinal column puts pressure on the nervous tissue, causing damage.

Clinical features

The incubation period for aseptic meningitis is 3 to 7 days from the time of infection. Most infected people either have no symptoms or develop only a cold or rash with low-grade fever. Those who progress to meningitis present with fever, severe headache, stiff neck, sensitivity to bright lights, drowsiness or confusion, and nausea and vomiting. Symptoms last from 7 to 10 days.

Diagnosis

Aseptic meningitis is diagnosed by clinical signs and symptoms indicating meningitis. A spinal tap is done immediately. Negative results for bacterial or fungal pathogens indicate viral meningitis. Identification of the specific viral pathogen is not done in the clinical setting.

Treatment

There are no antiviral agents that inhibit viral meningitis. Treatment for viral meningitis is symptomatic, including bed rest, fluids, and electrolytes to prevent dehydration and analgesics, like acetaminophen, to relieve fever and headache. Most patients recover completely on their own.

Prevention

- Adhering to good personal hygiene helps to reduce the risk of becoming infected. The most effective method of prevention is thorough and frequent hand washing.

- In day care centers and institutional settings, where enteroviruses may be easily spread, cleaning of contaminated surfaces and soiled articles must be done first with soap and water. After the initial cleaning, the surfaces should be disinfected with a dilute solution of chlorine-containing bleach to inactivate the virus.

Meningococcal Meningitis

The introduction and widespread use of the *Haemophilus influenzae* type b vaccine have significantly decreased *Haemophilus*-caused meningitis. Since its introduction, the primary causes of bacterial meningitis in adults have been *Streptococcus pneumoniae* (1.1 per 100,000) and *Neisseria meningitidis* (0.6 per 100,000).

Meningococcal meningitis is endemic in parts of Africa, India, and other developing nations. Periodic epidemics occur in sub-Saharan Africa, as well as among religious pilgrims traveling to Saudi Arabia for the hajj.

Cause of the disease

Neisseria meningitidis, a bacterial pathogen, is a gram-negative diplococcus that has an antiphagocytic capsule.

Transmission

Reservoir

About 4% of the adult population carry *Neisseria meningitidis* asymptomatically in the nasopharynx.

Mode of transmission

Transmission is via the droplet mode from coughing and sneezing.

Pathogenesis

Entry

The pathogen is inhaled via mucus droplets.

Attachment

The pathogen attaches to the nasopharynx.

Avoiding host defenses

Neisseria meningitidis has an antiphagocytic capsule and a protease that degrades immunoglobulin A, an antibody that is involved in mucosal immunity.

Damage

The pathogen invades the tissue of the nasopharynx, enters the bloodstream, and crosses the blood-brain barrier to enter the CNS. Indirect damage is caused by release of the endotoxin. The endotoxin induces a complex response that damages capillaries and tissues, resulting in necrotic lesions in various areas of the body, such as the skin, meninges, joints, and eyes.

Exit

The pathogen exits via respiratory droplets from coughing and sneezing.

Clinical features

Meningococcal meningitis begins with a mild fever and pharyngitis. Inflammation of the meninges leads to an intense headache and neck pain. Infrequently, a rash is present as a result of vascular dissemination. Untreated meningococcal meningitis leads to coma and death.

Diagnosis

Specimen

A cerebrospinal fluid specimen is obtained.

Test

The presence of gram-negative diplococci in stained smears is determined.

Treatment

β-Lactams, particularly penicillin, are effective against *Neisseria meningitidis*. In addition, hospital supportive measures may be needed to treat shock or disseminated intravascular coagulation.

Prevention

- Rifampin prophylaxis is used to prevent infection among close contacts of those with meningococcal meningitis. Rifampin also eliminates the pathogen from the nasopharynx of asymptomatic carriers.
- Vaccines are available to prevent meningitis caused by several different serotypes of *N. meningitidis*, including groups A, C, Y, and W-135.

Poliomyelitis

In the United States, no natural outbreaks of poliomyelitis (polio) have occurred for about 25 years. However, sporadic cases have occurred from rare complications of using the live attenuated oral polio vaccine. Currently, all polio vaccines contain an inactivated poliovirus, which should eliminate the vaccine-associated cases.

No outbreaks were reported in the Western Hemisphere from 1991 until a recent outbreak in Haiti and the Dominican Republic which was caused by low immunization rates. Clusters of the disease are still found in some areas in Africa, Southeast Asia, and the Indian subcontinent.

Cause of the disease

Polio is caused by poliovirus, a very small virus with a polyhedral capsid and single-stranded, positive-stranded RNA as genetic information.

Transmission

Reservoir

Asymptomatic carriers of poliovirus are the reservoir.

Mode of transmission

The virus is transmitted from person to person via the fecal-oral route.

Pathogenesis

Entry
The virus enters via ingestion of fecally contaminated food or water.

Attachment
The virus attaches to cells of the oropharynx, replicates, and is swallowed with saliva; it then attaches and replicates in cells of the intestine.

Avoiding host defenses
Poliovirus is stable under acid conditions, so it survives passage through the stomach. It is an intracellular pathogen that initially restricts infection to the epithelium, thus avoiding circulating antibodies and cells of the immune system.

Damage
The primary infection leads to viremia (viruses circulating in the blood). The virus can then attach to neurons, especially those of the anterior (motor) horn cells of the spinal cord.

Exit
The pathogen exits through the feces.

Clinical features
Over 95% of poliovirus infections are asymptomatic. About 4% cause a fever and a nonspecific illness without CNS involvement. Fewer than 1% of infections cause paralysis, with many of those infected recovering completely.

Poliomyelitis is a biphasic disease, with the first phase including fever, malaise, headache, sore throat, and vomiting. Viral meningitis symptoms occur 3 to 4 days later, including fever, headache, stiff neck, vomiting, and paralysis.

Diagnosis

Specimen
Feces or a throat swab is used as a specimen.

Tests
Tests consist of isolation of poliovirus from the pharynx or feces followed by deoxyribonucleic acid (DNA) sequencing to demonstrate a wild-type virus infection.

Treatment
There are no antiviral agents to inhibit the growth of poliovirus. Treatment includes symptomatic therapy.

Prevention
In 1961, Albert Sabin's live attenuated vaccine became the standard for prevention of poliomyelitis. It is a low-cost vaccine that can be delivered orally and provides mucosal immunity.

Rabies
Worldwide, canine rabies is still epidemic and a major source of human rabies. The World Health Organization estimates that as many as 35,000 deaths occur annually from rabies.

Cause of the disease
Rabies virus is an enveloped virus with a brick-shaped capsid containing single-stranded, negative-sense RNA.

Transmission

Reservoir
In the eastern United States, foxes and raccoons are the primary reservoirs for the pathogen. Skunks are the primary reservoir in the western United States.

Mode of transmission
Ninety percent of rabies cases in the United States are caused by bites from infected dogs.

Pathogenesis

Entry
The virus enters by the parenteral route via the bite of an infected animal.

Attachment
Initially, the rabies virus attaches to and replicates in muscle fibers.

Avoiding host defenses
Rabies virus replicates intracellularly, an environment protected from circulating antibodies and cells of the immune system.

Damage
Four to 13 weeks after infection and replication in muscle tissue, the virus enters the CNS. The cells of the limbic system are heavily affected, which may account for the aggressive behavior found in carnivores. The virus spreads through the CNS, paralyzing the swallowing reflex, and moves down the cranial nerves into the salivary glands, where the virus replicates to high density.

Exit
The virus exits when an infected animal bites a new host and infects it with virus-laden saliva.

Clinical features

Early signs and symptoms include malaise, chills, fever, headache, anorexia, myalgia, fatigue, and emotional lability. Later stages include paralysis of the swallowing reflex, hydrophobia, cardiac arrhythmia, paralysis, and death.

Diagnosis

Diagnosis is by postmortem histological examination of brain tissue using a direct immunofluorescent-antibody assay.

Treatment

Since the rabies virus takes about 4 weeks to enter the CNS, there is time to use postinfection vaccination to stimulate a sufficient immune response to clear the infection. The wound is carefully cleaned and dressed, followed by a series of injections of inactivated rabies virus grown in human cell cultures and the administration of human rabies immunoglobulins.

Prevention

- Rabies vaccination of domestic pets prevents the most common route of entry into the human population.
- Rabies vaccination of humans is needed for those whose occupations or hobbies put them at risk for rabies, such as animal control personnel and spelunkers in caves where infected bats live.

Tetanus

Tetanus is the ninth most common cause of death from infectious disease worldwide, with approximately 250,000 deaths annually, mostly in underdeveloped countries. Neonatal tetanus, from contamination of the cut umbilical cord with dirt, accounts for 50% of the tetanus-related deaths in developing countries. Tetanus results in approximately five deaths per year in the United States.

Cause of the disease

Clostridium tetani, a bacterial pathogen, is a gram-positive, rod-shaped bacterium that forms endospores. It is an obligate anaerobe that can produce a neurotoxin.

Transmission

Reservoir

Soil and the intestinal tracts of humans and animals are the reservoirs of the pathogen.

Mode of transmission

The pathogen is transmitted by direct contact with contaminated soil or feces.

Pathogenesis

Entry

The pathogen enters wounds that have a poor O_2 supply due to trauma, such as puncture wounds or those resulting from tissue being crushed.

Attachment

Attachment is not a necessary step for *Clostridium tetani*. When introduced into a suitably anaerobic site, the pathogen is able to germinate and produce the tissue-damaging toxin. The toxin produced by the pathogen binds to inhibitory motor neurons, resulting in muscles receiving only stimulatory signals.

Damage

The neurotoxin causes continuous muscle contraction.

Exit

The disease is noncommunicable.

Clinical features

After an incubation period of 4 to 10 days, muscle stiffness is followed by spasms of the jaw muscles, hence the former name "lockjaw." As the disease progresses, all voluntary muscles contract violently and repeatedly (tetanospasms). Death can result from cardiac and blood pressure changes.

Diagnosis

Diagnosis is made on clinical presentation, because the toxin is very potent and may cause tetanus without the ability to isolate the pathogen.

Treatment

Antitoxin is administered to inactivate the tetanus toxin, along with debridement of the damaged tissue from the original wound and treatment with penicillin.

Prevention

There is a highly effective vaccination used to prevent tetanus. The vaccine is prepared by inactivating the toxin with formaldehyde to create a toxoid.

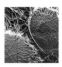

Outbreaks and Cases Requiring Application of Environmental and Industrial Microbiology Concepts

Mankind which began in a cave and behind a windbreak will end in the disease-soaked ruins of a slum.

H. G. WELLS, *The Fate of Man* (1939)

This section presents outbreaks in which preventing the spread of pathogens required an environmentally related solution. In addition, cases that allow students to investigate the microbes responsible for environmental damage are presented.

One key to maintaining public health is to ensure the safety of community drinking and recreational waters. Building water treatment facilities is expensive, and at times, the lack of public funds in some countries leads to poor maintenance of treatment facilities. Even in countries with well-developed public infrastructure, standards for water treatment can still fail to remove pathogens such as *Cryptosporidium parvum,* a chlorine-resistant protozoan pathogen that is not always removed by filtration systems during water treatment. Public recreational waters, such as pools and interactive fountains, can have design flaws or equipment failures that lead to contamination by fecal pathogens and outbreaks of diarrheal diseases.

Contaminated water can also transmit disease through air-conditioning systems. Some large buildings are cooled by air-conditioning systems that use cooling towers. If the water is contaminated with *Legionella* and some of the water leaks into the duct work, *Legionella* can be aerosolized throughout the facility, causing a large outbreak among susceptible individuals. Public health can also be compromised by the lack of a community effort to control disease vectors. Spraying of mosquitoes is important to prevent large outbreaks. Also, communities and home owners can reduce outbreaks by minimizing contact with rodents and other animals that can carry disease. This can be done by clearing garbage, wood piles, and brush near homes to reduce habitats and food sources.

Chemoautotrophic bacteria metabolize reduced inorganic molecules. In the process, they can cause direct damage by the oxidation of metals or the production of acidic end products. Although these microbes do not cause human illness, their control is important to reduce the billions of dollars in damage to public infrastructure in the United States alone. Leaching of metals caused by the metabolism of chemoautotrophic bacteria causes serious pollution as mine drainage enters waterways. Also, the accumulation of biofilms can decrease water flow through pipes, reducing the efficiency of water-cooled condensers and other industrial equipment. Bacterial metabolism can lead to corrosion of metal and the degradation of cement. As a result, city sewage systems that carry away sewage and rainwater must be replaced as the microbial metabolism causes the cement pipes to soften and leak. The investigation of methods to control biofilm growth and reduce microbially induced corrosion will continue to be a productive and expanding area of research.

Table VIII.1 Microbes associated with environmentally related microbiological issues

Organism/structure	Key physical properties	Environmental characteristics
Biofilm	Attaches and connects an interdependent microbial community to a surface	Biofilms anchor a bacterial community to indwelling prosthetic medical devices and prevent diffusion of antibiotics and disinfectants into biofilm bacteria, which may result in resistance. Biofilms adhere to surfaces, restricting the flow of fluids and promoting corrosion.
Bacteria		
Bacillus anthracis	Gram-positive endospore-forming bacillus; aerobic; produces an antiphagocytic capsule and tissue-damaging cytotoxins	Endospores can lie dormant in soil for decades.
Borrelia burgdorferi	Gram-negative spirochete	Vector-borne pathogen carried by the deer tick; disease prevention requires controlling deer and rodent populations
Enteric bacteria (pathogenic *Escherichia coli*, *Salmonella* spp., and *Shigella* spp.)	Gram-negative rods; oxidase negative; *E. coli* ferments lactose	Found in fecally contaminated drinking water and recreational waters; prevention requires water and/or sewage treatment
Legionella pneumophila	Fastidious gram-negative bacilli	Free living in aquatic environments; can contaminate water-cooled air-conditioning units
Rickettsia rickettsii	Obligate intracellular organism; very small	Vector-borne pathogen carried by ticks; disease prevention requires controlling the tick population
Sulfur-oxidizing bacteria	*Thiobacillus ferrooxidans*	Oxidation of pyrite by sulfur-oxidizing bacteria produces sulfuric acid; metabolism of sulfur-reducing bacteria also causes corrosion of concrete sewer pipes.

(continued)

Table VIII.1 (continued)

Organism/structure	Key physical properties	Environmental characteristics
Bacteria		
Sulfur-reducing bacteria	A diverse group with members among the *Deltaproteobacteria*, gram-positive bacteria, and *Archaea*	Microbially influenced corrosion of metals in pipes; control requires prevention of biofilm formation
Vibrio spp.	Gram-negative curved bacillus with a monopolar flagellum	Free-living in aquatic environments; control requires water treatment or filtration
Yersinia pestis	Gram-negative bacillus	Vector-borne pathogen carried by fleas; disease control requires controlling the rodent population
Protozoa		
Cryptosporidium parvum	Forms acid-fast, chlorine-resistant round cysts	Found in fecally contaminated drinking water; not killed by chlorine treatments or filtered by typical processes in water treatment facilities
Entamoeba histolytica	Forms round cysts and amoebae	Found in fecally contaminated drinking water; prevention requires water and sewage treatment
Giardia lamblia	Forms oval cysts and flagellated trophozoites	Found in fecally contaminated drinking water; prevention requires water and sewage treatment
Plasmodium falciparum	Sporozoum that infects red blood cells	Vector-borne pathogen carried by mosquitoes; disease prevention requires controlling the mosquito population
Viruses		
Dengue virus	Enveloped polyhedral capsid with single-stranded RNA	Vector-borne disease; prevention requires mosquito control
Hantaviruses	Enveloped helical capsid with single-stranded RNA	Vector-borne disease; prevention requires control of small-mammal populations

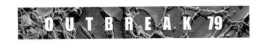
Gastroenteritis from an Interactive Water Fountain

FLORIDA, 1999

From 23 to 27 August 1999, the Volusia County, Florida, Health Department received reports of an outbreak of a gastrointestinal illness whose common exposure was play in an interactive water fountain at a beachside park that had opened 7 August. The most common symptoms of the 38 individuals affected were diarrhea (97%), abdominal cramps (90%), fever (82%), vomiting (66%), and bloody diarrhea (13%). Stool specimens indicated infection by either *Shigella* or *Cryptosporidium*.

The risk factors for acquiring a diarrheal illness were entering the fountain, fountain water ingestion, and consumption of food or drink at the interactive fountain. All ill people entered the fountain, and all but two ingested fountain water.

The fountain used recirculated water that drained from the wet deck/play area floor (no standing water) into an underground reservoir. The volume of recirculated water, the minimum flow rate through the recirculation system, and the turnover rate met the state code requirements for interactive water features. The recirculated water passed through a hypochlorite tablet chlorination system before being pumped back to the reservoir and then to several high-pressure fountain nozzles at ground level throughout the play area. No filtration system had been installed. The fountain was popular with diaper-wearing children and with toddlers, who frequently stood directly over the nozzles. Chlorine levels were not monitored, and the hypochlorite tablets, which were depleted after 7 to 10 days of use, had not been replaced after the park opened on 7 August.

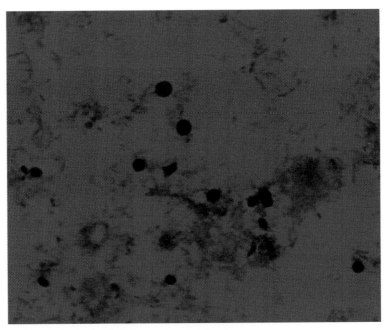

Figure 79.1 Acid-fast stain of a fecal smear.

QUESTIONS

1. What are the reservoirs for *Shigella* and *Cryptosporidium*?

2. Can the exact source of the pathogens be determined from the data presented? Explain why or why not.

3. Describe how you would have treated those affected by gastroenteritis.

4. If you had been the head of the Volusia County Health Department, what changes would you have required to stop the outbreak? To prevent future occurrences?

Dengue Fever Epidemics Return

BRAZIL, 2002

State health authorities reported an epidemic of dengue fever that affected nearly 44,000 people in Rio de Janeiro State, Brazil, during January and February of 2002. Unofficial estimates placed the number as high as 130,000 based on the expectation that many cases of dengue are often unreported. As a result of the large number of cases in and around Rio, there were 9-hour waits at hospitals and a shortage of blood from blood banks.

Dengue is a severe disease. Locally, it is referred to as "bonebreak fever" because it causes high fever, severe headaches, and intense joint pain. Dengue fever is usually not deadly, and most victims recover within a week.

The *Aedes* mosquito, which carries the dengue fever virus, was controlled in many areas of Brazil until the 1980s. The resurgence of the disease was the result of a combination of recent rains creating abundant pools and puddles for mosquito breeding and a high density of infected people. The rapid spread of the virus was expected to increase.

The impact of the epidemic was widespread, from politics to pop culture. Some people in Rio joked that the authorities were arguing whether mosquitoes were federal, state, or municipal insects. The epidemic entered the Brazilian presidential campaign, with two of the candidates blaming each other for allowing the disease to spread out of control. Several pop singers canceled their shows in the areas where the epidemic occurred. A samba using the epidemic as a theme was written.

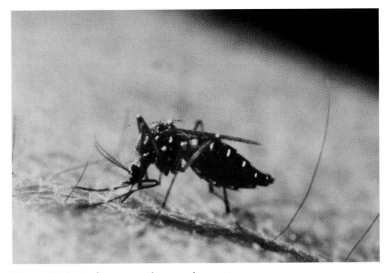

Figure 80.1 *Aedes aegypti* mosquito vector.

Even though the mortality of dengue fever is low, the large number of infections resulted in at least 18 deaths. Deaths are typically caused by a hemorrhagic complication of dengue that results when an individual is infected with two different strains of the virus.

QUESTIONS

1. What pathogen causes dengue fever?

2. What key environmental conditions led to this epidemic?

3. What personal activities would you have recommended so that individuals could reduce their risk of contracting dengue fever?

4. If you had been an advisor to the presidential candidates, what national, state, and local community efforts would you have recommended to eliminate dengue fever outbreaks in the future?

Acid Pollution in Waterways Due to Metal Leaching from Mine Tailings

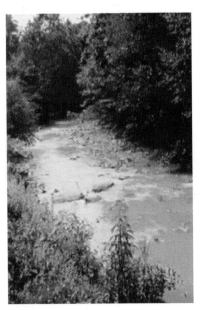

Figure 81.1 Mine drainage.

Pyrite mine tailings (iron- and sulfur-containing ore left over from mining operations) leach acid drainage into local waterways due primarily to the metabolic activity of *Thiobacillus ferrooxidans*. Abiotic oxidation of pyrite is slow; however, *T. ferrooxidans* catalyzes the oxidation of FeS_2, producing ferric ions and hydrogen ions. Iron ions (Fe^{3+}) and hydrogen ions leach into streams that drain the mine overburden. As a result of the H^+ release due to *T. ferrooxidans*, the pH of the mine drainage can fall below 3. Iron ions and other heavy-metal ions, such as zinc, copper, lead, arsenic, and manganese, are also leached into the mine drainage.

The pH of acid mine drainage is increased when it is diluted by fresh rainwater. When the pH rises above 3, iron ions precipitate out of the water and coat the stream bottom with a slimy orange sludge, iron(III) hydroxide [$Fe(OH)_3$]. This sludge tints the stream water an unnatural reddish-orange color.

QUESTIONS

1. How does *T. ferrooxidans* survive at pH 3?

2. How would the presence of heavy metals and a low pH affect the aquatic, microbial, and plant life downstream of the drainage?

3. How would a coating of $Fe(OH)_3$ sludge affect benthic microbes?

4. *T. ferrooxidans* is also used to economically bioleach gold and copper from low-grade ores for commercial gain. How is this process aided by the bacteria?

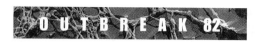

A Shigellosis Outbreak from a Wading Pool

IOWA, 2001

On 15 June 2001, local physicians reported 11 cases of diarrhea to a county health department. A preliminary investigation found that nine of these people had recently visited a large city park with a wading pool. Further investigation identified 69 others with *Shigella* infections. Of these, 45 (65%) were categorized as primary patients and 24 (35%) as secondary patients, who were infected through contact with a primary patient.

Illness among primary patients was primarily found in young children. The onset of illness among primary patients occurred between 12 and 14 June. Symptoms included diarrhea (100%), nausea (51%), vomiting (47%), bloody diarrhea (39%), and headache (29%). Seven (16%) patients were hospitalized. The onset of illness among the 24 secondary patients occurred from 15 to 22 June. The median age was 24 years; 58% of the patients were female. One person was hospitalized.

The pool, which had been in operation for approximately 60 years, was 40 feet in diameter and had a maximum depth of 14 inches. It was frequented by diaper-wearing children and by toddlers, and as many as 20 to 30 children might be in the pool at one time. The pool was a fill-and-drain system and was filled each morning with potable city water through a direct inlet pipe and a centrally located fountain; it was drained and left empty each evening. The pool had no recirculation or disinfection system (i.e., no pump, filter, or mechanical disinfection system). Residual water was also found in the pipes after the pool was drained. Each morning before it was filled, the pool was rinsed with a high-pressure washer, and it was scrubbed with a chlorine cleanser twice weekly. Chlorine levels were not monitored, and chlorine was not added to the pool water.

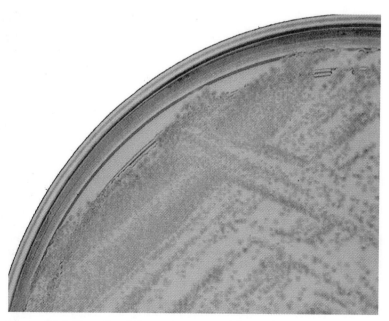

Figure 82.1 Growth of the pathogen on MacConkey agar.

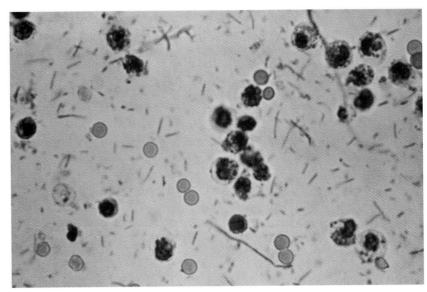

Figure 82.2 A light micrograph of a fecal smear.

After this outbreak, a community-wide outbreak of the pathogen occurred in several local day care centers.

QUESTIONS

1. What is the reservoir for *Shigella?*

2. Why were the secondary cases primarily found in women and shortly after the outbreak of primary cases?

3. How would you have changed the cleaning procedures or reengineered the wading pool to make it safe?

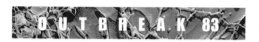

A Massive Outbreak of *Cryptosporidium* Infection Transmitted through the Public Water Supply

MILWAUKEE, WISCONSIN, 1993

Early in the spring of 1993, there was a widespread outbreak of acute watery diarrhea among the residents of Milwaukee. The median duration of illness was 9 days (range, 1 to 55 days). The median maximal number of stools per day was 12 (range, 1 to 90). Among 285 people surveyed who had laboratory-confirmed cryptosporidiosis, the clinical manifestations included watery diarrhea (93%), abdominal cramps (84%), fever (57%), and vomiting (48%). It was estimated that 403,000 people had watery diarrhea attributable to the outbreak.

Beginning on 23 March, there were marked increases in the turbidity of treated water at the city's southern water treatment plant. On 9 April, the plant was shut down. *Cryptosporidium* oocysts (the reproductive stage) were identified in water from ice made in southern Milwaukee during these weeks. During this period, there was a >100-fold increase in the rate of isolation of *Cryptosporidium*.

In the 2 years prior to the outbreak, cryptosporidiosis was listed as an underlying or contributing cause of death on the death certificates of four Milwaukee vicinity residents. In the 2 years following the outbreak, cryptosporidiosis was listed in 54 deaths. Of the individuals who died, 85% had acquired immune deficiency syndrome (AIDS).

During the outbreak, required tests for waterborne pathogens were negative.

QUESTIONS

1. Why did *Cryptosporidium* survive in the water treatment facilities?
2. Why was *Cryptosporidium* not detected by the required microbiological tests?
3. How is cryptosporidiosis treated?
4. What is the reservoir for *Cryptosporidium*?
5. Are current water treatment standards in the United States sufficient to prevent a future outbreak like this?

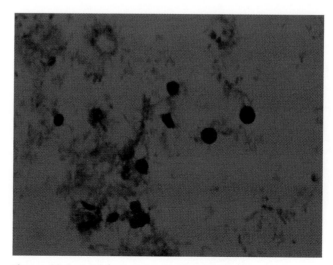

Figure 83.1 Acid-fast stain of a fecal smear.

Biofilm Fouling in Cooling Towers

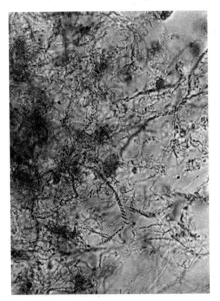

Figure 84.1 Biofilm formation in a cooling system.

The presence of microbial biofilms on surfaces may give rise to microbiologically influenced corrosion (MIC). Biofilms accumulate on all submerged industrial and environmental surfaces. A disinfectant's ability to control microbial growth, and thus MIC, is typically measured by evaluating its effect on planktonic bacteria (bacteria free in solution rather than attached to a surface), which often leads to an underestimate of the concentration required to control a biofilm. In one study, commercial formulations of chlorine were assayed for the ability to control microbial growth in cooling towers. Stainless steel plates were inserted in each tower basin for a period of 30 days before removal.

Parts per million	Colonies/cm^2 after 1 hour or treatment with:	
	Chlorine	Monochloramine
0	50,000	50,000
0.50	27,000	12,000
1.0	3,800	250
1.5	1,700	10

QUESTIONS

1. Is chlorine an effective treatment for killing microbes in biofilms in cooling towers? If so, at what concentration?

2. Why does basing the effectiveness of disinfectants on planktonic bacteria result in underestimating the dose required to kill biofilm bacteria?

3. Why is chlorine used to control microbial growth in a cooling tower rather than another biocide?

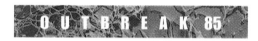

An Outbreak of Legionnaires' Disease from an Air-Conditioning Unit

BARROW, UNITED KINGDOM, 2002

An outbreak of Legionnaires' disease occurred in Barrow, United Kingdom, in 2002. Symptoms included fluid-filled lungs, fever, chills, cough, muscle aches, headaches, fatigue, diarrhea, and potentially kidney failure.

The disease killed an elderly man and infected 18 others in what could have been the United Kingdom's worst ever outbreak of legionellosis. Furthermore, 11 others were suspected of having the disease, and according to experts, as many as 130 more cases were possible. Untreated, *Legionella* pneumonia is typically lethal in about 15% of cases. Tens of thousands of people who had walked though the heart of the town in the previous weeks might also have been at risk of contracting the disease. As a result, health officials prepared to treat as many as 100 more cases of the disease over the next 10 days. All elective surgery at Furness General Hospital was cancelled for 2 days, and other hospitals in Kendal and Lancaster prepared to help.

A public health team was set up to search for the source of the infection. The only common feature was that all those with the disease had been in the Barrow town center recently. Suspicion focused on an air-conditioning unit housed on the roof of the council-owned civic center in the heart of the town near the main shopping street. The shopping center was opened in 1972 and was the only one in the town center that used a water-cooling system. The cooling system was fitted 40 feet up on the roof of the two-story complex, next to its rooftop car park. Each day, thousands of people walked past the center, called Forum 28, which housed a 550-seat theater, a restaurant, a bar, and a 280-seat concert hall. Researchers speculated that the system was in need of repair and was probably pumping out water droplets over a walkway leading to the town's main shopping arcade. The recent humid weather might have helped the pathogen to survive and flourish.

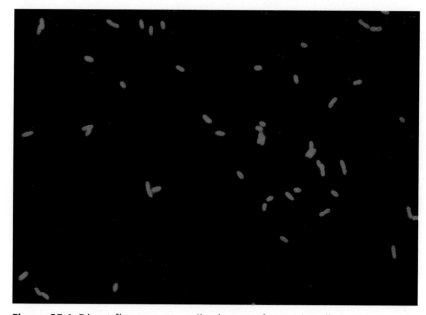

Figure 85.1 Direct fluorescent-antibody assay for *Legionella*.

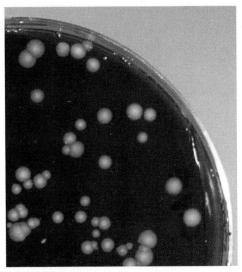

Figure 85.2 Growth of *Legionella* on charcoal agar.

QUESTIONS

1. What characteristics of *Legionella pneumophila* allow it to survive in air conditioner cooling towers?

2. How can *Legionella* be prevented from growing in the cooling towers?

3. What public health actions should have been taken to stop the outbreak?

Microbiologically Influenced Corrosion of Industrial Materials

EUROPE AND THE UNITED STATES

The damage caused by MIC is high. It is estimated that about 20% of all corrosion damage of metals and building materials is microbially influenced and enhanced. The annual costs of biodeterioration are in the billions of euros in Europe from the failure of metallic heat exchanger equipment, corroded concrete sewers, biologically attacked textiles, or decaying pieces of cultural property. In the United States, MIC degrades stainless steel heat exchangers over the course of about 8 years and causes approximately $55 million in damage each year. MIC damage to the production, transport, and storage of oil amounts to hundreds of millions of dollars per year in the United States, not including the costs of lost oil, environmental pollution, and soil remediation. The lifetime of household water heaters is determined by MIC. Shipyards, harbor installations, and offshore platforms are exposed to natural environments and suffer a high level of MIC. In addition, MIC is important in power plants, where heat exchangers generally use river water or groundwater as a cooling fluid.

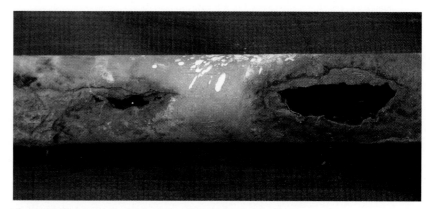

Figure 86.1 Corrosion on the surface of a pipe.

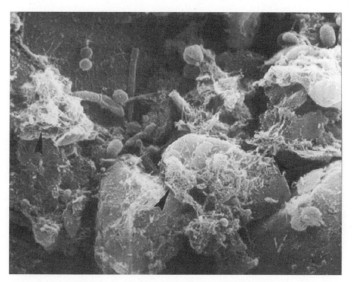

Figure 86.2 Biofilm growth on a metal surface.

QUESTIONS

1. Describe how microbes cause corrosion of metals.

2. How can manufacturing of heat exchangers in power plants be changed to decrease the effects of MIC?

3. What would be the consequences of MIC in buried pipelines carrying oil or water?

Increasing Production of Beer in the United States

Major U.S. beer-manufacturing plants operate 24 hours a day, 7 days a week, and routinely produce tens of millions of gallons of beer per year. The bottles and cans are rapidly transported upside down on conveyor belts before being filled. This prevents foreign materials from falling into the containers as they travel throughout the processing plant. However, it leads to a microbiological problem. Because the cans and bottles are upside down, the conveyor belts cannot be greased in the traditional way for fear of grease getting into the containers. Instead, the belts are lubricated with water sprayed from dozens of jets located along the belts. Due to the wet conditions and the availability of a nutrient source, microbiological organisms thrive and create a slimy biofilm on the surfaces of the conveyors. As a result, about every 3 days each line has to be shut down and cleaned for about 3 hours. The downtime can represent a serious loss of productivity and increases operating costs. Canning lines generally fill about 1,500 cans per minute with a wholesale value of $0.20 per can.

QUESTIONS

1. What is a biofilm?

2. What nutrients would the biofilm on the conveyors use for growth?

3. What would be the necessary characteristics of a biocide that could be used to prevent biofilm formation in the beer-manufacturing plants?

4. What cost savings would be realized if the conveyor had to be shut down and cleaned only once every 2 months instead of every third day?

5. What other bottling facilities would you expect to have similar problems?

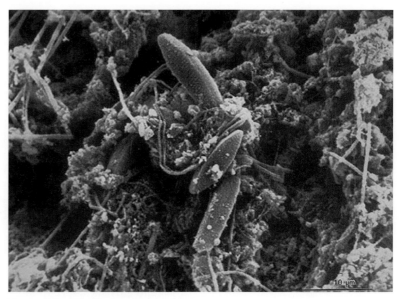

Figure 87.1 Biofilm growth.

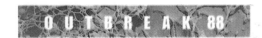
GLOBAL PERSPECTIVE

Four Successive Annual Outbreaks of Plague

MADAGASCAR, 1995

In March 1995, the first identified case of a deadly outbreak of plague occurred in Madagascar. Over the next 4 years, annual outbreaks resulted in 1,702 cases of plague.

All patients reported a high fever and enlarged lymph nodes in the cervical, axial, or inguinal regions. A total of 507 patients were admitted to the hospital; 40 (7.9%) of them died.

Conditions in hospitals in Mahajanga, Madagascar, were poor. A large proportion of treatment failures could have been avoided if patients had not waited 2 days or more before coming to the hospital. Moreover, the dates of onset seemed to be questionable for some serious cases; apparently families were often reluctant to admit that they had been negligent in managing the patient at home or that they had resorted to traditional healing practices before referring the patient to a hospital. Antibiotics used to treat the disease (streptomycin was the recommended treatment in Madagascar) had been totally effective. However, drug resistance might have developed, as one chloramphenicol-resistant isolate and one ampicillin-resistant isolate were identified in 1995 in the highlands.

The geographic distribution of cases according to districts is shown in Fig. 88.1. The incidence of the disease differed sharply according to districts: most patients (82.9%) lived in area 1, which included the most densely populated districts of the town. The southwestern part of the city (area 2) included the harbor and the old colonial town. Areas 3 and 4, the greener and less populous suburbs of Mahajanga, showed an intermediate incidence. The disease perimeter did not extend further than 10 to 15 km from town.

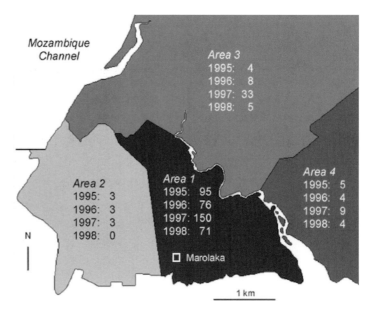

Figure 88.1 Incidence of laboratory-confirmed cases according to the patients' place of residence in Mahajanga, Madagascar.

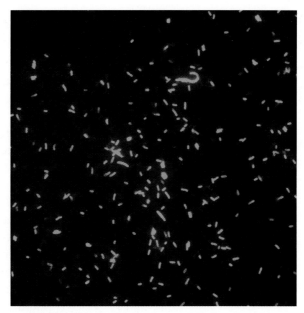

Figure 88.2 Direct fluorescent-antibody assay for *Yersinia pestis.*

A geomedical survey concluded that three different types of structures were present in the entire city of Mahajanga. Area 2 was almost comparable to a European city, with its wide paved streets, sewer network, store buildings with apartments in the upper floors, and low population density; areas 3 and 4 were semirural suburbs with low population density. In contrast, area 1, which was the epicenter of the outbreak, was densely populated with very poor people. This area also included the two largest markets, which generated the town's largest amount of garbage. No physical barrier separated area 1 from area 2, but socioeconomic conditions restricted contact between the populations.

An analysis of rat deaths was done for the 15 days preceding the onset of disease; 56.9% of people had found dead rats indoors or in the vicinity of their homes, while 43.1% had not noticed dead rats in their surroundings. Of the people who had noticed dead rats, 57.6% had found the dead rats inside their homes.

QUESTIONS

1. What pathogen causes plague?

2. What is the pathogen's natural reservoir?

3. How is the disease transmitted to humans?

4. Why was the outbreak focused in area 1 and not the other areas?

5. How would you have stopped this outbreak and prevented future outbreaks from occurring (take into account the very limited resources available to you)?

Biofilms

The Centers for Disease Control and Prevention and the National Institutes of Health estimate that 65% to 80% of all chronic infections can be attributed to microbial biofilms. Many of these chronic infections are caused by organisms such as *Candida albicans, Pseudomonas aeruginosa, Escherichia coli, Staphylococcus epidermidis,* and *Staphylococcus aureus.*

Structure

Bacterial biofilms consist of microorganisms attached to a surface by a slimy layer of extracellular polysaccharides. Mature biofilms have a complex organization. The extracellular polysaccharide matrix forms columns and knob-shaped pillars with an embedded interdependent community of bacteria. These structures contain channels and large spaces that allow the flow of liquid through the film to efficiently carry nutrients and oxygen to the cells and remove waste products.

Although a mature biofilm is a complex microbial ecosystem of interdependent bacteria, its formation requires two key steps: reversible attachment and irreversible attachment. Reversible attachment occurs when planktonic bacteria adhere to dissolved organic material that has stuck to a surface. External portions of the bacteria (such as pili or flagella) temporarily adhere to organic material left behind by the decomposition or excretion of organisms. Attachment may stimulate the bacterial cells to secrete a sticky polysaccharide that forms a matrix around the cells and glues them to the surface irreversibly.

Function

The bacterial cells secrete a polysaccharide matrix that aids the cells to survive hostile environments. Environmentally stressful conditions, such as desiccation or changes in pH and temperature, are modified by the biofilm matrix.

The biofilm can provide protection from some predatory protozoa. The matrix of the biofilm also acts to collect and concentrate essential nutrients found in the environment surrounding the biofilm. In a health care setting, the extracellular matrix restricts the diffusion of antibiotics and disinfectants, enabling the biofilm bacteria to survive conditions that effectively kill planktonic bacteria.

Benefits of biofilms

Biofilms have been used for decades in trickle tanks to treat sewage wastewater. Sewage is trickled through a large tank containing tons of rocks coated with biofilms. As the water trickles between the rocks, the aerobic bacteria digest the organic material in the feces to partially purify the water before it is released.

Problems caused by biofilms

Many industries continually fight the growth of biofilms to attempt to minimize damage to surfaces in contact with water. Metal water pipelines in cooling towers and heat exchangers are continuously corroded by biofilms. Thick biofilms also reduce water flow. Since biofilms adhere to plastic, they often form on inserted prosthetic medical devices and catheters, causing chronic infections. Often, removal of the medical device is the only solution to get rid of the infecting microbes. Biofilms also initiate the colonization of marine invertebrates on ships and submerged structures, leading to continuous damage in the marine industry. Biofilms can also ferment nutrients to acid end products. These acids cause cavities in teeth (plaque is a biofilm on teeth) and quickly corrode cement pipes used as storm drains and sewer pipes.

Treatment and control

Biofilms are much more resistant to antibiotics and disinfectants than planktonic bacteria due to the impermeability of the matrix to the chemicals. Medical devices are sometimes constructed with a coating of chemicals that inhibit biofilm formation.

High concentrations of chlorine or cationic surfactants are used to control biofilm growth in pipelines. Regular treatment is needed because of constant regrowth of the biofilms.

Cryptosporidiosis

Cryptosporidium parvum causes a self-limited diarrheal illness in healthy individuals, mostly children. Only recently has cryptosporidiosis been recognized as a cause of self-limited diarrhea in people with healthy immune systems and of severe prolonged diarrhea in patients with AIDS.

Cause of the disease

Cryptosporidium parvum is a eukaryotic protozoal pathogen with a complex life cycle that includes the formation of sporozoa and thick-walled oocysts that are acid-fast during staining (which indicates a cyst with a waxy protective coating).

Transmission

Reservoir

The pathogen can be carried by humans and a wide range of animals, including cattle, cats, deer, and horses.

Mode of transmission

The pathogen is spread by the fecal-oral route through contaminated drinking water, recreational water, and food.

Pathogenesis

Entry

Ingestion of approximately 100 infective oocysts in fecally contaminated material is sufficient for infection.

Attachment

The pathogen attaches to the epithelial cells of intestinal villi.

Avoidance of host defenses

Oocysts have acid-resistant capsules that allow them to pass through the low pH of the stomach without damage and to proceed into the intestines, where they attach.

Damage

After the ingestion of oocysts, asexual release of sporozoites is initiated. Sporozoites attach to and penetrate the intestinal mucosa, where they mature into other forms of the parasite and rupture the infected cells. Damaged tissue and inflammation prevent water absorption, which causes diarrhea.

Exit

Infective thick-walled oocysts are excreted through feces.

Clinical features

Symptoms (loose, watery diarrhea; stomach cramps; and a slight fever) may last 1 to 3 weeks and appear 2 to 10 days after infection. In individuals with poorly functioning immune systems, *Cryptosporidium* infection leads to a chronic watery diarrhea with severe cramps, weight loss, a low-grade fever, and severe dehydration.

Diagnosis

Specimen

A feces sample is obtained.

Tests

Acid-fast staining and detection of acid-fast oocysts by microscopy are used to identify the pathogen.

Treatment

People with a healthy immune system recover in 1 to 3 weeks without treatment. Oral fluids and electrolytes help to prevent dehydration from diarrhea.

In immunocompromised patients, such as AIDS patients, paromomycin is often used to inhibit the growth of the pathogen. Although paromomycin inhibits eukaryotic protein synthesis, it is not absorbed by the gastrointestinal (GI) tract, so oral administration preferentially inhibits *Cryptosporidium* in the GI tract.

Prevention

- Practice good hygiene.
- Wash hands thoroughly with soap and water (after using the toilet, changing diapers, handling animals, cleaning up feces, or handling anything contaminated with fecal matter and before eating or preparing food).
- Avoid drinking untreated water from lakes, streams, pools, hot tubs, or other water sources. Thick-walled oocysts can survive extreme environments, including high levels of chlorination.
- Peel or rinse fruits or vegetables to be eaten raw to prevent ingestion of a food that may be contaminated with feces.
- Drink bottled water without ice when traveling in places with poor sanitation.
- Boil contaminated water for at least 10 minutes or filter the water to remove any bacterial, protozoal, or viral pathogens.

Dengue Fever

Dengue is the most important mosquito-borne viral disease affecting humans. It is one of the top 10 killer infectious diseases worldwide. It is estimated that 2.5 billion people are at risk for acquiring dengue fever, and tens of millions of cases of dengue fever occur each year. The lethal version of the disease, dengue hemorrhagic fever, affects hundreds of thousands of people per year, with a case-fatality rate of about 5%.

Cause of the disease

The causative agent of dengue fever is a flavivirus, dengue virus. The virus has single-stranded ribonucleic acid (RNA) inside an enveloped icosahedral capsid (a protein shell with 20 sides). There are four different serotypes of dengue virus: DEN-1, DEN-2, DEN-3, and DEN-4.

Transmission

Reservoir

The virus survives in either a human-mosquito or a monkey-mosquito cycle. The disease is typically found in tropical and subtropical areas of the world.

Mode of transmission

Dengue fever is a vector-borne disease that is transmitted to humans by the bite of a female *Aedes aegypti* mosquito, a domestic day-biting mosquito that prefers to feed on humans.

Pathogenesis

Entry

The pathogen is introduced directly into the blood by the bite of an infected mosquito.

Attachment

The virus attaches to mononuclear phagocytes.

Avoiding host defenses

The virus is an intracellular pathogen that initially avoids circulating antibodies and cells of the immune system. The virus also destroys cells of the immune system.

Damage

Infection of monocytes results in an increase in the activation of complement and the release of kinins, which produce the systemic features of the disease. Dengue hemorrhagic fever is caused by a second infection by the dengue virus (especially DEN-2). The antibodies produced to fight off the first infection actually enhance the infection of monocytes during the second infection. The greater proportion of infected cells results in greater virus production. It is hypothesized that the infected monocytes release vasoactive mediators, resulting in the increased vascular permeability and hemorrhagic manifestations that characterize dengue hemorrhagic fever or dengue shock syndrome.

Clinical features

The incubation period is typically 5 to 8 days. Infection with dengue virus produces a spectrum of clinical illness ranging from a nonspecific viral syndrome to severe and fatal hemorrhagic disease.

Symptoms of dengue fever include sudden onset of fever that lasts for 2 to 7 days, severe headache, bone and joint pain, weakness, anorexia, nausea, vomiting, and a rash. Dengue hemorrhagic fever is characterized by dengue fever plus hemorrhagic manifestations: a tendency to bruise easily, bleeding nose or gums, and possibly internal bleeding, which may lead to failure of the circulatory system and shock, followed by death.

Diagnosis

Clinical

Dengue fever is often misdiagnosed as influenza, measles, typhoid fever, or malaria.

Laboratory

Specimen: A blood sample is taken.
Tests: The laboratory tests are detection of anti-dengue immunoglobulin M and immunoglobulin G by indirect enzyme-linked immunosorbent assay. Specific serotypes can be identified by indirect fluorescent-antibody testing.

Treatment

There are no antiviral medications to inhibit dengue virus. Analgesics with acetaminophen are used to reduce pain and fever. Aspirin and nonsteroidal anti-inflammatory drugs, such as ibuprofen, should be avoided because of their anticoagulant properties. Other symptomatic therapies include bed rest and either oral or intravenous fluids and electrolytes.

Prevention

- There is no vaccine for dengue fever.
- The focus for prevention is to eliminate the places where the mosquito lays her eggs—primarily artificial containers that hold water (e.g., plastic containers, 55-gallon drums, buckets, pet water bowls, flower vases, or used automobile tires).
- The risk of being bitten by mosquitoes indoors is reduced by utilization of air conditioning or windows and doors that are screened, application of mosquito repellents containing DEET, and wearing long-sleeved shirts and pants tucked into socks.

Legionnaires' Disease

A serious pulmonary infection attacked 235 people who were attending a convention of the American Legion in Philadelphia during the U.S. bicentennial celebration in July 1976—hence the name Legionnaires' disease and that of its causative organism, *Legionella pneumophila*. Since then, Legionnaires' disease has been recognized as the most common cause of atypical pneumonia in hospitalized patients. It is the second most common cause of community-acquired bacterial pneumonia.

Cause of the disease

The pathogen that causes Legionnaires' disease is *Legionella pneumophila*. It is a gram-negative aerobic bacillus that produces a capsule and has fastidious growth requirements.

Transmission

Reservoir

The pathogen is free-living in soil and stagnant water (25 to 42°C). *Legionella* can contaminate large air-conditioning systems that use water in cooling towers.

Mode of transmission

The pathogen is spread by inhalation of aerosolized droplets containing *Legionella*. The pathogen is not spread person to person. Most infections occur in patients who have compromised immunity and pulmonary function.

Pathogenesis

Entry

The pathogen enters by inhalation of aerosols containing *Legionella*.

Attachment

Legionella attaches to the alveolar sacs.

Avoiding host defenses

Legionella is phagocytized by alveolar macrophages but avoids destruction by preventing fusion with lysosomes. *Legionella* replicates inside the macrophage and causes cell lysis.

Damage

Legionella causes direct damage through cell lysis and indirect damage by inducing an inflammatory response and producing damaging enzymes and toxins. After lysing macrophages, the bacteria spread and continue to cause damage and inflammation, resulting in bronchial hemorrhaging and abscesses.

Clinical features

Most infections are asymptomatic or produce only mild symptoms. The disease has an incubation period of 2 to 10 days, normally lasting from 5 to 6 days. Symptoms include fever and chills, a nonproductive cough, difficulty breathing, confusion, headache, and muscle pain.

Diagnosis

Clinical

Diagnosis is by evidence of pneumonia, including rales (crackling sounds in the lungs, indicating fluid), and a chest X ray showing fluid in the lungs.

Laboratory testing

Specimen: A sputum or urine specimen is obtained.
Cultural testing: The organism grows slowly on a buffered cysteine-containing charcoal-yeast extract agar.
Noncultural testing: Indirect immunoflorescence microscopy and commercial rapid microagglutination tests are used.

Treatment

Macrolide antibiotics, such as erythromycin, have been commonly used to treat *Legionella*. Respiratory therapy is often required for seriously ill patients.

Prevention

- Perform regular maintenance and maintain adequate chlorination of ventilation systems and other potential reservoirs.
- Maintain water reservoir temperature at >60°C or <20°C.
- Avoid water stagnation.
- Avoid smoking and excessive alcohol consumption, which can lower resistance to the pathogen.

Shigellosis

Approximately 15,000 cases of shigellosis are reported annually in the United States. Shigellosis occurs worldwide, most frequently in areas with substandard hygiene in living conditions or in overcrowded areas with poor sanitation. It is also commonly found wherever war or natural disasters disrupt the public health infrastructure. Bacteremia occurs primarily in malnourished children and carries a mortality rate of 20% as a result of renal failure, hemolysis, thrombocytopenia (a decrease in the number of thrombocytes, needed for blood clotting), gastrointestinal hemorrhage, and shock. Hemolytic-uremic syndrome (HUS) may complicate infections with *Shigella* species and *Escherichia coli*. HUS has a mortality rate of >50%.

Cause of the disease

The disease is caused by *Shigella* species, including *Shigella dysenteriae* (which causes the most severe form of shigellosis) and *Shigella sonnei* (the most common species causing shigellosis in the United

States). A slender, gram-negative, rod-shaped bacterial pathogen, *Shigella* is a facultative anaerobic organism that produces H_2S from protein metabolism.

Transmission
Reservoir
The reservoir is the GI tract of humans.

Mode of transmission
The mode of transmission is person-to-person transmission by the fecal-oral route or from contaminated fomites or contaminated food.

Pathogenesis
Entry
The pathogen is most commonly transmitted by fecally contaminated water and unsanitary handling of food by food handlers. A small inoculum (10 to 200 organisms) is sufficient to cause infection.

Attachment
The bacteria attach to and penetrate the epithelial cells of the intestinal mucosa.

Avoiding host defenses
The bacteria infect epithelial cells and are not initially exposed to circulating antibodies or cells of the immune system.

Damage
After invasion, the bacteria multiply intracellularly. With this multiplication come local inflammation, fluid loss, and epithelial cell dysfunction, which result in tissue destruction. The pathogen can also release an exotoxin that causes local tissue destruction.

Exit
The pathogen exits in the feces.

Clinical features
Illness usually begins 1 to 4 days after the bacteria are swallowed and can last up to 7 days. Symptoms include watery or bloody diarrhea, an acute fever, abdominal cramps, nausea or vomiting, and blood, mucus, or pus in the stools. Shigellosis can also have serious complications, including severe dehydration due to excess fluid loss as a result of diarrhea, convulsions in young children, mucosal ulcerations, rectal bleeding, and HUS, which results from damage to the kidneys by the exotoxin release.

Diagnosis
Specimen
A feces sample is obtained.

Tests
The test is for growth on Hektoen enteric agar. *Shigella* colonies appear green without a black center because they do not produce H_2S as *Salmonella* does.

Treatment
Patients with mild symptoms tend to recover on their own. For more serious cases, a physician may prescribe an antibiotic to speed up the recovery process. Antibiotics are usually chosen after screening the pathogen for antibiotic resistance. Treatment with a drug to which *Shigella* is resistant only kills normal flora, allowing *Shigella* to utilize the nutrients and microenvironments previously occupied by the normal flora and leading to a more serious *Shigella* infection. Properly chosen antibiotics help kill the bacteria and shorten the duration of the illness.

In order to prevent dehydration, the patient should drink plenty of liquids to replace those lost through diarrhea and vomiting. The use of antidiarrheal agents can make the illness worse.

Prevention
- There is no vaccine to prevent shigellosis.
- Proper sanitation and hygiene are most important to prevent the spread of *Shigella*. Thoroughly washing the hands after using the toilet or before preparing food is important.
- When traveling to other countries where water sanitation may not be adequate, drink only treated or boiled water and eat only hot cooked foods or fruits you have peeled yourself.

Sulfur-Oxidizing Bacteria

Economic importance
Harmful effects
The mining of metal ores and coal brings millions of tons of pyrite (FeS_2)-containing material to the surface, where it interacts with oxygen and water to form an iron-rich acidic solution that leaches out of the piles of rock left over after the useful material has been harvested (mine tailings). The oxidation of pyrite by sulfur-oxidizing bacteria produces sulfuric acid, which drops the pH of the mine tailing runoff to 2.

In addition to the resulting death of aquatic organisms, due to low pH, the acid runoff also dissolves acid-soluble heavy metals and coats the ecosystem with yellow and brown iron precipitates, which are also toxic to aquatic organisms. As a result, the acid runoff from abandoned mining operations affects over 10,000 miles of waterways in the United States.

The corrosion of concrete sewer pipes requires both sulfate-reducing bacteria (SRB), found in anaerobic, nutrient-rich liquid sewage, and sulfide-oxidizing bacteria, found in the aerobic, moist headspace of the pipe. Under anaerobic conditions, the sulfur-reducing bacteria generate volatile H_2S, which diffuses into the air in the headspace. The sulfur-oxidizing bacteria growing in a biofilm on the concrete surface oxidize H_2S to sulfuric acid. The acid reacts with the calcium hydroxide binder to convert the hard concrete to a soft compound, calcium sulfate. Corrosion of concrete sewer pipes by biofilm-forming bacteria can occur at rates of over 4 millimeters per year, causing the life expectancy of the pipe to be reduced by approximately 20 years.

Beneficial effects

The sulfur-metabolizing organisms that cause so much damage to aquatic ecosystems can also be harnessed for industrial uses that help to minimize pollution damage. For example, sulfur-oxidizing bacteria can be used to remove sulfur compounds from coal before its burned, thus reducing the production of acid rain. They are also used to leach copper, uranium, and gold from ore. Over 30% of the copper and uranium in the United States is produced using microbially mediated leaching.

Key microbes

The spontaneous oxidation of pyrite slowly lowers the pH of the water runoff from mine tailings. The low pH provides an optimum condition for the growth of *Thiobacillus ferrooxidans,* which oxidizes inorganic sulfur- and iron-containing compounds. The energy derived from this process is used to drive CO_2 fixation by the chemoautotrophic bacteria. As the oxidation of pyrite proceeds, heat is released, causing the temperature of the tailings to increase. At high temperatures, the growth of *Sulfolobus* and *Acidianus,* thermophilic archaebacteria that can also oxidize pyrite, is favored.

Key processes

The following process is spontaneous in the presence of water and oxygen:

$$4FeS_2 \text{ (pyrite)} + 15O_2 + 14H_2O \rightarrow 4Fe(OH)_3 + 8H_2SO_4$$

In a microbially mediated process, *Thiobacillus ferrooxidans* can oxidize ferrous iron (Fe^{2+}) to ferric iron (Fe^{3+}) rapidly at low pH.

$$2Fe^{2+} + \tfrac{1}{2}O_2 + 2H^+ \rightarrow 2Fe^{3+} + H_2O$$

The ferric iron can then be utilized to produce more acid or can be used in the further oxidation of pyrite.

$$Fe^{3+} + 3H_2O \rightarrow Fe(OH)_3 + 3H^+$$

or

$$FeS_2 \text{ (pyrite)} + 14Fe^{3+} + 8H_2O \rightarrow 15Fe^{2+} + 2SO_4^{2-} + 16H^+$$

The dark-brown ferrous hydroxide precipitates out of solution and can coat the plants and benthos of aquatic ecosystems. The ferric iron remaining can react with sodium sulfate or potassium sulfate to form a yellow-brown precipitate that also damages the ecosystem.

Inhibition of damage

As the mine tailings are produced, the ore can be capped with a thick layer of clay to reduce its exposure to H_2O and oxygen. Alternatively, the tailings can be mixed with acid-neutralizing rocks. It may also be possible to engineer wetlands that produce sulfate-reducing bacteria that would neutralize the drainage from the tailings.

To stop corrosion in cement pipes used in wastewater removal, the environment is changed so that it no longer supports the activity of sulfate-reducing bacteria, the key microbe that causes the damage. This can be done by adding caustic soda to inhibit bacterial growth by raising the pH. Alternatively, damage can be reduced by providing the bacteria with ferric chloride. This serves as an alternate electron acceptor for the bacteria, which blocks its production of the sulfuric acid that causes the cement breakdown.

In cement sewer pipes, the growth of sulfate-oxidizing bacteria can be limited by raising the pH by the addition of caustic soda or by regularly providing the SRB with an alternate electron acceptor to SO_4^{2-} by adding ferric chloride or oxygen.

Sulfur-Reducing Bacteria

Economic importance

MIC of metals by biofilm-forming sulfate-reducing bacteria accounts for 15 to 30% of the corrosion failures in the gas and nuclear industries. It is a major cause of pipeline failures in water treatment, causing billions of dollars of damage requiring replacement of underground pipes in the United States.

Key microbes

SRB can use H_2 as an electron donor and SO_4^{2-} as an electron acceptor in anaerobic respiration to produce

H_2S. Aerobic respiration in eukaryotes uses reduced nicotinamide adenine dinucleotide (NADH) as an electron donor and O_2 as an electron acceptor to produce H_2O. The energy released by a series of redox reactions in both instances is used to produce an electrochemical gradient of H^+ to drive adenosine triphosphate (ATP) synthesis.

Key processes

Both types of corrosion are caused by bacteria that actively metabolize sulfur-containing compounds. Metals are degraded by SRB. Under anaerobic conditions, SRB use H_2 as an electron donor and sulfate as an electron acceptor.

$$4H_2 + SO_4^{2-} \rightarrow H_2S + 2\,OH^- + 2H_2O$$

This reduces the H_2 concentration and provides H_2S to drive the spontaneous breakdown of iron.

$$H_2S + Fe^{2+} \rightarrow FeS + H_2$$

and

$$Fe^{2+} + 2H_2O \rightarrow Fe(OH)_2 + H_2$$

The overall reaction for MIC of metal is as follows:

$$2Fe^{2+} + SO_4^{2-} + 2H_2 \rightarrow FeS + Fe(OH)_2 + 2(OH)^-$$

The biofilm matrix contributes to this process by promoting an anaerobic environment for the SRB. The biofilm contains a diverse group of microbes. Those near the surface actively metabolize O_2, resulting in an anaerobic environment for the SRB growing at the bottom of the biofilm on the metal surface. The biofilms also trap the corrosion products and organic acids at the metal-biofilm interface.

$$H_2SO_4 + Ca(OH)_2 \rightarrow CaSO_4 + 2H_2O$$

Inhibition of MIC

MIC cannot be prevented. The microbes that form the biofilms and perform the chemical reactions that result in metal corrosion are too universally distributed and well adapted for their growth and damage to be prevented. Nevertheless, reduction of MIC, through regular control activities, minimizes the damage and maximizes the life of metal pipes in the world's infrastructure.

One strategy to control MIC is to coat the metal surface with bacteriocidal chemicals. These chemicals inhibit microbial growth and metabolism and are effective until they dissolve or leach into the surrounding environment. Metal surfaces are coated with antimicrobial substances, such as copper, tin, quaternary ammonium compounds, and phenolics.

Another method used to minimize the damage from MIC is to remove the microenvironment that supports the growth of SRB. Oxidizing agents at high enough concentrations to diffuse through the polysaccharide matrix of the biofilm will effectively kill SRB. Disinfectants, such as chlorine or cationic surfactants, kill the biofilm bacteria. Regular treatment decreases corrosion caused by the continuous biofilm formation occurring in the pipes.

Plague

Worldwide, there are 1,000 to 2,000 cases of plague each year. Almost all of the cases reported during the 1990s were rural and occurred among people living in small towns and villages or agricultural areas.

Cause of the disease

Yersinia pestis, a bacterial pathogen, is a gram-negative rod-shaped bacterium with an antiphagocytic capsule. It is a facultative intracellular pathogen.

Transmission
Reservoir
Plague is a multisystem zoonosis that has an animal reservoir, primarily in the small-mammal population.

Mode of transmission
Plague is transmitted by the parenteral route from animal to animal and from animal to human by the bites of infective fleas. An uncommon mode of transmission is by inhaling infected droplets expelled by coughing from a person or animal with pneumonic plague.

Pathogenesis
Entry
The bite of an infected flea causes itching near the site of the break in the skin. Itching causes the feces carrying the pathogen from the flea to be introduced into the blood through scratching.

Attachment
The ability of *Yersinia pestis* to attach and enter a host cell is a key determinant of pathogenicity.

Avoiding host defenses
The pathogen synthesizes a capsule that is antiphagocytic.

Damage
The pathogen is carried to the lymph nodes that drain the area of the flea bite. The bacteria multiply in the nodes, cause inflammation, and spread. The patho-

gen produces coagulase and fibrinolysin, which degrade blood clots; an endotoxin, which can cause shock and disseminated intravascular coagulation; and V and W antigens, which enable the pathogen to cause an overwhelming septicemia.

Exit

If the pathogen travels to the lungs and causes pneumonia, it may be spread to another human via respiratory droplets.

Clinical features

There is an incubation period of 2 to 6 days after infection. Plague begins with a fever, headache, and general illness, followed by the development of painful, swollen regional lymph nodes (buboes). Plague septicemia follows, with rapid invasion of the bloodstream, producing severe illness, prostration, and extreme exhaustion. The pathogen may also spread to the lungs, causing an overwhelming pneumonia with high fever, cough, bloody sputum, and chills.

Diagnosis

Specimen

Blood or pus from an infected bubo is used as a specimen.

Tests

Gram staining is done to identify irregularly staining gram-negative rods that appear safety pin shaped. Direct fluorescent-antibody assays are used to confirm the diagnosis.

Treatment

Drug therapy begins as soon as plague is suspected. Several aminoglycosides are effective at treating plague. Aminoglycosides, such as streptomycin, are bacteriocidal and block the formation of 30S initiation complexes during the initiation of protein synthesis.

Where cost is important and the health care infrastructure is poorly developed, tetracyclines are also effective and can be delivered orally. Tetracyclines block aminoacyl-transfer RNA (tRNA) binding to 70S ribosomes during elongation in protein synthesis.

Prevention

- As soon as a diagnosis of suspected plague is made, the patient should be isolated to prevent spread to others.
- Those who have had contact with the plague patient must be traced and given prophylactic antibiotics.
- Insecticides can be used to control the flea population.
- Public health education can be used to instruct homeowners to eliminate food and shelter for rodents.
- Vaccination to prevent infection in at-risk groups should include people working with the plague bacterium in the laboratory or in the field and people working in plague-affected areas.

SECTION IX

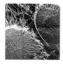 Bioterrorism Outbreaks

Our factory could turn out two tons of anthrax a day in a process as reliable and efficient as producing tanks, trucks, cars, or Coca-Cola.

KEN ALIBEK, former scientific head of the Soviet Union's bioweapon programs, *Biohazard* (1999)

In the past several hundred years, biological weapons (BWs) have been used occasionally as part of a military strategy whose main purpose was to incapacitate or kill opposing troops and civilian populations. Plague, anthrax, smallpox, and tularemia have been used with limited success, and in some cases, the biological weapons have infected those who intentionally released the agents.

In the last several decades, the use and development of biological weapons have greatly increased. Development has been led by countries that have used modern laboratory and genetic research tools to develop and test pathogens that are highly lethal, untreatable, and readily disseminated. State-sponsored research has been driven by fears of falling behind in the arms race; the relatively low levels of technology, cost, and expertise that are required to produce biological weapons; and the opportunity to be competitive with the world's superpowers.

The actual use of biological weapons has been limited to small sects and individual extremists, who have used them to advance their political or religious views. For these groups, biological weapons are attractive because, compared to many other acts of violence, they get more headlines in the media, affect more lives, and produce a general fear within the population that lasts longer.

Research on and use of offensive biological agents and toxins have been banned since the 1970s by an international treaty (Convention on the Prohibition of the Development, Production, and Stockpiling of Bacteriological and Toxin Weapons and on Their Destruction) that was signed by 103 countries, including the United States and the former Soviet Union. However, major research and development programs were covertly continued, expanded, and fully funded by countries such as the Soviet Union throughout the 1980s and much of the 1990s. The former Soviet Union's bioweapon development program employed tens of thousands of research scientists and technicians in over 40 BW production facilities, BW research facilities, and testing grounds. Despite the scope and duration of the program, the international community was unaware of the Soviet bioweapon technology or capacity until several scientists defected to Western countries.

Highly lethal pathogens that had no known treatment were weaponized. Tons of weapons grade *Bacillus anthracis,* smallpox virus, and plague were produced and stockpiled or placed into intercontinental ballistic missiles in place of nuclear warheads. With the collapse of the Soviet Union, the facilities were abandoned, leaving the most deadly pathogens in the world unsecured. Consequently, the Nunn-Lugar Act was passed by Congress to secure the weapons of mass destruction and help retool the factories for productive enterprises.

Besides the potential loss of life, biological weapons are unique in their ability to cause widespread panic. After a biological attack, health care systems quickly become overwhelmed with healthy individuals who are worried that they have been exposed. The general crisis that ensues has an adverse effect on the economy, as employers are less likely to invest in expansion and hire more employees.

This section focuses on understanding how the pathogens used as biological weapons are transmitted and how the diseases they cause are treated and prevented. An understanding of these diseases is the first step in developing effective strategies to identify the release of a bioterrorism agent and to provide a rapid and effective response.

Table IX.1 Infectious agents developed for use as bioweapons

Organism	Key physical properties	Disease characteristics
Bacteria		
Bacillus anthracis	Gram-positive bacillus; aerobic; produces an antiphagocytic capsule and tissue-damaging cytotoxins	Inhalation of weaponized anthrax spores causes highly lethal pneumonia and systemic infection.
Clostridium botulinum toxin	Anaerobic, gram-positive, endospore-forming bacillus that produces a potent neurotoxin, which causes muscle paralysis	Botulism, flaccid paralysis
Brucella spp.	Fastidious, gram-negative bacillus	Brucellosis can cause fever, lymphadenopathy, hepatosplenomegaly, and physiological problems.
Francisella tularensis	Fastidious, gram-negative bacillus	Tularemia causes skin ulcers, lymphadenopathy, fever, bacteremia, and pneumonia.
Yersinia pestis	Gram-negative bacillus	Localized lymphadenopathy (bubonic); highly lethal bacteremia and pneumonia
Viruses		
Filoviruses (Ebola virus, Marburg virus)	Enveloped helical capsid with single-stranded RNA	Hemorrhagic fever with high mortality; reservoir is not known
Smallpox virus	Enveloped brick-shaped capsid with double-stranded DNA	Smallpox causes a pustular rash with mortality rates of up to 30%.

An Accidental Release of Weaponized Anthrax

SVERDLOVSK, USSR, 1979

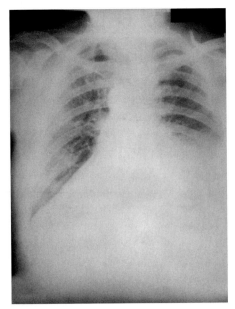

Figure 89.1 A chest X ray showing pneumonia and mediastinal widening.

In April and May 1979, an epidemic broke out in the city of Sverdlovsk in the Soviet Union (now Yekaterinburg, Russia). According to a report given by visiting Soviet doctors, the crisis began on the morning of 7 April, when Soviet officials were notified of a number of deaths over the previous weekend. Some deaths occurred outside the hospital, at home, in the street, and even in a field. Vladimir Nikiforov, the infectious disease chief at the Moscow Institute for the Advanced Training of Physicians, was flown out to Sverdlovsk and treated suspected victims with near-toxic doses of antibiotics.

The disease was anthrax. It began as a nonspecific flu-like illness characterized by fever, muscle aches, headache, a nonproductive cough, and mild chest discomfort. After a brief intervening period of improvement, there was rapid deterioration marked by high fever, difficulty breathing, lack of oxygen, and shock. Chest radiographs showed mediastinal widening (enlargement of the space between the lungs caused by tissue damage around the major blood vessels and heart) and pleural effusions (pus in the space between the lungs and body wall). The epidemic ran intensely from 4 to 19 April, the day the epidemic reached its peak with 10 new cases. There were 96 victims in all, according to Nikiforov. Most people who contracted the disease worked, lived, or attended daytime military reserve classes in the same area during the first week of April 1979. This restricted the sites where people were infected to a narrow zone, with its northern end in a military factory in the city and its other end near the city limits 4 kilometers to the south. Also, livestock died of a disease with similar symptoms in villages along the extended axis of this same zone out to a distance of 50 kilometers.

At the time, the Soviets claimed that the epidemic's source was bad meat, which caused an outbreak of intestinal anthrax. However, local people knew better. Those who were familiar with the outbreak noted that the personnel treating the supposed victims of food poisoning wore protective suits.

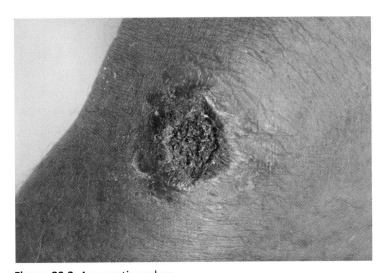

Figure 89.2 A necrotic eschar.

Although Western scientists suspected an airborne release of anthrax, most accepted the food-borne pathogen explanation. Raymond Zilinskas, a U.S. clinical microbiologist, summarized part of the logic in a 1980 report on the Sverdlovsk accident: "No nation would be so stupid as to locate a biological warfare facility within an approachable distance from a major population center."

In the 1990s, it was revealed that the city's bioweapon plant had accidentally released a plume of anthrax spores, causing the worst outbreak of inhalation anthrax ever recorded. On Friday, 30 March 1979, a clogged filter in the anthrax-drying plant at Compound 19 in Sverdlovsk was removed and not replaced, causing a fine dust of anthrax spores and chemical additive to be exhausted into the air for several hours, resulting in the anthrax outbreak.

QUESTIONS

1. What characteristics of *Bacillus anthracis* make it one of the most dangerous bioweapons?

2. Describe the pathogenesis of the organism.

3. Would you expect any long-term problems from this release of anthrax? Explain why or why not.

An Investigation of a Brucellosis Outbreak as Bioterrorism

NEW HAMPSHIRE, 1999

Several days before being admitted to a hospital, a 38-year-old woman who resided in New Hampshire experienced malaise, headache, fever, chills, diarrhea, and irritability. On 25 March 1999, she was admitted to hospital A in New Hampshire, where she was diagnosed with brucellosis. Her disease progressed over 3 days to respiratory failure requiring mechanical ventilation. On day 22, after 3 weeks of intensive care, the patient was transferred to hospital B in Boston, Massachusetts. Hospital personnel interviewed family members, who reported no history of traditional risk factors for exposure to a pathogen that would typically account for her clinical presentation.

On day 24, the patient's family reported to hospital personnel that the patient's illness might have been caused by exposure to "laboratory flasks" and "cultures" kept in her apartment by her boyfriend. He was described as a foreign national studying marine biology who was formerly affiliated with a local university but had recently returned to his country of citizenship. On day 25, the patient's family brought laboratory flasks, petri dishes, and culture media to hospital B from the patient's apartment. Several contained an unidentified clear liquid, and some were marked with dates from the 1980s. Infection control staff at hospital B were notified of the laboratory-type materials on day 27.

On day 28, the Centers for Disease Control and Prevention (CDC) and the New Hampshire Department of Health and Human Services (NHDHHS) were notified. The NHDHHS had received no reports of brucellosis through its passive surveillance system. In response to the case report, the NHDHHS contacted hospital infection control nurses but identified no other cases of unusual febrile illness in southern New Hampshire during the preceding few weeks.

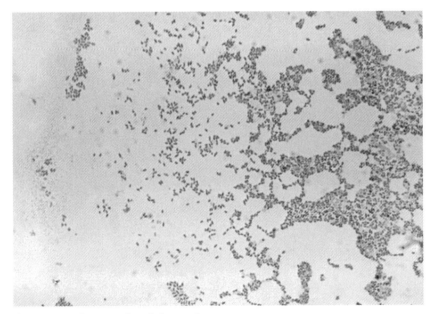

Figure 90.1 Gram stain of the pathogen.

On day 33, at hospital B, the patient died from adult respiratory distress syndrome. An autopsy was requested by public health authorities; however, the possibility of a biological terrorism threat created concern on the part of the hospital pathology staff, and the autopsy was postponed.

QUESTIONS

1. Besides *Brucella*, list several diseases and their pathogens that could have been grown in the apartment and that might have accounted for the woman's signs and symptoms.

2. How would you have established whether the woman's disease was caused by an intentional infection with *Brucella*?

3. How would you detect future cases of brucellosis?

4. How is *Brucella* transmitted?

5. If this were a bioterrorism event, what would be two high-priority activities that you would publicly implement to help minimize the threat? Briefly explain your reasoning.

A Tularemia Outbreak

MULTISTATE, 2002

An outbreak of tularemia, an illness with high mortality, was observed in captured wild prairie dogs (*Cynomys ludovicianus*) at a commercial exotic animal distributor in Texas. Before shipments were halted on 1 August 2002, approximately 250 of an estimated 3,600 prairie dogs that passed through the Texas facility had died. The sick animals were believed to be part of a single shipment of prairie dogs that were caught in South Dakota starting on 18 May and shipped to the Texas distributor on 16 June. Prairie dogs were shipped by the Texas facility and by a South Dakota trader to wholesalers, retailers, and individuals in Arkansas, Florida, Illinois, Michigan, Mississippi, Nevada, Ohio, Texas, Washington, and West Virginia and exported to Belgium, the Czech Republic, Japan, The Netherlands, and Thailand. Unusually high numbers of sick or dead prairie dogs were reported from Texas and the Czech Republic.

There were some reports of human illness following the handling of prairie dogs. After 2 to 6 days, individuals experienced a sudden onset of a high fever, chills, headaches and muscle aches, and a feeling of weakness. In addition, chest discomfort and a dry cough were common.

The CDC laboratory tests of blood and sputa revealed *Francisella tularensis*, a small, aerobic, gram-negative coccobacillus. Identification was completed in a specialized high-level biosafety laboratory.

Due to the potential for global spread of the outbreak, the World Health Organization and the European Union Disease Surveillance Network became involved in the investigation. *Francisella tularensis* is also a potential bioweapon and is among the CDC's top six agents of concern. This outbreak was not a bioterrorist attack.

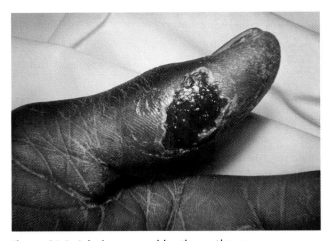

Figure 91.1 A lesion caused by the pathogen.

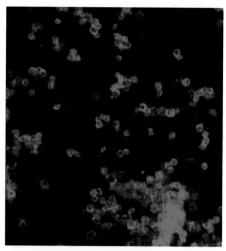

Figure 91.2 Direct fluorescent-antibody assay for *Francisella tularensis.*

QUESTIONS

1. What characteristics of the pathogen make it a highly dangerous bioterrorism agent?

2. Why are special precautions taken in handling this pathogen in the laboratory?

3. Describe how you would have managed this outbreak.

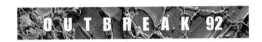

Bioterrorist Release of Anthrax Bacteria by a Religious Cult

KAMEIDO, JAPAN, 1993

In July 1993, a liquid suspension of *Bacillus anthracis* was aerosolized from the roof of an eight-story building in Kameido, a suburb of Tokyo, Japan, by the religious group Aum Shinrikyo. Forty-one nearby residents reported foul odors to local environmental-health authorities. The foul odors were thought to be causing appetite loss, nausea, and vomiting in some exposed people.

On the morning of 1 July, residents reported loud noises and an intermittent mist emanating from one of two cooling towers on the building's roof (Fig. 92.1); 118 complaints about the foul odors were received. The day was rainy and cloudy, with no direct sunlight and a mild wind. The same day, residents in the neighborhood reported a "gelatin-like, oily, gray-to-black" fluid due to the mist from the cooling towers collecting on the side of the building. Environmental officials collected samples of the fluid and stored them in a refrigerator (4°C) for later testing.

Because of the complaints, officials requested permission to inspect the building's interior, but the Aum Shinrikyo members refused. Officials checked the building's surroundings, collected air samples, and began to observe activity at the building, but other than the nuisance posed by the odor, no readily apparent risk to human health could be found.

Intermittent misting continued until demands from local residents forced the cult to agree to cease using the rooftop device and to clean and vacate the building. No equipment remained when officials inspected the building on 16 July, although they noted black stains on the walls.

This incident was largely forgotten until the cult launched a sarin gas attack on the Tokyo subway system in 1995: 3,800 people became

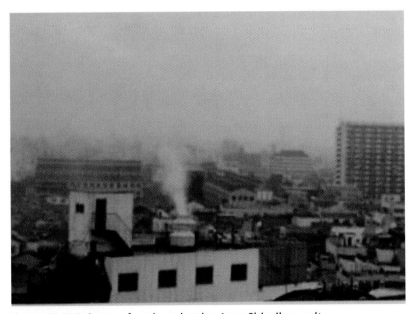

Figure 92.2 Release of anthrax by the Aum Shinrikyo cult.

ill, with nearly 1,000 requiring hospitalization and 12 deaths. Police investigations then uncovered the true nature of the incident of mist and foul odors in 1993—Aum Shinrikyo cult members testified that the odors were caused by their efforts to aerosolize a liquid suspension of *Bacillus anthracis* in an attempt to cause an inhalation anthrax epidemic. They believed this epidemic would trigger a world war and lead to their deity, Asahara, ruling the world.

In November 1999, the one remaining fluid sample, collected as part of the 1993 investigation, was tested for microbiologic pathogens at Northern Arizona University in Flagstaff, Arizona. Provisional microscopy examination of the fluid stained by malachite green-safranin showed bacterial spores, a large amount of debris, and vegetative (nonsporulating) bacterial cells. Aliquots of the fluid were streaked on sheep blood agar plates and incubated aerobically at 37°C. After overnight growth, the plates were found to contain a mixed bacterial flora; approximately 10% of the colonies were similar in appearance to *B. anthracis*. The suspect colonies were non-hemolytic and had the "gray-ground-glass" appearance typical of *B. anthracis*. A representative selection of 48 colonies of the *B. anthracis*-like agent were purified by single-colony streaking and then subjected to genetic analysis using the polymerase chain reaction (PCR). The primers were specific for sites unique to *B. anthracis* and its plasmids, which carry genes coding for anthrax toxin and capsule production.

Analysis of the 48 suspect colonies confirmed them to be *B. anthracis*, and all had the same genotype. The gene for the plasmid coding for the anthrax capsule consistently failed to be identified. All colonies contained the toxin-encoding plasmid. This genotype was identical to that of the Sterne 34F2 strain, used commercially in Japan to vaccinate animals against anthrax.

QUESTIONS

1. How could the weather have affected the attempt to cause an inhalation anthrax outbreak?

2. Why is the ability to form endospores important for the pathogen to be able to be used as a bioweapon?

3. What role does a capsule play in a microbe's pathogenesis?

4. What role do exotoxins play in a microbe's pathogenesis?

5. Could inhalation anthrax have been the cause of appetite loss, nausea, and vomiting in some exposed people?

6. What would be your top priority in preventing this type of terrorism attack today?

7. What would be your second priority?

A Death from Ebola Hemorrhagic Fever at a Former Bioweapon Laboratory

RUSSIA, 2004

The former Soviet Union had an active state-supported bioweapon research and production program from the 1970s through the mid-1990s. One branch of the program was called VECTOR—the State Research Center for Virology and Biotechnology. At VECTOR, molecular biologists worked to develop lethal viruses into effective biological weapons. They chose pathogens for which there was no known treatment or vaccine. Since the breakup of the former Soviet Union into independent countries, the U.S. government and private companies have been providing aid to countries with former bioweapon laboratories so that the facilities can be converted to peaceful research. About $10 million has been spent at VECTOR facilities.

While working to develop a vaccine against Ebola virus, a Russian scientist at a VECTOR laboratory in Siberia accidentally stuck herself with a needle contaminated with the virus. The scientist contracted Ebola hemorrhagic fever and died. Although the accident occurred on 5 May 2004, VECTOR officials did not report it to the World Health Organization for over a week.

Internationally, this raised significant concern. Not only was the international community concerned that one of the most lethal pathogens known to man might have been spread, but the delay also meant that other international experts were unable to provide advice on treatment that might have been lifesaving.

U.S. aid to former bioweapon programs is controversial, because it is hard to verify that the resources contributed are used for peaceful projects. However, these programs may keep former bioweapon researchers employed and prevent them from seeking employment with terrorist-supported states that are seeking to develop weapons of mass destruction. American experts said the accident had not occurred in a laboratory receiving U.S. government or private money for research.

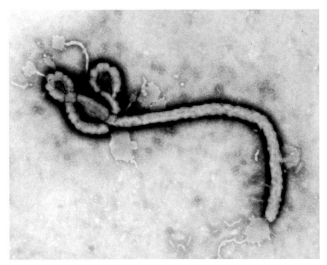

Figure 93.1 A transmission electron micrograph of the viral pathogen.

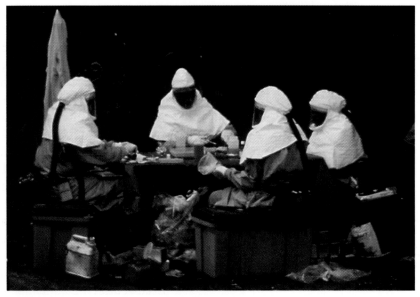

Figure 93.2 Field testing for the pathogen.

QUESTIONS

1. What are the potential benefits of American aid to convert VECTOR's bioweapon facilities to peaceful research? What are the potential hazards?

2. What tissue(s) does the pathogen damage that leads to hemorrhaging?

3. How would you have prevented this outbreak from spreading to other scientists at VECTOR?

4. What precautions need to be taken when working with this deadly virus?

5. Compare this pathogen with smallpox virus as a potential biological weapon. Which would be more dangerous as a weapon of mass destruction?

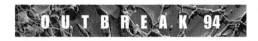

An Inexpensive and Simple Botulism Bioweapon

WASHINGTON, D.C., 2003

Easy to find and easy to produce, botulism toxin is the most poisonous natural substance on Earth. In the hands of a bioterrorist, a single gram could kill 1 million people. Anthony Fauci of the National Institutes of Health has stated that preventing the use of botulism toxin is one of the nation's highest priorities.

The toxin easily poisons those who eat it, and experts fear terrorists could infect the nation's food supply and sicken thousands, making the 2001 anthrax attacks by mail seem minor by comparison. The government has only enough antitoxin available to treat the victims of a small attack—one official put the inventory at more than 1,000 doses—and the special treatment needed for children is produced only by a California program now in jeopardy because of the state's budget shortfall.

Unlike smallpox, the most widely publicized bioterrorism threat, botulism is not contagious, and with medical treatment, the vast majority of those affected survive. But while smallpox no longer exists in the wild, botulism toxin is easily acquired. The organism, *Clostridium botulinum,* is found in soil and, along with its spores, can contaminate poorly prepared food. About 120 Americans contract botulism each year. Roughly three in four are infants, who can contract it by eating small amounts of raw honey.

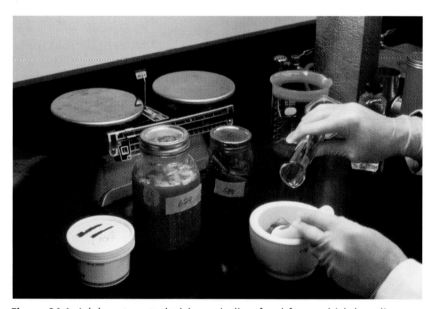

Figure 94.1 A laboratory technician grinding food from which botulism toxin will be extracted.

Disseminating botulism toxin may not be particularly difficult, though one would need basic microbiology skills. Heating food long enough at a high enough temperature kills the organism, but milk and other dairy products are not heated long enough during processing to inactivate the toxin. If botulism toxin were introduced into the milk supply, it might not be inactivated during the processing stage. There is also concern about the vulnerability of tankers transporting milk.

QUESTIONS

1. What are the clinical signs and symptoms of botulism?

2. What medical conditions is botulism toxin used for today?

3. How would you plan to prevent widespread panic if a release of botulism toxin occurred?

State-Sponsored Bioweapon Research

FORMER SOVIET UNION, 1990s

In 1972, the Biological Weapons Convention was held. The resolution it produced (the Convention on the Prohibition of the Development, Production, and Stockpiling of Bacteriological and Toxin Weapons and on Their Destruction) prohibiting research on and development of offensive biological weapons was eventually signed by 103 nations, including the United States and the former Soviet Union. Despite agreeing to the convention, the Soviet government initiated a well-funded, technologically advanced biological weapons program.

Ken Alibek, the scientific chief of the Soviet Union's biological weapons program at its peak, oversaw much of the research and development at the 47 different bioweapon factories located in 29 different cities. When the program was operating at full capacity in the late 1980s, more than 60,000 people were engaged in research, testing, production, and equipment design throughout the country. Alibek stated, "Money was never a problem. As late as 1990, when Soviet leader Mikhail Gorbachev was promising the world major cutbacks in our arsenals, I was authorized to spend the equivalent of $200 million, plus $470 million for new buildings. The total figure spent that year on biological weapons development was close to a billion dollars." The Soviet government decided that the best agents were those for which there was no known cure. This led to a constant race against new developments in the bioweapon laboratories. Every time a new treatment or vaccine was developed, scientists designed new ways to overcome its effects.

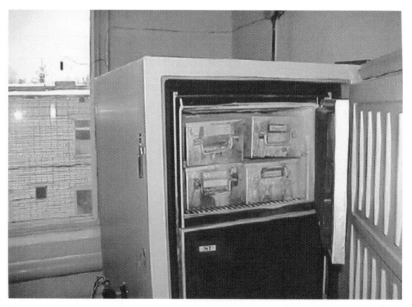

Figure 95.1 An unsecured freezer containing agents used as biological weapons.

Alibek stated that the working stockpiles of bioweapons included 20 tons of weaponized smallpox, a weaponized anthrax production capacity of 4,500 tons per year, tularemia and plague bacteria resistant to 10 different antibiotics, and even combination bioweapons. These weapons combined pathogens in unique ways to make the bioweapons more lethal and very difficult to trace or to determine the cause of the death. For example, Sergei Popov, a former bioweapon researcher in the Soviet Union, constructed a combination pathogen that initially caused legionellosis. Several days after apparently recovering from the *Legionella* infection, the infected individual would then come down with lethal encephalitis that would initially present as similar to multiple sclerosis. As a result, diagnosis of the actual pathogen that caused the disease would be very difficult.

Alibek stated, "The threat of a biological attack has increased as the knowledge developed in our labs—of lethal formulations that took our scientists years to discover—has spread to rogue regimes and terrorist groups. Bioweapons are no longer restricted to the two superpowers that polarized the world during the Cold War. They are cheap, easy to make, and easy to use. In the coming years, they will become very much a part of our lives."

QUESTIONS

1. Explain why agents of anthrax, tularemia, plague, and smallpox are among the most feared microbes that could potentially be used in a bioterrorism attack.

2. Alibek states that bioweapons are "cheap, easy to make, and easy to use." Do you agree with his assessment? Explain your reasoning.

3. Provide two or three reasons why countries today would support state-sponsored bioweapon research using all modern laboratory and genetic research tools.

4. What international policies and activities should the United States support in order to reduce the risk of countries' supporting or constructing bioweapons?

An Outbreak of Weaponized Smallpox

ARALSK, USSR, 1971

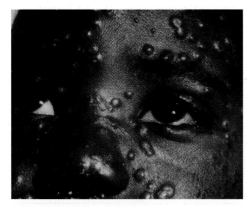

Figure 96.1 A pustular rash.

During the summer of 1971, a previously unreported outbreak of smallpox is now known to have occurred in Aralsk, a city of approximately 50,000 people on the northern shore of the Aral Sea in the then-Soviet republic of Kazakhstan. On or about 15 July 1971, a biological research vessel called the *Lev Berg* set sail from Aralsk on an extended voyage. The ship was scheduled to stop at two dozen research stations scattered around the Aral Sea and planned to return to its homeport on 8 August 1971. On board the *Lev Berg* was a young fisheries expert, patient 1, who was responsible for, among other things, casting nets and collecting various species of fish and plants for archiving. As the youngest member of the crew, she was the one working most frequently on deck. She spent most of her time casting nets to catch fish, which she then took to the small laboratory below deck to archive samples, perform simple analysis, and make notations in the laboratory journal. The main purpose of the *Lev Berg* expedition was to assess the ecological damage to the sea as a result of water diversion from rivers normally feeding the Aral Sea to irrigate cotton fields. By her personal account, at no time was she allowed to leave the ship during its voyage.

During the trip, the ship inadvertently strayed close to Vozrozhdeniye Island, a site of BW field testing by the Soviet Ministry of Defense. Pyotr Burgasov, a former chief sanitary physician of the Soviet Union, was interviewed in November 2001. He stated that on Vozrozhdeniye Island in the Aral Sea, the strongest formulations of BWs were tested. The *Lev Berg* came within 15 kilometers of the island (it was not supposed to come any closer than 45 kilometers) during a BW test in which 400 grams of weaponized smallpox virus was exploded on the island.

Patient 1 became ill shortly after arriving home in Aralsk on 11 or 12 August. She experienced fever, headache, and muscle aches. She

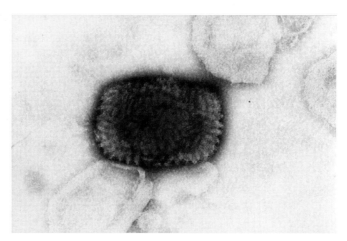

Figure 96.2 A transmission electron micrograph of the viral pathogen.

was nursed by her mother and visited by the local general practitioner, who noted that she had a fever of 39°C and a cough. The doctor prescribed antibiotics and aspirin but did not make a definitive diagnosis. Shortly thereafter, a diffuse rash covered her entire body and her fever broke. Patient 1 had been vaccinated against smallpox, as had the other members of her family.

On 27 August, patient 1's 9-year-old brother, patient 2, came down with a fever and a skin rash. A pediatrician diagnosed hives, a skin eruption often considered to be an allergic reaction. Patient 2 was treated with tetracycline and aspirin and recovered completely over the next 2 weeks. Patient 2 had classic smallpox symptoms: a very high temperature for 3 days, followed by a pustular rash which covered his whole body with pustules about 2 to 3 millimeters in diameter. The rash lasted 2 weeks and then crusted over. After the rash disappeared, he had smallpox scars that disappeared after about 2 years.

Over the next 3 weeks, physicians in Aralsk saw eight additional patients, six adults and two children. The two children, who were unvaccinated against smallpox, developed hemorrhagic complications and died. One unvaccinated adult, the 23-year-old schoolteacher of patient 2, also died from the hemorrhagic variant of the disease. The other five infected adults had been vaccinated against smallpox.

QUESTIONS

1. How is smallpox spread?

2. Why is smallpox potentially more dangerous than almost any other bioweapon?

3. Describe the morbidity and mortality of the disease.

4. Describe how the spread of the disease has been prevented in the past. Would this strategy have worked for the outbreak described? If not, propose an alternative method for disease containment.

APPLICATION

Assume that it is 1971 and you are the scientific head of the former Soviet Union's secret bioweapon program. You have been assigned to head up the government's effort to prevent the spread of this outbreak. Your top objective is to minimize the number of deaths from disease. You have at your disposal all the authority and resources of the government of the Soviet Union.

1. What action will be your first priority? Explain your reasoning.

2. What action will be your second priority? Explain your reasoning.

Anthrax

Anthrax is found in three potentially fatal forms: cutaneous anthrax infects the skin of animals and humans that have come in contact with anthrax endospores, gastrointestinal (GI) anthrax causes serious damage to the GI tract when animals eat infected food, and inhalation anthrax causes life-threatening pneumonia. In today's world, inhalation anthrax is an indication of the use of biological weapons.

Cause of the disease

Anthrax is caused by *Bacillus anthracis*, a bacterial pathogen. *Bacillus anthracis* is a large, aerobic, nonmotile, gram-positive rod that forms an antiphagocytic capsule. The genus *Bacillus* is capable of forming spores that can survive for long periods under harsh conditions.

Transmission

Humans can become infected by coming into contact with the spores of infected animals that enter through the skin, mucous membranes, or respiratory tract. The most common means of infection for humans is contact with anthrax spores found on animal products, such as hides, bristles, or wool.

Reservoir

Bacillus anthracis is found in the soil where animals that have died of anthrax have decomposed.

Mode of transmission

Cutaneous anthrax is transmitted by direct contact with endospore-contaminated material—infected tissue, the carcass of a dead animal, or contaminated soil. Gastrointestinal anthrax is transmitted by ingestion of contaminated food. Inhalation anthrax is transmitted by airborne particles less than 5 micrometers in diameter. This normally requires the technologically demanding process of preparing the endospores for use as a biological weapon.

Pathogenesis

Entry

The endospores enter the body by way of the skin, mucous membranes, or respiratory tract.

Attachment

The spores germinate and attach to the tissues that they have entered.

Avoiding host defenses

The pathogen produces an antiphagocytic capsule that enables it to avoid phagocytosis.

Damage

The pathogen produces two toxins—the edema factor causes large amounts of fluid to be lost from the capillaries, while the lethal factor causes cell death, leading to necrosis (dead tissues) and hemorrhaging.

Exit

The pathogen is not typically spread person to person, since infection is normally from the soil reservoir.

Clinical features

Symptoms vary, depending on how the disease was contracted, but in all cases, symptoms usually arise within 7 days of infection.

Cutaneous anthrax symptoms

Skin infection begins as a raised, itchy bump that looks similar to an insect bite. Within 1 or 2 days, the bump develops into a painless ulcer (an eschar), usually 1 to 3 centimeters in diameter. Also, lymph nodes in the area begin to swell. In about 20% of untreated cases, the pathogen enters the bloodstream and causes a fatal infection.

Inhalation anthrax symptoms

The symptoms of inhalation anthrax initially resemble those of a common cold. After several days, the symptoms progress to severe breathing problems and shock. Pulmonary anthrax usually results in death 1 to 2 days after the onset of symptoms.

Intestinal anthrax symptoms

The major symptom of intestinal anthrax is inflammation of the intestinal tract. The initial signs—nausea, loss of appetite, vomiting, and fever—are followed by abdominal pain and severe diarrhea. Intestinal anthrax is lethal in about 40% of cases.

Diagnosis

Clinical features aid in diagnosis. The spreading, necrotic eschar indicates cutaneous anthrax. Inhalation anthrax is characterized by overwhelming pneumonia. A chest X ray shows not only fluid in the lungs, but also a widening of the mediastinal cavity (the space between the lungs where the heart and major blood vessels are located) caused by large amounts of fluid released from the infected mediastinal lymph nodes.

Bacillus anthracis can be identified by a rapid hemagglutination test. However, diagnosis must be confirmed by a positive blood culture showing gram-positive, endospore-forming rods.

Treatment

A number of antibiotics given in large doses are effective. Ciprofloxacin, a fluoroquinolone, kills *Bacillus anthracis* by inhibiting deoxyribonucleic acid (DNA) gyrase activity, thus preventing DNA replication by the pathogen.

Prevention

- People in high-risk occupations should be given a series of anthrax immunizations that lead to immunity. Animals can also be vaccinated.
- Infected animals should be isolated.
- Carcasses of dead animals should be incinerated.

Botulism Toxin

Botulism toxin in solution is colorless, odorless, and as far as is known, tasteless. Botulism toxin is the most poisonous substance known. A single gram of crystalline toxin, evenly dispersed and inhaled, would kill more than 1 million people. The lethal dose of botulism toxin has been estimated to be 0.70 to 0.90 micrograms if inhaled and 70 micrograms if eaten.

Cause of the disease

Botulism toxin is produced by *Clostridium botulinum*, a bacterium that can be isolated from the soil relatively easily by someone with basic microbiology skills. The toxin itself is composed of two polypeptide chains linked together to form an enzyme. Botulism toxin is very poisonous because the enzyme continues to catalyze damage to the nervous system until it is destroyed.

Transmission

Although large-scale dissemination of botulism toxin requires significant technological capabilities, as a bioterrorism agent it would most likely be used to deliberately contaminate food or be released from a small aerosol container in crowded areas.

Pathogenesis

Entry

Intentionally released botulism toxin would enter through the GI tract or be inhaled into the respiratory tract.

Attachment

Botulism toxin binds to the neuronal-cell membrane at the nerve terminus and enters the neuron by endocytosis.

Avoiding host defenses

The concentration of botulism toxin required to cause serious illness or death is too low to stimulate an immune response.

Damage

Botulism toxin cleaves proteins in the neuron to enzymatically prevent acetylcholine release. Unless it can release acetylcholine, the neuron cannot stimulate muscle contraction.

Clinical features

Typically, cases present 12 to 72 hours after the toxin is ingested. Patients with botulism typically present with difficulty seeing, speaking, and/or swallowing. As paralysis extends beyond the cranial nerves controlling the head, generalized weakness becomes prominent. As a result of difficulty swallowing and loss of the protective gag reflex, patients may require mechanical ventilation. In untreated persons, death results from airway obstruction (paralysis of the pharyngeal muscles) and inability to inhale (diaphragmatic paralysis). Botulism intoxication does not cause a fever.

Diagnosis

Clinical diagnosis of botulism is confirmed by specialized laboratory testing that often requires days to complete. The standard laboratory diagnostic test for clinical specimens and foods is the mouse bioassay. In that test, mice are given the specimen that may contain the botulism toxin. A control group is also given an antitoxin. A positive test is indicated when the mice without the antitoxin show paralysis and the control group mice, given the antitoxin, are normal.

Treatment

Recovery results from new motor axons' growing to make new connections with the muscles. Since this process takes weeks or months to complete, paralysis can last a significant time. Therapy for botulism intoxication consists of supportive care and passive immunization with equine antitoxin. Botulism patients require supportive care that often includes feeding by parenteral nutrition, mechanical ventilation, and treatment of secondary infections.

Prevention

- Botulism toxin is rapidly inactivated by chlorination and aeration used to treat water. The toxin is readily inactivated by heat (≥85°C for 5 minutes). Therefore, adequate heating during cooking prevents botulism.

- Decontamination can take place naturally: it is estimated that deliberately released botulism toxin would decay and be harmless in about 2 days. Contaminated objects or surfaces should be cleaned with 0.1% hypochlorite bleach solution if they cannot be avoided for the hours to days required for natural degradation.

Brucellosis

Because *Brucella* is an extremely infectious pathogen and can be delivered as an aerosol, it became the first agent weaponized in the former U.S. offensive BW program. By 1955, the United States was producing *Brucella suis*-filled cluster bombs for the Air Force at the Pine Bluff Arsenal in Arkansas. Development of brucellae as a weapon was halted in 1967, and President Richard Nixon later banned development of all biological weapons on 25 November 1969.

Cause of the disease

The pathogenic agents for brucellosis are *Brucella* species, bacterial pathogens. *Brucella* is an aerobic gram-negative coccobacillus.

Transmission

Reservoir

Brucellosis is a zoonosis. *Brucella* has reservoirs in many different animals. The *Brucella* species that are transmitted to humans include *Brucella abortus* (cattle), *Brucella melitensis*, *Brucella ovis* (sheep and goats), *Brucella suis* (pigs), and rarely *Brucella canis* (dogs).

Mode of transmission

Brucellosis is a zoonotic infection transmitted from animals to humans by ingestion of infected food products, direct contact with an infected animal, or inhalation of aerosols. Worldwide, it is most commonly transmitted through abrasions of the skin from handling infected mammals. In the United States, the disease occurs more frequently by ingestion of unpasteurized milk or dairy products. It is also possible to introduce *Brucella* by inhalation of contaminated droplets. Transmission by this route is very rare.

Pathogenesis

Entry

Brucellae can gain entry into humans through breaks in the skin, mucous membranes, and conjunctiva and through the respiratory and GI tracts.

Attachment

Brucella is engulfed by polymorphonuclear leukocytes and macrophages.

Avoiding host defenses

Brucella is not destroyed by phagocytes. Instead, *Brucella* prevents fusion of the phagosome and lysosome.

Damage

Brucellae are transported into the lymphatic system and may replicate there locally; they also may replicate in the kidney, liver, spleen, breast tissue, or joints, causing both localized and systemic infections. Damage causes an inflammatory reaction, central necrosis, and lesions and abscesses that can be distributed in many different organs. Infection can lead to a fatal septicemia.

Exit

Typically, *Brucella* exits through infected tissue.

Clinical features

Brucellosis has a 1- to 3-week incubation period. In humans, brucellosis can cause a range of symptoms that are similar to the flu and may include fever, sweats, headaches, back pains, and physical weakness. Severe infections of the central nervous system or the lining of the heart may occur.

Brucellosis can also cause long-lasting or chronic symptoms that include recurrent fevers, joint pain, and fatigue. The symptoms can result in relatively long-term disability. This potential for long-lasting infection that can disable workers in either military or civilian occupations makes *Brucella* an appealing choice for a biological weapon.

Diagnosis

Brucella is highly infectious in the laboratory via aerosolization; handling cultures warrants biosafety level 3 precautions.

Specimen

A blood or bone marrow specimen is obtained.

Test

Indirect enzyme-linked immunosorbent assays can be used to measure antibodies against *Brucella* from blood samples taken 2 weeks apart.

Treatment

A 6-week therapy of doxycycline and rifampin has been used to treat brucellosis and prevent relapse of the disease. Monotherapy relapse rates approach 40%. Doxycycline blocks elongation of protein synthesis on 70S bacterial ribosomes. Rifampin inhibits ribonucleic acid (RNA) synthesis by blocking sigma factor activity in identifying promoters.

Prevention

Prevention focuses on elimination of domestic and feral animal reservoirs and detection of *Brucella* in foods.

Ebola Hemorrhagic Fever

From the scraps of information he had been able to obtain about the situation in Sudan and Zaire, they were dealing with a plague virus that was tremendously lethal and that could be spreading from person to person in a manner not previously seen with such a lethal virus. The cardinal issue was now lucid, if starkly frightening. Is this virus going to turn out to be transmitted by sneezing and coughing in a manner similar to influenza. If you have an infection that is virtually fatal, as this turned out to be, and transmitted by that mechanism, now, suddenly you have a threat to the entire human species.

Karl Johnson, head of the Special Pathogens Branch of the CDC, on his way to investigate the first Ebola hemorrhagic fever outbreak in Zaire

Cause of the disease

Ebola virus is the causative agent of Ebola hemorrhagic fever. It is an enveloped virus with a helical capsid that is twisted like a shepherd's crook. The virus contains single-stranded, negative-stranded RNA for genetic information.

Transmission

Reservoir

The exact origin, locations, and natural habitat of Ebola virus remain unknown. Researchers believe that the virus has a reservoir in an animal host that is native to the African continent. The virus has been acquired from ill chimpanzees in the jungles of the Congo and Gabon.

Mode of transmission

The pathogen is primarily transmitted by direct contact with infected fluids, such as blood, secretions, organs, or semen of infected people. Health care workers have frequently been infected while attending patients.

Pathogenesis

The pathogenesis of Ebola virus has not been completely characterized. The disease is rare and occurs in remote areas of Africa. Due to the extreme danger of working with the virus, research is done only in a level IV biohazard facility.

Damage is caused by destruction of endothelial tissue. As a result, capillaries throughout the body are damaged, leading to massive tissue damage and fluid loss from all internal organs.

Clinical features

The incubation period ranges from 2 to 21 days after infection. Ebola hemorrhagic fever is often characterized by the sudden onset of fever, weakness, muscle pain, headache, and sore throat, followed by vomiting, diarrhea, rash, limited kidney and liver functions, and both internal and external bleeding.

Diagnosis

Laboratory tests for Ebola hemorrhagic fever are done in high-level biohazard facilities using enzyme-linked immunosorbent assays to identify viruses or antibodies to the virus in the blood. PCR can also be used to detect Ebola virus genetic information.

Treatment

No specific treatment exists for Ebola hemorrhagic fever. Severe cases require intensive supportive care, as patients are frequently dehydrated from excessive internal bleeding and are in need of careful monitoring of blood components to attempt to balance fluid, electrolytes, and blood components by using intravenous therapy.

Prevention

- Containment: patients with suspected cases should be isolated from other patients, and strict barrier nursing techniques should be practiced. Hospital staff should have individual gowns, gloves, and masks. Gloves and masks must not be reused unless they are disinfected.

- Prompt burial: patients who die from the disease should be promptly buried or cremated.

- Contact tracing: since the primary mode of person-to-person transmission is contact with contaminated blood, secretions, or body fluids, any person who has had close physical contact with patients should be kept under strict surveillance, i.e., body temperature checks twice a day, with immediate hospitalization and strict isolation recommended for individuals with temperatures above 38.3°C (101°F).

- Casual contacts should be placed on alert and asked to report any fever.
- Surveillance of suspected case patients should continue for 3 weeks after the date of their last contact. Hospital personnel who come into close contact with patients or contaminated materials without barrier nursing attire must be considered exposed and put under closely supervised surveillance.

Engineered Biological Weapons

Development

The sciences of microbiology and weapon development were first seriously linked during World War II, when offensive biological weapons were developed for use. Development at that time focused on natural diseases that were incapacitating and/or lethal and that could be easily introduced into the opposing civilian populations or troops. Plague was introduced into China by the Japanese, and tularemia was used against German troops. BWs were used as part of an overall national military strategy. Their main purpose was the incapacitation or death of the opposing troops and civilian population. Not surprisingly, the release of BWs often backfired and also infected those implementing the BWs. Many countries developed BWs as part of the massive military weapon development that followed World War II. For many countries, this continued until 1972, when President Nixon proposed the international elimination of offensive BWs. The Convention on the Prohibition of the Development, Production, and Stockpiling of Bacteriological and Toxin Weapons and on Their Destruction was signed by President Ford in 1975 and was eventually signed by 103 nations.

Since then, experimentation on BWs has continued. For the countries that have adhered to the ban on the development of offensive BWs, research has focused on how to defend against them. For those that secretly continued BW development, all the resources of modern science and some of the best and most creative scientists have been used to develop BWs that have only been limited by the imagination of their designers.

Rationale

These programs have been driven by a fear of falling behind in the arms race and the attractiveness of a weapon of mass destruction that requires relatively low levels of technology, expertise, and cost. In addition, countries with an effective BW program are immediately competitive with the offensive capabilities of the world's superpowers.

Agents

The key BW agents include those described as category A. They include the agents of anthrax (Bacillus anthracis), plague (Yersinia pestis), smallpox (variola major virus), tularemia (Francisella tularensis), botulism (Clostridium botulinum toxin), and viral hemorrhagic fevers (Ebola and Marburg viruses). These biological agents are the most feared for several reasons. They are all potentially weapons of mass destruction. The U.S. Office of Technology Assessment estimates that 130,000 to 3 million deaths could occur after a release of 100 kilograms of aerosolized anthrax over Washington, D.C., making the attack as lethal as a hydrogen bomb. They can also (i) be easily disseminated or transmitted from person to person, (ii) result in high mortality rates and have the potential for major public health impact, (iii) cause public panic and social disruption, and (iv) require special action for public health preparedness.

Motives

Current motives for BW use and development appear to be changing. Instead of major offensive programs sponsored by technologically developed countries to keep pace in the arms race, BWs are increasingly being used by small sects and individual extremists to advance political and religious views. As a result, they gain attention for their extremist views or inflict revenge or punishment for perceived cultural faults and opposing political or religious views. Modern BW use gets more news coverage, affects more lives, and lasts longer than other acts of violence. It is not necessary for BWs to cause deaths in order for them to have a major impact. BW release causes economic depression, social anxiety, and panic and overwhelms the health care system with the "worried well," people who fear they have been exposed or infected.

Plague

Worldwide, there are 1,000 to 2,000 cases of plague each year. Almost all of the cases reported from 1995 to 2005 were rural and occurred among people living in small towns and villages or agricultural areas.

Cause of the disease

Yersinia pestis, a bacterial pathogen, is a gram-negative, rod-shaped bacterium with an antiphagocytic capsule. It is a facultative intracellular pathogen.

Transmission

Reservoir

Plague is a multisystem zoonosis that has an animal reservoir primarily in the small mammal population.

Mode of transmission

Plague is transmitted by the parenteral route from animal to animal and from animal to human by the bites of infective fleas. An uncommon mode of transmission is the inhalation of infected droplets expelled by coughing from a person or animal with pneumonic plague.

Pathogenesis

Entry

The bite of infected fleas causes itching near the site of the break in the skin. Scratching causes the feces carrying the pathogen from the fleas to be introduced into the blood.

Attachment

The ability of *Yersinia pestis* to attach to and enter a host cell is a key determinant of pathogenicity.

Avoiding host defenses

The pathogen synthesizes a capsule that is antiphagocytic.

Damage

The pathogen is carried to the lymph nodes that drain the area of the flea bite, where the bacteria multiply, cause inflammation, and spread. The pathogen produces the following virulence factors: coagulase, which causes blood clots to form, and fibrinolysin, which degrades blood clots; the endotoxin, which can cause shock and disseminated intravascular coagulation; and V and W antigens, which enable the pathogen to cause an overwhelming septicemia.

Exit

If the pathogen spreads to the lungs and causes pneumonia, it may be spread to another human via respiratory droplets.

Clinical features

There is an incubation period of 2 to 6 days after initial infection. Plague begins with a fever, headache, and general illness, followed by the development of painful, swollen regional lymph nodes (buboes).

Plague septicemia follows, with rapid invasion of the bloodstream, producing severe illness, prostration, and extreme exhaustion. The pathogen may also spread to the lungs, causing overwhelming pneumonia with high fever, cough, bloody sputum, and chills.

Diagnosis

Specimen

A sample of blood or pus from an infected bubo is obtained.

Tests

Gram staining is used to identify irregularly staining gram-negative rods that appear to be safety pin shaped. Direct fluorescent-antibody assays are used to confirm the diagnosis.

Treatment

Drug therapy begins as soon as plague is suspected. Several aminoglycosides are effective at treating plague. Aminoglycosides, such as streptomycin, are bacteriocidal and block the formation of 30S initiation complexes during the initiation of protein synthesis.

Where costs are important and the health care infrastructure is poorly developed, tetracyclines are also effective and can be delivered orally. Tetracyclines block aminoacyl-transfer RNA (tRNA) binding to 70S ribosomes during the elongation of protein synthesis.

Prevention

- As soon as a diagnosis of suspected plague is made, the patient should be isolated to prevent spread to others.
- Those who have had contact with the plague patient should be traced and given prophylactic antibiotics.
- Insecticides can be used to control the flea population.
- Public health education can be used to instruct home owners to eliminate food and shelter for rodents.
- Vaccination is required to prevent infection in at-risk groups, including people working with the plague bacterium in the laboratory or in the field and people working in plague-affected areas.

Smallpox

Naturally occurring smallpox has been eradicated worldwide through an international vaccination effort by the World Health Organization Global Commission for Smallpox Eradication. However, smallpox is still an important infectious disease because of the weaponization of the smallpox virus as part of offensive bioweapon research done in the former Soviet Union. As a result, use of the smallpox virus as a bioterrorism weapon is a significant concern.

Cause of the disease

The pathogenic agent of smallpox is the variola virus, an orthopoxvirus. The virus has double-stranded DNA as genetic information and an enveloped, brick-shaped capsid.

Transmission

Reservoir

Variola virus infects only humans.

Mode of transmission

Transmission occurs by the droplet mode or through fomites contaminated with pus or respiratory secretions from an infected individual.

Pathogenesis

Entry

The virus enters via the respiratory route.

Attachment

Variola virus attaches to tissues of the oropharynx, nasopharynx, and lower respiratory tract.

Avoiding host defenses

The virus initially avoids circulating antibodies and cells of the immune system because it is an intracellular pathogen.

Damage

Initially, the virus is carried to and replicates in the lymph organs. After 1 to 2 weeks, the virus is disseminated through the blood to other organs and to capillaries under the skin. The pustular rash occurs as the body's inflammatory response defends against the pathogen.

Exit

The virus exits through mucus droplets during coughing and through the pustules that form on the skin.

Clinical features

The smallpox virus enters the throat and the respiratory tract. Virus entry is followed by a 1- to 2-week incubation period. A sudden onset of fever, backache, headache, and malaise occurs before the classic eruption of the rash. A red rash appears in the mouth, and vesicles appear around the face, forearms, hands, and the trunk and legs. These break down to release large amounts of virus. Vesicles eventually evolve into pustules, which crust over by the 14th day of the rash, leaving behind deep pigmented areas.

Diagnosis

The clinical presentation of smallpox is unique and diagnostic. A case of smallpox today would be confirmed by genetic testing at a biosafety level 4 laboratory facility.

Treatment

Currently, there is no effective antiviral treatment for smallpox. Antibiotics are given to reduce the likelihood of secondary bacterial infections that can lead to hemorrhaging and gangrene. Supportive care is given to increase patient comfort.

Prevention

- The last known case of naturally occurring smallpox was in the town of Merka, Somalia, in 1977. By 1979, the officially declared eradication had been achieved throughout the world. Eradication was achieved by widespread surveillance for rapid case detection, quarantine of infected individuals, and vaccination and isolation of all people who were exposed to the disease.
- A vaccination program was renewed in 2003 for those individuals who would be first responders to a bioweapon attack.

Tularemia

Tularemia is a bacterial zoonosis with reservoirs in many mammals. The causative agent can survive for weeks under a variety of environmental conditions. Naturally occurring cases are limited to rural areas. The agent is one of six category A bioweapons because of its highly infectious nature, its virulence (disease-causing ability), and its ability to enter human hosts through a variety of routes.

Cause of the disease

Francisella tularensis, a bacterial pathogen, is a small, aerobic, gram-negative coccobacillus that is a facultative intracellular pathogen. Pathogenic strains have a capsule that prevents their digestion within macrophages.

Transmission

Reservoir

Francisella tularensis has widely diverse animal hosts, habitats, and vectors. It can survive in contaminated water, soil, and vegetation. Its hosts include voles, mice, water rats, squirrels, rabbits, and prairie dogs, and it can be introduced by tick, fly, and mosquito vectors.

Mode of transmission

The pathogen is one of the most infectious bacteria known. It can be transmitted as a vector-borne pathogen, through direct contact with contaminated material or organisms, or through the ingestion and inhalation of aerosols.

Pathogenesis

Entry

The pathogen enters the skin, mucous membranes, gastrointestinal tract, and/or lungs.

Attachment

The pathogen attaches to a variety of tissues.

Avoiding host defenses

The pathogen is protected from destruction by its capsule after it is engulfed by macrophages. It then multiplies within the macrophages and is carried to regional lymph nodes before it is disseminated to organs throughout the body.

Damage

The pathogen causes direct tissue death (necrosis) with the formation of large amounts of pus. The extensive inflammation caused by the infection damages capillaries, leading to hemorrhaging.

Clinical features

Tularemia can have several distinct clinical presentations, depending on the route of entry and the tissues infected. Clinical features can include cutaneous ulcers with swollen regional lymph nodes; conjunctivitis with swelling around the eyes; pharyngitis or tonsillitis with swelling of the lymph nodes in the neck; intestinal pain, vomiting, and diarrhea; pneumonia; and/or fever.

In naturally occurring cases, the case-fatality rate is about 2%. When the pathogen is inhaled as a result of a bioterrorism attack, the case-fatality rate would be about 40%.

Diagnosis

Clinical diagnosis is supported by evidence or history of a tick or deerfly bite, exposure to tissues of a mammalian host of *Francisella tularensis*, or exposure to potentially contaminated water.

Francisella tularensis may be identified by direct examination of blood, secretions, pus samples, or biopsy specimens using direct fluorescent-antibody or immunohistochemical stains. Since tularemia is highly infectious, clinical laboratories need to practice special safety procedures.

Treatment

Aminoglycosides, such as streptomycin and gentamicin, are commonly used. Aminoglycosides block the formation of the 30S initiation complex during protein synthesis.

Prevention

- In the United States, a live attenuated vaccine derived from the avirulent live vaccine strain has been used to protect laboratory personnel who routinely work with *Francisella tularensis*.

- Avoiding contact with sick animals or carcasses reduces the risk of exposure to tularemia.

APPENDIX A

Antimicrobial Agents

Table 1 Antibacterial agents: inhibitors of bacterial cell wall synthesis

Chemical class	Target	Mechanism of action	Common use
β-Lactams (e.g., penicillins, cephalosporins)	Penicillin-binding protein	Blocks cross-bridge linkage, preventing peptidoglycan synthesis	Gram-positive rods and cocci
Glycopeptides (e.g., vancomycin)	Peptidoglycan precursor translocation enzyme	Prevents movement of peptidoglycan precursor across the membrane to the outside of the cell	Drug of last resort for multiple-drug-resistant gram-positive rods and cocci or acute life-threatening infections
Peptides (e.g., bacitracin)	Lipid carrier of peptidoglycan precursor	Blocks release of peptidoglycan precursor from lipid carrier	Topical antibiotic for infections by gram-positive bacteria

Table 2 Antibacterial agents: inhibitors of macromolecule synthesis

Chemical class	Target	Mechanism of action	Common use
Quinolones (e.g., ciprofloxacin)	DNA replication	Blocks DNA gyrase activity	Anthrax
Rifampins	mRNA synthesis	Blocks recognition of promoter by RNA polymerase sigma factor	Mycobacteria; *Neisseria meningitidis* prophylaxis
Aminoglycosides (e.g., streptomycin, gentamicin)	Initiation of protein synthesis	Blocks formation of 30S initiation complex	Mycobacteria; *Klebsiella pneumoniae*
Tetracyclines	Elongation of protein synthesis	Blocks aminoacyl-tRNA binding to the ribosome A site	Intracellular pathogens *Rickettsia* and *Chlamydia*
Chloramphenicol	Elongation of protein synthesis	Blocks peptide bond formation	Second-line therapy for treating meningitis and anaerobe infections
Macrolides (e.g., azithromycin, erythromycin)	Completion of protein synthesis	Stimulates peptidyl-tRNA dissociation, causing premature termination of protein synthesis	*Chlamydia, Mycoplasma*; an alternative to the β-lactams

Table 3 Antibacterial agents: inhibition of essential and unique pathways

Chemical class	Target	Mechanism of action	Common use
Sulfonamides (e.g., sulfamethoxazole)	Synthesis of an essential enzyme cofactor, tetrahydrofolic acid, needed for enzymes used to synthesize purines and pyrimidines	Competitive inhibition of dihydropteroate synthetase, an enzyme necessary for tetrahydrofolic acid synthesis (a *para*-aminobenzoic acid analog)	In combination with trimethoprim to target gram-negative enteric bacteria
Trimethoprim	Synthesis of an essential enzyme cofactor, tetrahydrofolic acid, needed for enzymes used to synthesize purines and pyrimidines	Competitive inhibition of dihydrofolate reductase, an enzyme necessary for tetrahydrofolic acid synthesis (a dihydrofolic acid analog)	In combination with sulfonamides to target gram-negative enteric bacteria

Table 4 Antiviral agents

Chemical class	Target	Mechanism of action[a]	Common use
Amantidine	Entry	Specific inhibitor of influenza A virus entry	Reduces severity and duration of influenza A virus infections
Nucleoside analogs (e.g., acyclovir)	Nucleic acid replication	Analogs of deoxythymidine; phosphorylated in herpesvirus-infected cells and block DNA synthesis	Treatment of herpesvirus infections: cold sores, genital herpes, serious complications of chicken pox
Nucleoside analogs (e.g., azidothymidine)	Nucleic acid replication	Analogs of deoxythymidine; have high affinity for reverse transcriptase	Used in combination with other antivirals to treat HIV disease
Nucleoside analogs (e.g., 3-thiocytidine)	Nucleic acid replication	Analogs of deoxycytidine; high affinity for reverse transcriptase	Used in combination with other antivirals to treat HIV disease
Nucleoside analogs (e.g., ribavirin)	Gene expression	Analogs of deoxyguanine; block mRNA capping in RSV-infected cells	RSV-caused bronchiolitis
Protease inhibitors (e.g., indinavir, nelfinavir)	Viral assembly	Block HIV protease activity	Used in combination with other antivirals to treat HIV disease

[a]RSV, respiratory syncytial virus; HIV, human immunodeficiency virus.

Table 5 Antiprotozoal and antifungal agents

Chemical class	Target	Mechanism of action[a]	Common use
Azoles (e.g., miconazole)	Fungal cell membrane	Inhibit synthesis of ergasterol, an essential membrane steroid	Treatment of vaginal yeast infections, athlete's foot, and other surface skin infections by molds
Polyenes (e.g. amphotericin B, nystatin)	Fungal cell membrane	Bind to ergasterol in membranes of fungi and form a pore, causing cell lysis	Treatment of systemic fungal infections and topical treatment for vaginal yeast infections
Aminoquinolines (e.g., chloroquine, phospho-chloroquine, quinine)	*Plasmodium* preferentially concentrates aminoquinoline analogs	Multiple potential pathways to cause damage (DNA damage, toxic complex formed, alters internal pH)	Treatment and prophylaxis for malaria
Paromomycin	Antiprotozoal agent by inhibiting protein synthesis on 80S ribosomes	Stimulates peptidyl-tRNA dissociation, causing premature termination of protein synthesis (since paromomycin is not absorbed systemically, it selectively targets the protozoa in the GI tract)	Used to treat GI tract infections by protozoa
Nitroimidazoles (e.g., metronidazole)	Antiprotozoal and antianaerobe agents; DNA structure is altered, leading to breakage	Metronidazole causes DNA damage only in a reductive environment, such as is found in the GI tract when pathogenic microbes use up most available oxygen.	Anaerobic bacteria; GI tract infections by *Giardia* and *Entamoeba*
Tetracycline	Antimalarial agent that inhibits protein synthesis on 70S ribosomes (including mitochondrial ribosomes of *Plasmodium*)	Blocks binding of aminoacyl-tRNA to the A site of the ribosome	Antimalarial agent for drug-resistant *Plasmodium*
Pyramethamine	Antimalarial agent that blocks synthesis of an essential enzyme cofactor, tetrahydrofolic acid	Structural analog of dihydrofolic acid; acts as a competitive inhibitor to block synthesis of tetrahydrofolic acid	Antimalarial agent for drug-resistant *Plasmodium*

[a]GI, gastrointestinal.

APPENDIX B

References for Study Questions

The answers for the questions following each outbreak description can be obtained from the reference material provided at the end of each chapter. The list below provides references in which the source material for the outbreak descriptions can be found. Several questions at the ends of outbreaks do not have specific answers but require the student to investigate the socioeconomic, political, and/or religious factors involved and to provide a reasonable rationale for their choice. Like most of life's real problems, there is more than one possible solution—choosing the best among the many good and bad possibilities is the real challenge. The references can be used to find out how outbreaks are contained and prevented by the experts at the Centers for Disease Control and Prevention.

To locate online journals, such as the *Morbidity and Mortality Weekly Report* and *Emerging Infectious Diseases,* students should use the Centers for Disease Control and Prevention website at http://www.cdc.gov. This site contains easily identifiable links to the journals' home pages. Both the *Morbidity and Mortality Weekly Report* and *Emerging Infectious Diseases* have simple and effective search engines in which students can enter either the authors, the article title, or the volume of the journal to access the full text of these articles. Students can access articles that are contained in other scientific journals or newspapers at their college libraries. URLs are provided for materials from sources that may not be easily obtained at a college library.

SECTION I
Outbreaks and Cases Emphasizing Concepts in Basic Microbiology

OUTBREAK 1 Tuberculosis

Munsiff, S. S., T. Bassoff, B. Nivin, J. Li, A. Sharma, P. Bifani, B. Mathema, J. Driscoll, and B. N. Kreiswirth. 2002. Molecular epidemiology of multidrug-resistant tuberculosis, New York City, 1995–1997. *Emerg. Infect. Dis.* 8:1230–1238.

OUTBREAK 2 Mycoplasmal Pneumonia

Smyth, L., S. Swope, L. Wiser, G. T. Reed, E. D. Peterson, R. A. French, F. W. Smith, T. J. Halpin, P. J. Somani, M. Emig, R. R. Liu, K. Storms, G. P. Melcher, M. J. Dolan, J. Schuermann, D. M. Simpson, S. F. Kondracki, C. K. Csiza, R. A. Duncan, G. S. Birkhead, and D. L. Morse. 1993. Outbreaks of *Mycoplasma pneumoniae* respiratory infection—Ohio, Texas, and New York, 1993. *Morb. Mortal. Wkly. Rep.* 42:937–939.

OUTBREAK 3 Biofilm-Forming Bacteria

Nouwen, J. L., A. van Belkum, S. de Marie, J. Sluijs, J. J. Wielenga, J. A. Kluytmans, and H. A. Verbrugh. 1998. Clonal expansion of *Staphylococcus epidermidis* strains causing Hickman catheter-related infections in a hemato-oncologic department. *J. Clin. Microbiol.* 36:1095–1137.

OUTBREAK 4 Gonorrhea

Bethea, R. P., S. Q. Muth, J. J. Potterat, D. E. Woodhouse, J. B. Muth, N. E. Spencer, and R. E. Hoffman. 1991. Gang related outbreak of penicillinase producing *Neisseria gonorrhoeae* and other sexually transmitted diseases—Colorado Springs, Colorado, 1989–1991. *Morb. Mortal. Wkly. Rep.* 42:25–28.

OUTBREAK 5 *Pseudomonas aeruginosa* Infections

Beckett, G., D. Williams, G. Giberson, K. F. Gensheimer, K. Gershman, P. Shillam, R. E. Hoffman, R. Merry, H. Savalox, and L. Fawcett. 2000. *Pseudomonas* dermatitis folliculitis associated with pools and hot tubs—Colorado and Maine, 1999–2000. *Morb. Mortal. Wkly. Rep.* 49:1087–1091.

OUTBREAK 6 Anthrax

Shireley, L., T. Dwelle, D. Streitz, and L. Schuler. 2001. Human anthrax associated with an epizootic among livestock—North Dakota, 2000. *Morb. Mortal. Wkly. Rep.* 50:677–680.

OUTBREAK 7 Salmonellosis

Zansky, S., B. Wallace, D. Schoonmaker-Bopp, P. Smith, F. Ramsey, J. Painter, A. Gupta, P. Kalluri, and S. Noviello. 2001. Outbreaks of multidrug-resistant *Salmonella typhimurium* associated with veterinary facilities—Idaho, Minnesota, and Washington, 1999. *Morb. Mortal. Wkly. Rep.* 50:701–704.

OUTBREAK 8 Pertussis

Plott, K., F. B. Pascual, K. M. Bisgard, C. Vitek, T. V. Murphy, and C. R. Curtis. 2002. Pertussis deaths—United States, 2000. *Morb. Mortal. Wkly. Rep.* 51:616–618.

OUTBREAK 9 *Staphylococcus aureus* Infections

Miller, D., V. Urdaneta, A. Weltman, and S. Park. 2002. *Staphylococcus aureus* resistant to vancomycin—United States, 2002. *Morb. Mortal. Wkly. Rep.* 51:565–567.

OUTBREAK 10 Influenza

Christensen, S. E., R. C. Wolfmeyer, S. M. Suver, C. D. Hill, and S. F. F. Britton. 2001. Influenza B virus outbreak on a cruise ship—Northern Europe, 2000. *Morb. Mortal. Wkly. Rep.* 50:137–140.

OUTBREAK 11 Acquired Immune Deficiency Syndrome

Coles, F. B., G. S. Birkhead, P. Johnson, P. F. Smith, R. Berke, P. Allenson, and M. Clark. 1999. Cluster of HIV-positive young women—New York, 1997–1998. *Morb. Mortal. Wkly. Rep.* 48:413–416.

OUTBREAK 12 Rubella

Langvardt, D., G. Pezzino, M. Mayer, C. Miller, J. Weston, C. Allensworth, R. Raymond, and R. C. Jones. 2001. Rubella outbreak—Arkansas, 1999. *Morb. Mortal. Wkly. Rep.* 50:1137–1139.

OUTBREAK 13 Rotavirus

Ashley, D., E. Hedmann, K. Lewis-Bell, E. Ward, J. Bryce, R. M. Turcios, D. Tuller, M. A. Widdowson, J. S. Bresee, S. Adams, S. Monroe, J. R. Gentsch, R. I. Glass, and T. K. Fischer. 2003. Outbreak of severe rotavirus gastroenteritis among children—Jamaica, 2003. *Morb. Mortal. Wkly. Rep.* 52:1103–1105.

OUTBREAK 14 Cryptosporidiosis

Regan, J., R. McVay, M. McEvoy, J. Gilbert, R. Hughes, T. Tougaw, E. Parker, W. Crawford, J. Johnson, J. Rose, S. Boutros, S. Roush, T. Belcuore, C. Rains, J. Munden, L. Stark, E. Hartwig, M. Pawlowicz, R. Hammond, D. Windham, and R. Hopkins. 1996. Outbreak of cryptosporidiosis at a day camp—Florida, July–August 1995. *Morb. Mortal. Wkly. Rep.* 45:442–444.

OUTBREAK 15 Enterohemorrhagic *E. coli*

Bergmire-Sweat, D., L. Marengo, P. Pendergrass, K. Hendricks, M. Garcia, R. Drumgoole, T. Baldwin, K. Kingsley, B. Walsh, S. Lang, L. Prine, T. Busby, L. Trujillo, D. Perrotta, A. Hathaway, B. Jones, A. Jaiyeola, and S. Bengtson. 2000. *Escherichia coli* O111:H8 outbreak among teenage campers—Texas, 1999. *Morb. Mortal. Wkly. Rep.* 49:321–324.

OUTBREAK 16 Influenza

Chotpitayasunondh, T.; S. Lochindarat; P. Srisan; K. Chokepaibulkit; J. Weerakul; M. Maneerattanaporn; P. Sawanpanyalert; World Health Organization, Thailand; and Centers for Disease Control and Prevention International Emerging Infections Program, Thailand. 2004. Cases of influenza A (H5N1)—Thailand, 2004. *Morb. Mortal. Wkly. Rep.* 53:100–103.

SECTION II
Outbreaks of Diseases of the Respiratory Tract

OUTBREAK 17 Legionellosis
BBC News. 13 July 2001. Legionnaires' sweeps Spanish city. [Online.] http://news.bbc.co.uk/2/hi/europe/1437275.stm.

OUTBREAK 18 Respiratory Syncytial Virus Pneumonia and Bronchiolitis
George, J. 2 July 1998. Visitors descend on Keewatin as RSV outbreak wanes. *Nunatsiaq News.* [Online.] http://www.nunatsiaq.com/archives/nunavut980731/nvt80703_05.html.

OUTBREAK 19 Tuberculosis
Patterson, S., D. Bugenske, C. Pozsik, E. Brenner, R. Bellew, D. Drociuk, S. Rabley, and J. Gibson. 2000. Drug-susceptible tuberculosis outbreak in a state correctional facility housing HIV-infected inmates—South Carolina, 1999–2000. *Morb. Mortal. Wkly. Rep.* 49:1041–1044.

OUTBREAK 20 Otitis Media
Addison, A., L. Addison, H. Perry, J. Jenkins, S. Lance-Parker, K. Arnold, S. Kramer, and P. Blake. 2002. Multidrug-resistant *Streptococcus pneumoniae* in a child care center—Southwest Georgia, December 2000. *Morb. Mortal. Wkly. Rep.* 50:1156–1158.

OUTBREAK 21 Measles
Izurieta, H., M. Brana, P. Carrasco, V. Dietz, G. Tambini, C. A. de Quadros, O. Barrezueta, N. López, D. Rivera, L. López, M. Villegas, E. Maita, C. Garcia, D. Pastor, C. Castro, J. Boshell, O. Castillo, G. Rey, F. de la Hoz, D. Caceres, M. Velandia, W. Bellini, J. Rota, P. Rota, F. Lievano, and C. Lee. 2002. Outbreak of measles—Venezuela and Colombia, 2001–2002. *Morb. Mortal. Wkly. Rep.* 51:757–760.

OUTBREAK 22 Chicken Pox
Winquist, A. G., A. Roome, and J. Hadler. 2001. Varicella outbreak at a summer camp for human immunodeficiency virus infected children. *Pediatrics* 107:67–72.

OUTBREAK 23 Diphtheria
Regional Office for Europe and Global Program on Vaccines and Immunization, World Health Organization; Regional Office for Eastern Europe and Central Asia and Child Survival Unit, United Nations Children's Fund; Childhood and Respiratory Diseases Branch, Division of Bacterial and Mycotic Diseases, National Center for Infectious Diseases, Centers for Disease Control and Prevention; International Health Program Office; and Child Vaccine Preventable Disease Branch, Division of Epidemiology and Surveillance, National Immunization Program, Centers for Disease Control and Prevention. 1995. Diphtheria epidemic—new independent states of the former Soviet Union, 1990–1994. *Morb. Mortal. Wkly. Rep.* 44:177–181.

OUTBREAK 24 Mononucleosis
Diaz, L., S. Miranda, J. C. Nunez, E. I. Ponce, M. V. Ramos, H. Pedroga, and J. V. Rullan. 1991. Pseudo-outbreak of infectious mononucleosis—Puerto Rico, 1990. *Morb. Mortal. Wkly. Rep.* 40:552–555.

OUTBREAK 25 Lobar Pneumonia
Bresnitz, E., C. Grant, S. Ostrawski, C. Morris, J. Calabria, B. Reetz, and S. Clugston. 2001. Outbreak of pneumococcal pneumonia among unvaccinated residents of a nursing home—New Jersey, April 2001. *Morb. Mortal. Wkly. Rep.* 50:707–710.

OUTBREAK 26 Influenza
Barry, J. M. 2004. *The Great Influenza*, p. 297–337. Viking Penguin, London, United Kingdom.

World Health Organization. 28 January 2004. "We must take urgent action now to stop the further spread of the avian influenza to newer areas and to humans," says WHO. [Online.] http://w3.whosea.org/EN/Section316/Section503/Section1549_6147.htm.

OUTBREAK 27 Strep Throat
Crum, N. F., B. R. Hale, D. A. Bradshaw, J. D. Malone, H. M. Chun, W. M. Gill, D. Norton, C. T. Lewis, A. A. Truett, C. Beadle, J. L. Town, M. R. Wallace, D. J. Morris, E. K. Yasumoto, K. L. Russell, E. Kaplan, C. Van Beneden, and R. Gorwitz. 2003. Outbreak of group A streptococcal pneumonia among Marine Corps recruits—California, November 1–December 20, 2002. *Morb. Mortal. Wkly. Rep.* 52:106–109.

OUTBREAK 28 Measles
Kline, D., H. Dakkak, A. Cami, F. Abduliahu, L. Cela, K. Venovska, Y. Mokuo, M. Duprat, D. Panev, D. Mikic, Z. Desovski, S. Stefanoski, B. Ancevska, N. Janeva, and C. Maroto Camino. 1999. Vaccination campaign for Kosovar Albanian refugee children—former Yugoslav Republic of Macedonia, April–May, 1999. *Morb. Mortal. Wkly. Rep.* 48:799–803.

SECTION III
Outbreaks of Diseases of the Gastrointestinal Tract

OUTBREAK 29 Salmonellosis
Reporter, R., L. Mascola, L. Kilman, A. Medina, J. Mohle-Boetani, J. Farrar, D. Vugia, M. Fletcher, M. Levy, O. Ravenholt, L. Empey, D. Maxson, P. Klouse, A. Bryant, R. Todd, M. Williams, G. Cage, and L. Bland. 2000. Outbreaks of *Salmonella* serotype Enteritidis infection associated with eating raw or undercooked shell eggs—United States, 1996–1998. *Morb. Mortal. Wkly. Rep.* 49:73–79.

OUTBREAK 30 Cryptosporidiosis
Veverka, F., N. Shapiro, M. K. Parish, S. York, W. Becker, F. Smith, C. Allensworth, T. Baker, P. Iwen, and T. Safranek. 2001. Protracted outbreaks of cryptosporidiosis associated with swimming pool use—Ohio and Nebraska, 2000. *Morb. Mortal. Wkly. Rep.* 50:406–410.

OUTBREAK 31 Enterohemorrhagic *E. coli*
Novello, A. 1999. Public Health Dispatch: outbreak of *Escherichia coli* O157:H7 and *Campylobacter* among attendees of the Washington County Fair—New York, 1999. *Morb. Mortal. Wkly. Rep.* 48:803.

OUTBREAK 32 Amoebiasis

Kreidl, P., P. Imnadze, L. Baidoshvili, and D. Greco. 1999. Investigation of an outbreak of amoebiasis in Georgia. *Euro Surveill.* 4:103–104.

OUTBREAK 33 Typhoid Fever

Katz, D. J., M. A. Cruz, and M. J. Trepka. 2002. An outbreak of typhoid fever in Florida associated with an imported frozen fruit. *J. Infect. Dis.* 186:234–239.

OUTBREAK 34 Giardiasis

Colvin, H., B. Thomas, D. Bruce, and M. Crawford. 22 October 1982. Giardia outbreak in a day care nursery—Juneau. *State of Alaska Epidemiology Bulletin 21.* [Online.] http://www.epi.hss .state.ak.us/bulletins/docs/b1982_21.htm.

OUTBREAK 35 Shigellosis

Los Angeles County Health Department; San Diego County Health Department; California Department of Health Services; Multnomah County Health Department; Clackamas County Health Department; Oregon Health Division; Public Health—Seattle and King County; Washington Department of Health; and Foodborne and Diarrheal Diseases Branch, Division of Bacterial and Mycotic Diseases, National Center for Infectious Diseases, Centers for Disease Control and Prevention. 2000. Public Health Dispatch: outbreak of *Shigella sonnei* infections associated with eating a nationally distributed dip—California, Oregon, and Washington, January 2000. *Morb. Mortal. Wkly. Rep.* 49:60–61.

OUTBREAK 36 Listeriosis

Philadelphia Department of Public Health; New York City Department of Health and Mental Hygiene; Pennsylvania Department of Health; New York State Department of Health; New Jersey Department of Health and Senior Services; Delaware Health and Social Services; Maryland Department of Health and Mental Hygiene; Connecticut Department of Public Health; Michigan Department of Community Health; Massachusetts Department of Public Health; Food Safety and Inspection Service, U.S. Department of Agriculture; and Division of Bacterial and Mycotic Diseases, National Center for Infectious Diseases, Centers for Disease Control and Prevention. 2002. Public Health Dispatch: outbreak of listeriosis—Northeastern United States, 2002. *Morb. Mortal. Wkly. Rep.* 51:950–951.

OUTBREAK 37 Botulism

Rifkin, G., K. Sibounheuang, L. Peterson, K. Kelly, C. Langkop, D. Kauerauf, E. Groeschel, B. Adam, C. Austin, and S. Bornstein. 2000. Foodborne botulism from eating home-pickled eggs—Illinois, 1997. *Morb. Mortal. Wkly. Rep.* 49:778–780.

OUTBREAK 38 Enterohemorrhagic *E. coli* Infections

Shillam, P., A. Woo-Ming, L. Mascola, R. Bagby, C. Lohff, S. Bidol, M. G. Stobierski, C. Carlson, L. Schaefer, L. Kightlinger, S. Seys, K. Kubota, P. S. Mead, and P. Kalluri. 2002. Multistate outbreak of *Escherichia coli* O157:H7 infections associated with eating ground beef—United States, June–July 2002. *Morb. Mortal. Wkly. Rep.* 51:637–639.

OUTBREAK 39 Hepatitis A

Dato, V., A. Weltman, K. Waller, M. A. Ruta, A. Highbaugh-Battle, C. Hembree, S. Evenson, C. Wheeler, and T. Vogt. 2003. Hepatitis A outbreak associated with green onions at a restaurant—Monaca, Pennsylvania, 2003. *Morb. Mortal. Wkly. Rep.* 52:1155–1157.

OUTBREAK 40 Viral Gastroenteritis

Fletcher, M., M. E. Levy, and D. D. Griffin. 2000. Foodborne outbreak of group A rotavirus gastroenteritis among college students—District of Columbia, March–April 2000. *Morb. Mortal. Wkly. Rep.* 49:1131–1133.

OUTBREAK 41 Cholera

McLean, V. 21 July 1994. Doctors fear cholera epidemic among Rwandans. *USA Today,* p. 7.

SECTION IV
Outbreaks of Sexually Transmitted Diseases

OUTBREAK 42 Syphilis

Goodman, R. D. 19 October 1999. *Frontline:* The lost children of Rockdale County. [Online.] http://www.pbs.org/wgbh/pages/ frontline/shows/georgia/etc/script.html.

OUTBREAK 43 Chancroid

Greenwood, J. R., T. Prendergast, L. R. Ehling, C. Zavala, and J. Chin. 1982. Epidemiologic notes and reports. Chancroid—California. *Morb. Mortal. Wkly. Rep.* 31:173–175.

OUTBREAK 44 Acquired Immune Deficiency Syndrome

Ross, S. 20 April 2004. LA County Health Department seeks records; threatens regulation. *Adult Video News.* [Online.] http://www.avn.com/index.php?Primary_Navigation=Articles &Action=View_Article&Content_ID=81269.

OUTBREAK 45 Gonorrhea

Ohye, R.; V. Lee; P. Whiticar; P. Effler; H. Domen; G. Hoff; J. Joyce; R. Archer; M. Hayes; J. Hale; K. Holmes; L. Doyle; G. Procop; Epidemiology and Surveillance Branch, Division of STD Prevention, National Center for HIV, STD, and TB Prevention; Bacterial STD Branch, Division of AIDS, STD, and TB Laboratory Research, National Center for Infectious Diseases; and EIS officers, Centers for Disease Control and Prevention. 22 September 2000. Fluoroquinolone resistance in *Neisseria gonorrhoeae*, Hawaii, 1999, and decreased susceptibility to azithromycin in *N. gonorrhoeae*, Missouri, 1999. *Morb. Mortal. Wkly. Rep.* 49:833–837.

OUTBREAK 46 Genital Warts and Cervical Cancer

Armstrong, L. R., H. I. Hall, P. A. Wingo, and S. Kassim. 2002. Invasive cervical cancer among Hispanic and non-Hispanic women—United States, 1992–1999. *Morb. Mortal. Wkly. Rep.* 51:1067–1070.

OUTBREAK 47 Chlamydial Sexually Transmitted Diseases

van de Laar, M. J. W., H. M. Götz, O. de Zwart, W. I. van der Meijden, J. M. Ossewaarde, H. B. Thio, J. S. A. Fennema, J. Spaargaren, H. J. C. de Vries, S. M. Berman, J. R. Papp, and K. A. Workowski. 2004. Lymphogranuloma venereum among men who have sex with men—Netherlands, 2003–2004. *Morb. Mortal. Wkly. Rep.* 53:985–988.

OUTBREAK 48 Syphilis

DeNoon, D. 25 July 2000. Virtual meeting plus real sex equals disease. *WebMD Medical News Archive.* [Online.] http://my.webmd.com/content/article/27/1728_59915.htm.

OUTBREAK 49 Acquired Immune Deficiency Syndrome

Joint United Nations Program on HIV/AIDS and World Health Organization. 2002. *AIDS Epidemic Update, December, 2002,* p. 19–20.

SECTION V

Outbreaks of Diseases of the Skin, Eyes, and Deep Tissue

OUTBREAK 50 *Staphylococcus aureus* Skin Infections

Khurshid, M. A., T. Chou, R. Carey, R. Larsen, C. Conover, and S. L. Bornstein. 2000. *Staphylococcus aureus* with reduced susceptibility to vancomycin—Illinois, 1999. *Morb. Mortal. Wkly. Rep.* 48:1165–1167.

OUTBREAK 51 *Pseudomonas aeruginosa* Skin Infections

Beckett, G., D. Williams, G. Giberson, K. F. Gensheimer, K. Gershman, P. Shillam, R. E. Hoffman, R. Merry, H. Savalox, and L. Fawcett. 2000. *Pseudomonas* dermatitis/folliculitis associated with pools and hot tubs—Colorado and Maine, 1999–2000. *Morb. Mortal. Wkly. Rep.* 49:1087–1091.

OUTBREAK 52 Ringworm

Layman, C. 4 March 1993. Ringworm pins wrestlers. *State of Alaska Epidemiology Bulletin* 9. State of Alaska Health and Social Services, Juneau, Alaska. [Online.] http://www.epi.hss.state.ak.us/bulletins/docs/b1993_09.htm.

OUTBREAK 53 Pneumococcal Conjunctivitis

Leighton, C., D. Piper, J. Gunderman-King, V. Rea, K. Gensheimer, J. Randolph, R. Danforth, L. Webber, E. Pritchard, G. Beckett, V. Shinde, R. Facklam, C. Whitney, N. Hayes, and B. Flannery. 2003. Pneumococcal conjunctivitis at an elementary school—Maine, September 20–December 6, 2002. *Morb. Mortal. Wkly. Rep.* 52:64–66.

OUTBREAK 54 Measles

Division of Global Migration and Quarantine, National Center for Infectious Diseases, and Epidemiology and Surveillance Division, National Immunization Program, Centers for Disease Control and Prevention. 2004. Measles among children adopted from China: update. *Morb. Mortal. Wkly. Rep.* 53:459.

OUTBREAK 55 Hepatitis

Balter, S., M. Layton, K. Bornschlegel, P. F. Smith, M. Crutcher, S. Mallonee, J. Fox, P. Scott, T. Safranek, D. Leschinsky, K. White, J. F. Perz, I. T. Williams, B. P. L. Chiarello, A. L. Panlilio, M. Phillips, M. Marx, A. Macedo de Oliveira, D. Comstock, N. Malakmadze, T. Samandari, and T. M. Vogt. 2003. Transmission of hepatitis B and C viruses in outpatient settings—New York, Oklahoma, and Nebraska, 2000–2002. *Morb. Mortal. Wkly. Rep.* 52:901–906.

OUTBREAK 56 Group A *Streptococcus* Infections

CNN. 3 May 2004. Hospital reports flesh-eating bacteria cases. [Online.] http://www.cnn.com/2004/HEALTH/05/03/flesh.eating.bacteria/index.html.

OUTBREAK 57 Group A *Streptococcus* Infections

Barry, M. A., K. Matthews, P. Tormey, B. T. Matyas, S. M. Lett, J. A. Ida, D. M. Hamlin, P. Kludt, K. Yih, and A. DeMaria, Jr. 1997. Outbreak of invasive group A *Streptococcus* associated with varicella in a childcare center—Boston, Massachusetts, 1997. *Morb. Mortal. Wkly. Rep.* 46:944–948.

OUTBREAK 58 *Staphylococcus aureus* Skin Infections

Hopper, L. 1 November 2003. Increase in staph infections bewilders local physicians. *Houston Chronicle*, p. A1.

OUTBREAK 59 Gas Gangrene

U.N. Office for the Coordination of Humanitarian Affairs. 31 December 2004. Earthquake and tsunami: Indonesia, Maldives, Sri Lanka, Thailand, Seychelles, Somalia. OCHA Situation Report no. 8. [Online.] http://ochaonline.un.org/webpage.asp?Page=813.

SECTION VI

Outbreaks of Multisystem Zoonoses and Vector-Borne Diseases

OUTBREAK 60 Typhus

Raoult, D., V. Roux, J. B. Ndihokubwayo, G. Bise, D. Baudon, G. Marte, and R. Birtles. 1997. Epidemic typhus (jail fever) outbreak in Burundi. *Emerg. Infect. Dis.* 3:357–360.

OUTBREAK 61 Malaria

Hussain, S. Z. 21 May 2002. Malaria, gastroenteritis hit Assam, 70 dead. *Health-India*. Available online at http://www.indialists.org/pipermail/health-india/2002-May.txt.

OUTBREAK 62 West Nile Virus Encephalitis

Chow, C. C., S. P. Montgomery, D. R. O'Leary, R. S. Nasci, G. L. Campbell, A. M. Kipp, J. A. Lehman, K. Olson, P. Collins, and A. A. Marfin. 2002. Provisional surveillance summary of the West Nile virus epidemic—United States. *Morb. Mortal. Wkly. Rep.* 51:1129–1136.

OUTBREAK 63 Yellow Fever

Hall, P., M. Fojtasek, J. Pettigrove, N. Sisley, J. Perdue, K. Hendricks, S. Stanley, D. Perrotta, A. A. Marfin, G. L. Campbell,

R. S. Lanciotti, L. R. Petersen, P. E. Rollin, T. G. Ksiazek, M. S. Cetron, D. Sharp, and K. G. Julian. 2002. Fatal yellow fever in a traveler returning from Amazonas, Brazil, 2002. *Morb. Mortal. Wkly. Rep.* 51: 324–325.

OUTBREAK 64 Hantavirus Pulmonary Syndrome

Craig, W., K. Cook, J. Carney, S. Schoenfeld, B. Wilcke, and T. Algeo. 2001. Hantavirus pulmonary syndrome—Vermont, 2000. *Morb. Mortal. Wkly. Rep.* 50:603–635.

OUTBREAK 65 Rocky Mountain Spotted Fever

Levy, C., J. Burnside, T. Tso, S. Englender, M. Auslander, S. Billings, K. Bradley, J. Bos, L. Burnsed, J. Brown, D. Mahoney, K. Chamberlain, M. Porter, C. Duncan, B. Johnson, R. Ethelbah, K. Robinson, M. Wessel, S. Savoia, C. Garcia, J. Dickson, D. Kvamme, D. Yost, M. Traeger, J. Krebs, C. Paddock, W. Shieh, J. Guarner, S. Zaki, D. Swerdlow, J. McQuiston, W. L. Nicholson, and L. Demma. 2004. Fatal cases of Rocky Mountain spotted fever in family clusters—three states, 2003. *Morb. Mortal. Wkly. Rep.* 53:407–410.

OUTBREAK 66 Ebola Hemorrhagic Fever

Oyok, T., C. Odonga, E. Mulwani, J. Abur, F. Kaducu, M. Akech, J. Olango, P. Onek, J. Turyanika, I. Mutyaba, H. R. S. Luwaga, G. Bisoborwa, A. Kaguna, F. G. Omaswa, S. Okware, A. Opio, J. Amandua, J. Kamugisha, E. Mukoyo, J. Wanyana, C. Mugero, M. Lamunu, G. W. Ongwen, M. Mugaga, C. Kiyonga, Z. Yoti, A. Olwa, M. deSanto, M. Lukwiya, P. Bitek, P. Louart, C. Maillard, A. Delforge, C. Levenby, E. Munaaba, J. Lutwama, S. Banonya, Z. Akol, L. Lukwago, E. Tanga, and L. Kiryabwire. 2001. Outbreak of Ebola hemorrhagic fever—Uganda, August 2000–January 2001. *Morb. Mortal. Wkly. Rep.* 50:73–77.

OUTBREAK 67 Leptospirosis

Hahn, C.; L. Mascola; R. Cader; D. Haake; D. Vugia; C. Easman; J. Keystone; B. Connor; GeoSentinel Global Surveillance Network of the International Society of Travel Medicine; Council of State and Territorial Epidemiologists; J. Purdue; K. Hendricks; J. Pape; L. McFarland; World Health Organization; M. Eyeson-Annan; P. Buck; H. Artsob; M. Evans; R. Salmon; B. Smyth; T. Coleman; V. Cardenas; Division of Applied Public Health Training, Epidemiology Program Office; Meningitis and Special Pathogens Branch, Division of Bacterial and Mycotic Diseases; Surveillance and Epidemiology Branch, Division of Quarantine, National Center for Infectious Diseases; Centers for Disease Control and Prevention Eco-Challenge Investigation Team; and EIS officers, Centers for Disease Control and Prevention. 2001. Update: outbreak of acute febrile illness among athletes participating in Eco-Challenge-Sabah 2000—Borneo, Malaysia, 2000. *Morb. Mortal. Wkly. Rep.* 50:21–24.

OUTBREAK 68 Dengue Fever

Feliciano de Melecio, C., H. Horta, R. Barea, A. Casta-Velez, A. Ayala, C. Vargas-Nunez, C. Deseda, R. Hunter-Mellado, J. Morales-Morales, I. Figueroa, O. Reyes, B. Munoz, M. A. Mercado, and E. German. 1998. Dengue outbreak associated with multiple serotypes—Puerto Rico, 1998. *Morb. Mortal. Wkly. Rep.* 47:952–956.

OUTBREAK 69 Lyme Disease

State Health Departments and Bacterial Zoonoses Branch, Division of Vector-Borne Infectious Diseases, National Center for Infectious Diseases, Centers for Disease Control and Prevention. 1999. Lyme disease—United States. *Morb. Mortal. Wkly. Rep.* 50:181–185.

OUTBREAK 70 Plague

Guiyoule, A., G. Gerbaud, C. Buchrieser, M. Galimand, L. Rahalison, S. Chanteau, P. Courvalin, and E. Carniel. 2001. Transferable plasmid-mediated resistance to streptomycin in clinical isolate of *Yersinia pestis. Emerg. Infect. Dis.* 7:43–48.

World Health Organization and Division of Quarantine, National Center for Prevention Services, and Bacterial Zoonoses Branch, Division of Vector-Borne Infectious Diseases, National Center for Infectious Diseases, Centers for Disease Control and Prevention. 1994. International notes update: human plague—India, 1994. *Morb. Mortal. Wkly. Rep.* 43:761–762.

SECTION VII
Outbreaks of Diseases of the Central Nervous System

OUTBREAK 71 Polio

Ministry of Health, Country Office, Praia, Cape Verde; Intercountry Office for West Africa, Abidjan, Cote d'Ivoire; Intercountry Office for Southern Africa and Regional Office for Africa, Harare, Zimbabwe; Institute Pasteur, Dakar, Senegal; National Institute of Virology, Johannesburg, South Africa; Vaccines and Other Biologicals Department, World Health Organization; and Division of Quarantine and Respiratory and Enteric Viruses Branch, Division of Viral and Rickettsial Diseases, National Center for Infectious Diseases, and Vaccine Preventable Disease Eradication Division, National Immunization Program, Centers for Disease Control and Prevention. 2000. Public Health Dispatch: outbreak of poliomyelitis—Cape Verde, 2000. *Morb. Mortal. Wkly. Rep.* 49:1070.

OUTBREAK 72 Botulism

Horn, A., K. Stamper, D. Dahlberg, J. McCabe, M. Beller, and J. P. Middaugh. 2001. Botulism outbreak associated with eating fermented food—Alaska, 2001. *Morb. Mortal. Wkly. Rep.* 50: 680–682.

OUTBREAK 73 Rabies

University of Alabama at Birmingham Hospital; Jefferson County Health Department; Alabama Department of Public Health; Arkansas State Department of Health; Oklahoma State Department of Health; Regional and local health departments; Division of Healthcare Quality Promotion, Texas Department of Health; and Division of Viral and Rickettsial Diseases, National Center for Infectious Diseases, Centers for Disease Control and Prevention. 2004. Update: investigation of rabies infections in organ donor and transplant recipients—Alabama, Arkansas, Oklahoma, and Texas, 2004. *Morb. Mortal. Wkly. Rep.* 53:615–616.

OUTBREAK 74 Tetanus

Orengo, J. C., Y. García, A. Rodríguez, J. Rullán, M. H. Roper, P. Srivastava, T. V. Murphy, and F. Alvarado-Ramy. 2002. Tetanus—Puerto Rico, 2002. *Morb. Mortal. Wkly. Rep.* 51:613–615.

OUTBREAK 75 Viral Meningitis

Waite, D., P. Beckenhaupt, L. LoBianco, P. Mshar, A. Nepaul, K. Marshall, T. Brennan, J. L. Hadler, W. A. Nix, M. Pallansch, and E. M. Begier. 2003. Aseptic meningitis outbreak associated with echovirus 9 among recreational vehicle campers—Connecticut, 2003. *Morb. Mortal. Wkly. Rep.* 53:710–713.

OUTBREAK 76 Creutzfeldt-Jakob Disease

Faiola, A. 5 February 2005. Japan says man died of mad cow disease. *Washington Post*, p. A16.

OUTBREAK 77 Meningococcal Meningitis

Rowland, R. 25 August 2000. Michigan authorities seek party-goers exposed to meningitis. [Online.] http://archives.cnn.com/2000/US/08/24/rave.meningitis/.

OUTBREAK 78 Meningococcal Meningitis

Fine, A., M. Layton, A. Hakim, and P. Smith. 2000. Serogroup W-135 meningococcal disease among travelers returning from Saudi Arabia—United States, 2000. *Morb. Mortal. Wkly. Rep.* 49:345–346.

SECTION VIII

Outbreaks and Cases Requiring Application of Environmental and Industrial Microbiology Concepts

OUTBREAK 79 Cryptosporidiosis

Minshew, P.; K. Ward; Z. Mulla; R. Hammond; D. Johnson; S. Heber; R. Hopkins; and Division of Bacterial and Mycotic Diseases and Division of Parasitic Diseases, National Center for Infectious Diseases, Division of Applied Public Health Training, Epidemiology Program Office, and an EIS Officer, Centers for Disease Control and Prevention. 2000. Outbreak of gastroenteritis associated with an interactive water fountain at a beachside park—Florida, 1999. *Morb. Mortal. Wkly. Rep.* 49:565–568.

OUTBREAK 80 Dengue Virus

Muello, P. 3 March 2002. Dengue fever is sickening thousands. *Milwaukee Journal Sentinel.*

OUTBREAK 81 Sulfur-Oxidizing Bacteria

Stone, R. 2005. Radiation hazards: Kyrgyzstan's race to stabilize buried ponds of uranium waste. *Science* 307:198–200.

OUTBREAK 82 Shigellosis

Lohff, C. J., G. M. Nissen, M. L. Magnant, M. P. Quinlisk, C. L. Tieskoetter, P. L. Kowalski, P. A. Buss, T. A. Link, M. R. Corrigan, J. P. Viner, A. J. Behnke, M. S. DeMartino, and A. K. Houston. 2001. Shigellosis outbreak associated with an unchlorinated fill-and-drain wading pool—Iowa, 2001. *Morb. Mortal. Wkly. Rep.* 50:797–800.

OUTBREAK 83 Cryptosporidiosis

MacKenzie, W. R., N. J. Hoxie, M. E. Proctor, M. S. Gradus, K. A. Blair, D. E. Peterson, J. J. Kazmierczak, D. G. Addiss, K. R. Fox, J. B. Rose, and J. P. Davis. 1994. A massive outbreak in Milwaukee of *Cryptosporidium* infection transmitted through the public water supply. *N. Engl. J. Med.* 331:161–167.

OUTBREAK 84 Sulfur-Reducing Bacteria

Üretgen, I. T. 2004. Comparison of the efficacy of free residual chlorine and monochloramine against biofilms in model and full scale cooling towers. *Biofouling* 20:81–85.

OUTBREAK 85 Legionellosis

García-Fulgueiras, A., C. Navarro, D. Fenoll, J. García, P. González-Diego, T. Jiménez-Buñuales, M. Rodriguez, R. Lopez, F. Pacheco, J. Ruiz, M. Segovia, B. Balandron, and C. Pelaz. 2003. Legionnaires' disease outbreak in Murcia, Spain. *Emerg. Infect. Dis.* 9:915–921.

OUTBREAK 86 Sulfur-Oxidizing and Sulfur-Reducing Bacteria

Center for Biofilm Engineering. 2005. The CBE industry program. [Online.] http://www.erc.montana.edu/Ind-Col99-SW/index.htm.

OUTBREAK 87 Biofilm-Forming Bacteria

Halox Technologies. June 2005. Microbiological control and biofilm elimination in bottling and canning. Halox case history. [Online.] http://www.haloxtech.com/CaseHistory.asp.

OUTBREAK 88 Plague

Boisier, P., L. Rahalison, M. Rasolomaharo, M. Ratsitorahina, M. Mahafaly, M. Razafimahefa, J. M. Duplantier, L. Ratsifasoamanana, and S. Chanteau. 2002. Epidemiologic features of four successive annual outbreaks of bubonic plague in Mahajanga, Madagascar. *Emerg. Infect. Dis.* 8:43–48.

SECTION IX

Bioterrorism Outbreaks

OUTBREAK 89 Anthrax

Smart, J. K. 1997. History of chemical and biological warfare: an American perspective, p. 67–68. *In* R. Zaitchuk, F. Edward, and R. F. Bellamy (ed.), *Textbook of Military Medicine: Medical Aspects of Chemical and Biological Warfare.* Office of the Surgeon General, Department of the Army, Washington, D.C.

OUTBREAK 90 Brucellosis

Greenblatt, J., C. Hopkins, A. Barry, and A. DeMaria. 2000. Suspected brucellosis case prompts investigation of possible bioterrorism-related activity—New Hampshire and Massachusetts, 1999. *Morb. Mortal. Wkly. Rep.* 49:509–512.

OUTBREAK 91 Tularemia

Lindley, C., S. Avashia, K. Hendricks, J. Rawlings, J. Buck, J. Kool, K. Gage, M. Schriefer, D. Dennis, M. Chu, J. Peterson, J. Montenieri, D. Kim, T. Demarcus, and M. Cetron. 2002. Public

Health Dispatch: outbreak of tularemia among commercially distributed prairie dogs, 2002. *Morb. Mortal. Wkly. Rep.* **51:** 688, 699.

OUTBREAK 92 Anthrax

Takahashi, H., P. Keim, A. F. Kaufmann, C. Keys, K. L. Smith, and K. Taniguchi. 2004. *Bacillus anthracis* incident, Kameido, Tokyo, 1993. *Emerg. Infect. Dis.* **10:**117–120.

OUTBREAK 93 Ebola Hemorrhagic Fever

Miller, J. 25 May 2004. Scientist dies in Ebola accident at former weapons lab. *New York Times.*

OUTBREAK 94 Botulism Toxin

Associated Press. 25 March 2003. Is nation ready for botulinum attack? Experts fear trouble ahead. http://www.cnn.com/2003/HEALTH/03/25/botulinum.toxin.ap/index.html.

OUTBREAK 95 Engineered Biological Weapons

Alibek, K. 1999. *Biohazard: the Chilling True Story of the Largest Covert Biological Weapons Program in the World—Told from Inside by the Man Who Ran It.* Random House, New York, N.Y.

OUTBREAK 96 Smallpox

Brown, D. 16 June 2002. Soviets had '71 smallpox outbreak. *Washington Post,* p. A25.

Figure Credits

Figure 1.1 Source: Lewis Tomalty and Gloria Delisle; from the Microbe Library, American Society for Microbiology (http://www.microbelibrary.org).

Figure 2.1 Reprinted from A. Yáñez, L. Cedillo, O. Neyrolles, E. Alonso, M.-C. Prévost, J. Rojas, H. L. Watson, A. Blanchard, and G. H. Cassell, *Emerg. Infect. Dis.* 5:164–167, 1999.

Figure 3.1 Source: Mahmoud Yassien and Nancy Khardori; from the Microbe Library, American Society for Microbiology (http://www.microbelibrary.org).

Figure 4.1 Source: J. Michael Miller; from the Microbe Library, American Society for Microbiology (http://www.microbelibrary.org).

Figure 4.2 Source: Public Health Image Library (PHIL), Centers for Disease Control and Prevention (CDC).

Figure 5.1 Photograph by the author.

Figure 5.2 Source: PHIL, CDC.

Figure 6.1 Source: Larry Stauffer, Oregon State Public Health Laboratory; from PHIL, CDC.

Figure 6.2 Source: Larry Stauffer, Oregon State Public Health Laboratory; from PHIL, CDC.

Figure 7.1 Photograph by the author.

Figure 7.2 Source: Gilda L. Jones (CDC); from PHIL.

Figure 8.1 Source: PHIL, CDC.

Figure 9.1 Source: PHIL, CDC.

Figure 9.2 Source: Cara Calvo.

Figure 10.1 Photograph by the author.

Figure 11.1 Source: Edwin P. Ewing, Jr. (CDC); from PHIL.

Figure 12.1 Source: Edwin P. Ewing, Jr. (CDC); from PHIL.

Figure 12.2 Source: PHIL, CDC.

Figure 13.1 Source: Erskine Palmer (CDC); from PHIL.

Figure 14.1 Source: Peter Drotman (CDC); from PHIL.

Figure 15.1 Source: Cara Calvo.

Figure 15.2 Photograph by the author.

Figure 16.1 Source: Erskine Palmer (CDC); from PHIL.

Figure 17.1 Source: William Cherry (CDC); from PHIL.

Figure 17.2 Source: Jim Feeley (CDC); from PHIL.

Figure 18.1 Source: H. Craig Lyerla (CDC); from PHIL.

Figure 19.1 Source: Lewis Tomalty and Gloria Delisle; from the Microbe Library, American Society for Microbiology (http://www.microbelibrary.org).

Figure 19.2 Source: PHIL, CDC.

Figure 20.1 Photograph by the author.

Figure 20.2 Source: PHIL, CDC.

Figure 21.1 Source: PHIL, CDC.

Figure 21.2 Source: PHIL, CDC.

Figure 22.1 Source: Joe Miller (CDC); from PHIL.

Figure 23.1 Source: PHIL, CDC.

Figure 24.1 Photograph by the author.

Figure 24.2 Photograph by the author.

Figure 25.1 Source: Thomas Hooten (CDC); from PHIL.

Figure 25.2 Photograph by the author.

Figure 26.1 Source: National Museum of Health and Medicine, Armed Forces Institute of Pathology, Washington, D.C.

Figure 27.1 Source: PHIL, CDC.

Figure 27.2 Source: Cara Calvo.

Figure 28.1 Source: PHIL, CDC.

Figure 28.2 Source: PHIL, CDC.

Figure 29.1 Photograph by the author.

Figure 29.2 Source: PHIL, CDC.

Figure 30.1 Source: Peter Drotman (CDC); from PHIL.

Figure 31.1 Source: Cara Calvo.

Figure 31.2 Photograph by the author.

Figure 32.1 Source: PHIL, CDC.

Figure 33.1 Source: PHIL, CDC.

Figure 33.2 Source: Charles N. Farmer, Armed Forces Institute of Pathology; from PHIL, CDC.

Figure 34.1 Source: Mae Melvin (CDC); from PHIL.

Figure 35.1 Photograph by the author.

Figure 35.2 Source: PHIL, CDC.

Figure 36.1 Photograph by the author.

Figure 37.1 Source: George Lombard (CDC); from PHIL.

Figure 37.2 Source: Larry Stauffer, Oregon State Public Health Laboratory; from PHIL, CDC.

Figure 38.1 Source: Cara Calvo.

Figure 38.2 Photograph by the author.

Figure 39.1 Source: Betty Partin (CDC); from PHIL.

Figure 40.1 Source: Erskine Palmer (CDC); from PHIL.

Figure 40.2 Photograph by the author.

Figure 41.1 Source: William A. Clark (CDC); from PHIL.

Figure 41.2 Source: PHIL, CDC.

Figure 41.3 Source: PHIL, CDC.

Figure 42.1 Source: Susan Lindsley (CDC); from PHIL.

Figure 43.1 Source: Joe Miller (CDC) and N. J. Fiumara; from PHIL.

Figure 43.2 Source: Joe Miller (CDC); from PHIL.

Figure 44.1 Source: Edwin P. Ewing, Jr. (CDC); from PHIL.

Figure 45.1 Source: PHIL, CDC.

Figure 45.2 Source: Susan Lindsley (CDC); from PHIL.

Figure 46.1 Reprinted from L. R. Armstrong, H. I. Hall, P. A. Wingo, and S. Kassim, *Morb. Mortal. Wkly. Rep.* 51:1067–1070, 2002.

Figure 46.2 Reprinted from L. R. Armstrong, H. I. Hall, P. A. Wingo, and S. Kassim, *Morb. Mortal. Wkly. Rep.* 51:1067–1070, 2002.

Figure 46.3 Source: PHIL, CDC.

Figure 46.4 Source: Joe Miller (CDC); from PHIL.

Figure 47.1 Source: Vester Lewis (CDC); from PHIL.

Figure 48.1 Source: Edwin P. Ewing, Jr. (CDC); from PHIL.

Figure 48.2 Source: Susan Lindsley (CDC); from PHIL.

Figure 49.1 Source: Michael Jensen, World Health Organization.

Figure 49.2 Source: Michael Jensen, World Health Organization.

Figure 50.1 Source: PHIL, CDC.

Figure 51.1 Photograph by the author.

Figure 51.2 Source: PHIL, CDC.

Figure 52.1 Source: Lucille K. Georg (CDC); from PHIL.

Figure 52.2 Source: Libero Ajello (CDC); from PHIL.

Figure 53.1 Photograph by the author.

Figure 53.2 Source: PHIL, CDC.

Figure 53.3 Source: Joe Miller (CDC); from PHIL.

Figure 54.1 Source: PHIL, CDC.

Figure 54.2 Source: PHIL, CDC.

Figure 56.1 Source: PHIL, CDC.

Figure 56.2 Source: Cara Calvo.

Figure 57.1 Source: PHIL, CDC.

Figure 57.2 Source: Cara Calvo.

Figure 58.1 Source: PHIL, CDC.

Figure 58.2 Source: Margaret Johnson; from the Microbe Library, American Society for Microbiology (http://www.microbelibrary.org).

Figure 59.1 Source: Don Stalons (CDC); from PHIL.

Figure 60.1 Source: David Walker and Vsevolod Popov; from the Microbe Library, American Society for Microbiology (http://www.microbelibrary.org).

Figure 60.2 Source: Dennis D. Juranek (CDC); from PHIL.

Figure 60.3 Source: PHIL, CDC.

Figure 61.1 Source: Mae Melvin (CDC); from PHIL.

Figure 61.2 Source: Pierre Virot, World Health Organization.

Figure 62.1 Source: Jim Gathany (CDC); from PHIL.

Figure 62.2 Source: Cynthia Goldsmith (CDC); from PHIL.

Figure 63.1 Source: PHIL, CDC.

Figure 63.2 Source: PHIL, CDC.

Figure 64.1 Source: National Center for Infectious Diseases, CDC; from PHIL.

Figure 64.2 Source: PHIL, CDC.

Figure 64.3 Source: D. Loren Ketai (CDC); from PHIL.

Figure 65.1 Source: PHIL, CDC.

Figure 65.2 Source: PHIL, CDC.

Figure 66.1 Source: C. Goldsmith (CDC); from PHIL.

Figure 66.2 Source: PHIL, CDC.

Figure 67.1 Source: Martin Hicklin (CDC); from PHIL.

Figure 68.1 Source: Division of Vector-Borne Infectious Diseases, National Center for Infectious Diseases, CDC (http://www.cdc.gov/ncidod/dvbid/dengue/map-distribution-2005.htm).

Figure 68.2 Source: PHIL, CDC.

Figure 69.1 Source: Edwin P. Ewing, Jr. (CDC); from PHIL.

Figure 69.2 Source: Michael L. Levin (CDC); from PHIL.

Figure 70.1 Source: Jack Poland (CDC); from PHIL.

Figure 70.2 Source: PHIL, CDC.

Figure 70.3 Source: Jack Poland (CDC); from PHIL.

Figure 71.1 Source: J. Esposito and F. A. Murphy (CDC); from PHIL.

Figure 71.2 Source: P. Virot, World Health Organization.

Figure 72.1 Source: Larry Stauffer, Oregon State Public Health Laboratory; from PHIL, CDC.

Figure 73.1 Source: Daniel P. Perl (CDC); from PHIL.

Figure 74.1 Source: PHIL, CDC.

Figure 74.2 Source: PHIL, CDC.

Figure 76.1 Source: Animal and Plant Health Inspection Service, U.S. Department of Agriculture; from PHIL, CDC.

Figure 76.2 Source: Animal and Plant Health Inspection Service, U.S. Department of Agriculture; from PHIL, CDC.

Figure 77.1 Source: M. S. Mitchell (CDC); from PHIL.

Figure 78.1 Source: D. Brodsky (CDC); from PHIL.

Figure 78.2 Source: PHIL, CDC.

Figure 79.1 Photograph by the author.

Figure 80.1 Source: PHIL, CDC.

Figure 81.1 Source: PHIL, CDC.

Figure 82.1 Photograph by the author.

Figure 82.2 Source: PHIL, CDC.

Figure 83.1 Photograph by the author.

Figure 84.1 Source: Judy Bowen; from the Microbe Library, American Society for Microbiology (http://www.microbelibrary.org).

Figure 85.1 Source: William Cherry (CDC); from PHIL.

Figure 85.2 Source: Jim Feeley (CDC); from PHIL.

Figure 86.1 Photograph by the author.

Figure 86.2 Source: Donald Gibbon and Rodney Donlan; from the Microbe Library, American Society for Microbiology (http://www.microbelibrary.org).

Figure 87.1 Source: Donald Gibbon and Rodney Donlan; from the Microbe Library, American Society for Microbiology (http://www.microbelibrary.org).

Figure 88.1 Reprinted from P. Boisier, L. Rahalison, M. Rasolomaharo, M. Ratsitorahina, M. Mahafaly, M. Razafimahefa, J. M. Duplantier, L. Ratsifasoamanana, and S. Chanteau, *Emerg. Infect. Dis.* 8:311–316, 2002.

Figure 88.2 Source: Larry Stauffer, Oregon State Public Health Laboratory; from PHIL, CDC.

Figure 89.1 Source: Arthur E. Kay (CDC); from PHIL.

Figure 89.2 Source: James H. Steele (CDC); from PHIL.

Figure 90.1 Source: PHIL, CDC.

Figure 91.1 Source: Larry Stauffer, Oregon State Public Health Laboratory; from PHIL, CDC.

Figure 91.2 Source: D. Sellers (CDC and Emory University); from PHIL.

Figure 92.1 Reprinted from H. Takahashi, P. Keim, A. F. Kaufmann, C. Keys, K. L. Smith, K. Taniguchi, S. Inouye, and T. Kurata, *Emerg. Infect. Dis.* (http://www.cdc.gov/ncidod/EID/vol10no1/03-0238.htm, 14 January 2004).

Figure 93.1 Source: Frederick A. Murphy (CDC); from PHIL.

Figure 93.2 Source: Ethleen Lloyd (CDC); from PHIL.

Figure 94.1 Source: V. R. Dowell (CDC); from PHIL.

Figure 95.1 Source: U.S. Senate (http://lugar.senate.gov/photos/nunn-lugar.html).

Figure 96.1 Source: PHIL, CDC.

Figure 96.2 Source: Kenneth L. Herrmann (CDC); from PHIL.

Index